Third International Conference on Myopia

Documenta Ophthalmologica
Proceedings Series volume 28

Editor H.E. Henkes

Dr W. Junk Publishers   The Hague—Boston—London   1981

Third International Conference
on Myopia
Copenhagen, August 24-27, 1980

Edited by H. C. Fledelius, P. H. Alsbirk
and E. Goldschmidt

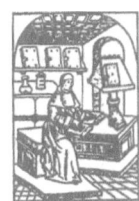

Dr W. Junk Publishers   The Hague—Boston—London   1981

Distributors:

for the United States and Canada

Kluwer Boston, Inc.
190 Old Derby Street
Hingham, MA 02043
USA

for all other countries

Kluwer Academic Publishers Group
Distribution Center
P.O. Box 322
3300 AH Dordrecht
The Netherlands

Library of Congress Cataloging in Publication Data   CIP

International Conference on Myopia (3rd : 1980 :
    Copenhagen, Denmark)
    Third International Conference on Myopia,
Copenhagen, August 24-27, 1980.

    (Documenta ophthalmologica.   Proceedings
series ; v. 28)
    1. Myopia--Congresses.   I. Fledelius, H. C.
II. Alsbirk, P. H.   III. Goldschmidt, Ernst Walter
Matthias, 1933-   .   IV. Series. [DNLM: 1. Myopia
--Congresses.   W3 DO637 v. 28 1980 / WW 320 I61
1980t]
RE938.I57 1980   617.7'55   81-5778
                                               AACR2

ISBN-13: 978-94-009-8664-0   e-ISBN-13: 978-94-009-8662-6
DOI: 10.1007/978-94-009-8662-6

Cover design: Max Velthuijs

Dr W. Junk Publishers, P.O. Box 13713, 2501 ES The Hague, The Netherlands.

PREFACE

Considering the high incidence of myopia – and its inherent morbidity – it may wonder that the item is dealt with only sporadically in recent literature, and almost never at international conferences.

However, there was a First International Conference on Myopia in New York 1964, and the Second was held in Yokohama 1978, affiliated to the XXIII World Congress of Ophthalmology. Here it was attempted to set outlines for future myopia research, and, as a practical implicaton, the arrangement of the Third International Conference on Myopia was entrusted to Danish ophthalmologists.

This conference took place in Copenhagen, August 24–27, 1980. To make the scope the widest possible, the conference was, as was the predecessing in Japan, open not only to ophthalmologists, but 'to all being active in the various aspects of myopia research'.

The conference report gives a picture of the Copenhagen meeting. Furthermore, a platform or current status of myopia research has hereby been established. The editors have made it their main task to arrange the papers, and to bring them in a form suited for print, while criticism by editorial referees has been considered inappropriate. The papers give an impression of the ambiguity still prevailing in the field, and although 'trends' are obvious, a final consensus of Conference was not arrived at. To document this state of affairs, however, is considered a useful task.

We further intended to publish the most fruitful discussions, given in relation to the papers presented, but we have decided to omit this due to heterogeneity of the available material. These contributions are, however, collected in an informal supplementum, which will be sent to the conference participants and – on written request (Myopia Conference Secretariat, E 2061, Rigshospitalet, DK-2100 Copenhagen Ø) – to those specially interested.

The conference report has been sponsored by grants from the International Society for Myopia Research and the Tuborg Foundation. The editors are grateful for this support.

Copenhagen, December 1980   THE EDITORS

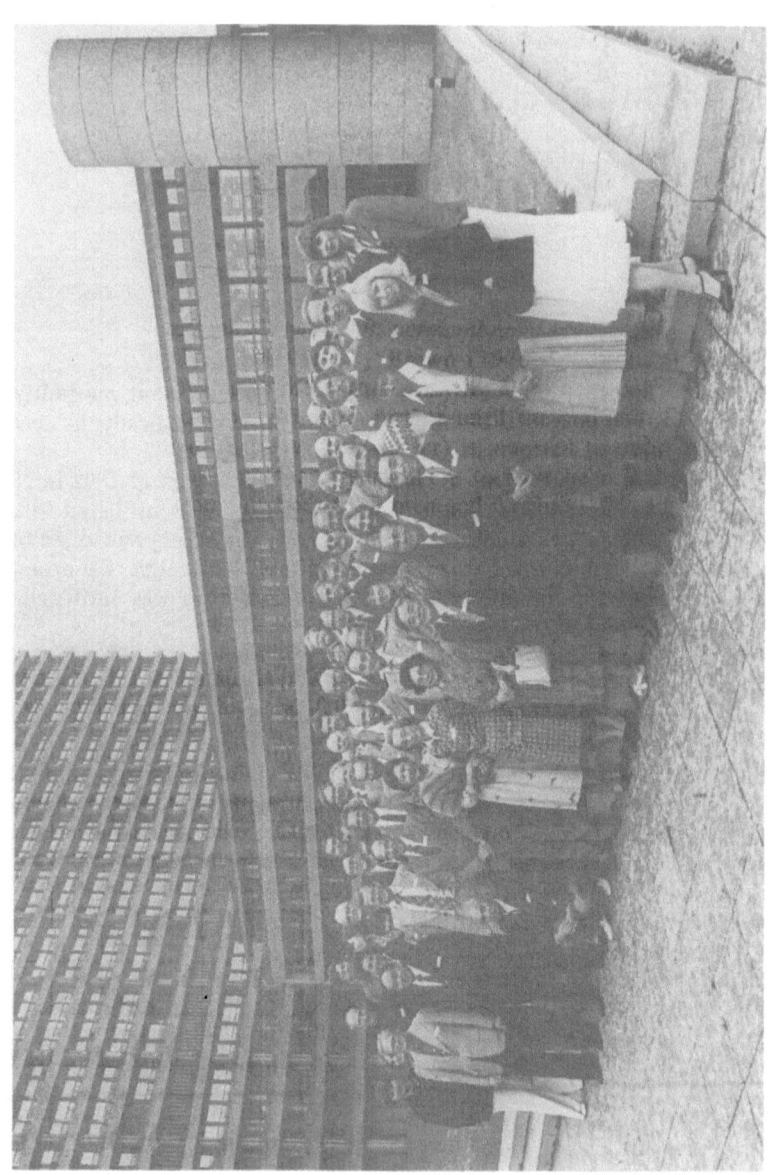

INTRODUCTION AND WELCOME

Myopia is known in all races, but the frequency varies considerably. Variation also appears within limited population groups, and a great deal of research on the subject has therefore been concerned with the fundamental questions: Why do some people become myopic, but others not? Is myopia caused by external factors or is it hereditary? Is myopia a product of civilization – an environmental disease the reasons for which we do not know – or is it genetically determined and affected only to a limited degree by external conditions?

These problems have been given a leading role in ophthalmological research for more than a century, and there is hardly another field in ophthalmology that has given rise to more violent and passionate discussion. Occasionally the debate has been characterized by strong polemics, with mutual accusations of scientific irresponsibility. Honest attempts to achieve an approximation between adherents to the different schools of thought have been rare, due in part, no doubt, to tradition, orthodoxy and semantic problems.

Just how confused the entire complex of problems is may be revealed by a glance through (even) modern ophthalmic textbooks, where recent discoveries (e.g. within laboratory myopia, genetics and epidemiology) and re-discoveries (regarding myopia and near work) are hardly noticed. It therefore seems necessary to try to evaluate the classical theories against the results from this 'new wave' in myopia research.

There is an increasing demand of qualified and open-minded research leading to a deeper understanding of myopia pathogenesis. We devote the conference to this purpose. A hearty welcome to Copenhagen!

ERNST GOLDSCHMIDT M.D.,
Professor in Ophthalmology,
Chairman of The Conference,
Odense, Denmark

Thank you very much for holding the 3rd International Conference on Myopia. We are so happy to find such a large attendance here, and we deeply appreciate the painstaking and strenuous efforts made by the organizing committee.

Denmark has a very long history of studies on myopia. It was as early as in 1883 that Dr. Tscherning found school myopia to be weak myopia, thus laying, as pioneer, the foundation of our studies of myopia. Dr. Bjerrum, who is famous all over the world for his discovery of scotoma due to glaucoma, reported on the incidence of myopia in 1886. In the 1900s, Dr. Blegvad discovered how myopia tends to develop. These findings are all very important achievements, and represent a brilliant and outstanding tradition of studies, borne by the scholars in the past as well as by the doctors present here today.

It is indeed significant that this academic conference is held in Denmark, a country so closely associated with studies of myopia. We expect that this conference will surely mark another remarkable step in the progress of our studies of myopia.

Thank you for your attention.

TIKASI SATO, M.D.,
President of the International Society for
Myopia Research (ISMR),
Yokohama, Japan

CONTENTS

Session VII. Complications in high myopia
    (Moderator: Dr. T. Sato, M.D.)

Session VIII. On prophylaxis and treatment of myopia
    (Moderator: Professor F.A. Young, Ph.D.)

PROPORTION OF MYOPIA IN VISUAL SCREENING OF SCHOOL CHILDREN

L. LAATIKAINEN AND H. ERKKILÄ

(Helsinki, Finland)

ABSTRACT

The prevalence of myopia in late childhood seems to have increased in Finland during the last decades. Eighty per cent of school children with decreased visual acuity and more than half of those annually referred to an ophthalmologist have myopia. Myopia is therefore the main target of the visual screening at school age, and it comprises a great proportion of the work done at the school eye clinics.

INTRODUCTION

The main purpose of visual screening in early childhood is the detection of amblyopia. At school age myopia gradually becomes the commonest cause of decreased visual acuity and the main target of the screening. In Finland visual screening of school children is performed by the school nurse on every child at the age of 7–8, 9–10, 11–12, and 14–15 years. It includes testing of the visual acuity for distance as well as general inspection in order to detect strabismus. Children with decreased visual acuity of less than 0.8 in one or both eyes, obvious strabismus or subjective symptoms related to reading are referred to an ophthalmologist for further eye examination.

In order to estimate the need for ophthalmological health service at school age and to find out the prevalence of refractive errors, strabismus and other ocular abnormalities in school children we performed an ophthalmological survey on 411 children by examining 23 whole classes of pupils representing these age groups (Laatikainen & Erkkilä 1980a). In this paper the proportion and clinical significance of myopia in the survey are presented. For comparison, some statistics from the routine school eye clinic are given.

SUBJECTS AND METHODS

All children were examined by the authors. Visual acuity for distance was tested using the Snellen chart. Cover test and Titmus stereo test were performed, and refraction was determined both before and 40–50 min after the instillation of 1% cyclopentolate twice in each eye. Here refractive errors are expressed in spherical equivalents of the cycloplegic values.

RESULTS

In the four age groups studied, each of them consisting of about 100 children, the prevalence of myopia increased successively. In the youngest age group myopia occurred in less than 2% of the eyes whereas in the oldest group myopia of 0.5 D or more was found in 22% of the eyes (Table 1). In 13 cases myopia was monocular. Therefore the percentual figures of myopic children were slightly higher than those of myopic eyes (Table 1). Twenty three of the 47 myopic pupils were girls and 24 were boys. The age distribution of the myopic girls and boys did not differ significantly. Eighteen of the 411 children (4.4%) had had a low birth weight of 2500 g or less. One of them had myopia.

Table 1. Prevalence of myopia in 411 non-selected school children.

Age	Myopic eyes (%)	Myopic children (%)
7–8 (n = 81)	1.9	2.5
9–10 (n = 109)	6.4	7.3
11–12 (n = 111)	7.2	9.0
14–15 (n = 110)	21.8	24.5
Total	9.9	11.4

Table 2. Degree of myopia in 411 non-selected school children.

| Age | Number of eyes | | | |
	-0.5 to -1.25 D.	-1.5 to -2.25 D.	-2.5 to -3.25 D.	-3.5 D.
7–8	3	–	–	–
9–10	8	–	6	–
11–12	8	7	1	–
14–15	28	12	3	5
Total	47	19	10	5

In the youngest age group the degree of myopia was less than 1.5 D in all cases, in the other groups about half of the myopic eyes were less than 1.5 D. At the age of 14 years myopia of 3.5 D or more was found in five of the 48 myopic eyes (Table 2). One of the 47 myopic children had astigmatism of 1 D or more. In this case both eyes were astigmatic. The frequency of astigmatism in the myopic group (2.5%) was slightly lower than in the total series (3.6%).

Thirteen of the 47 myopic children (28%) had monocular myopia. The age distribution of the monocular myopes did not differ from that of all myopic pupils. Most monocular cases were mild. Thus anisometropia of

2

more than 1 D. was found in five of these 13 children – in the group of binocular myopia, anisometropia was found in one of the 34 children. All the monocular myopes had binocular vision. Subnormal recordings at the Titmus test, at the level of 200 seconds of arc of disparity, were found only in those who in addition to monocular myopia had anisometropia of about 2 D or more. One child with monocular myopia had intermittent esotropia, and one had microstrabismus and mild functional amblyopia with the visual acuity of 0.6. Three of the 34 binocular myopes had manifest strabismus, but none of them had amblyopia.

In this survey 43 of the 55 children (78%) with visual acuity of less than 0.8 in one or both eyes, and 64% of all fulfilling the criteria for further eye examination, were myopic. The corresponding percentages in the first year statistics at the routine school eye clinic were 76 and 57%.

DISCUSSION

According to the results of the survey it could be expected that 10% of all school children would annually fail at the screening of the visual acuity (Laatikainen and Erkkilä 1980b). Almost 80% of them would have myopia. The proportion of myopic children at the routine school eye clinic corresponded with these results.

At the survey the prevalence of myopia at the age of seven years corresponded with that reported from Finland in 1927 by Heinonen. On the contrary, the 22% prevalence of myopic eyes in the age group of 14 years exceeded considerably the 14% prevalence found by Heinonen in this age group in 1934. Thus it seems that the incidence of myopia in late childhood has increased during the last decades. The reason for this cannot be ascertained on the basis of this study.

In the pathogenesis of myopia genetic factors (Sorsby et al. 1966) and the amount of accommodation (near work) (Richler and Bear 1980) have been considered the most important. The children examined were randomly selected representing all social classes. Therefore great differences in the genetic pattern of these two series cannot be expected. It is possible that the amount of near work had slightly increased in this age group although both series were composed of school children.

Another possible explanation for increased prevalence of myopia in late childhood is that increase in the axial length of the eye – uncompensated by correlated growth of the cornea and lens – is related to the greater and more rapid general growth of the children due to better nutrition and general health of the population. This is supported by earlier findings that myopia develops earlier in girls than in boys (Young et al. 1954; Sorsby et al. 1961; Goldschmidt 1968) although this was not confirmed in the present study. This theory could also explain at least part of the increase in the prevalence of myopia after the introduction of formal education in Eskimo and Amerind populations (Young et al. 1969; Woodruff and Samek 1977). Prematurity has also been considered as a cause of myopia. In this series low birth weight did not increase the prevalence of myopia.

3

Monocular myopia of mild degree was common but it was not found to disturb binocular vision significantly unless anisometropia of about 2 D was present. Thus it seems justified to leave mild monocular myopia in children uncorrected unless strabismus is present. Manifest strabismus was found in five of the 47 myopic children and one of them had mild amblyopia due to microstrabismus.

REFERENCES

Goldschmidt, E., On the etiology of myopia. An etiological Study. Acta Ophthalmol., Suppl. 98 (1968).

Heinonen, O., Untersuchungen betreffend die Refraktion des Auges, speziell mit Berücksichtigung einiger Spezialfragen. Acta Soc. Med. 'Duodecim', 9 (3): 1 (1927).

Heinonen, O., Weitere Studien über die Schulmyopie. Acta Ophthalmol. 12: 110 (1934).

Laatikainen, L. & Erkkilä, H., Refractive errors and other ocular findings in school children. Acta Ophthalmol. 58: 129 (1980a).

Laatikainen, L. & Erkkilä, H., Visual screening of school children. Acta Ophthalmol. 58: 137 (1980b).

Richler, A. & Bear, J.C., Refraction, nearwork and education. A population study in Newfoundland. Acta Ophthalmol. 58: 468 (1980).

Sorsby, A., Benjamin, B. & Sheridan, M., Refraction and its components during the growth of the eye from the age of three. Spec. Rep. Ser. No. 301, Med. Res. Council, London (1961).

Sorsby, A., et al., Family studies on ocular refraction and its components. J. Med. Genet. 3: 269 (1966).

Woodruff, M.E. & Samek, M.J. A study of the prevalence of spherical equivalent refractive states and anisometropia in Amerind populations in Ontario. Can. J. Publ. Hlth. 68: 414 (1977).

Young, F.A., et al., The Pullman Study, a visual survey of Pullman school children. Am. J. Optom. 31: 192 (1954).

Young, F.A., et al., The transmission of refractive errors with Eskimo families. Am. J. Optom. 46: 676 (1969).

Author's address:
H. Erkkilä, M.D.
University Eye Hospital
Haartmaninkatu 4 C
00290 Helsinki 29
Finland

THE DISTRIBUTION OF MYOPIA IN MAN AND MONKEY

F.A. YOUNG

(Pullman, Washington and Houston, Texas, USA)

ABSTRACT

A recently published national probability sample of the refractive characteristics of the United States population 4—74 years indicates that adults 18—44
have the greatest amount of myopia. This distribution plus one taken in
1928 on Washington, D.C. school children six years and older are compared
with refraction distributions of three groups of monkeys — wild, open space
monkeys, laboratory caged monkeys, and near-visual space monkeys. The
children and wild monkey distributions are virtually identical. The adults
and laboratory caged monkeys are very similar. The near-visual space
monkeys are significantly (0.01 level) more myopic than any of the other
groups.

INTRODUCTION

For a number of years we have been examining the refractive characteristics
of humans and sub-human primates when these groups have been subjected
to different visual environments in the hopes of determining the relative
contribution of heredity and environment to the development of myopia.

A considerable amount of data have been gathered on randomly selected
monkeys placed in different visual environments such as (a) a near-point
visual environment which restricts the monkey from seeing beyond 16- to
20- in. from the eyes through the use of translucent but not transparent
cages; (b) standard laboratory cages in standard size laboratory rooms which
effectively restricts the animal to an 8- to 10-ft distance visual environment
and (c) the natural visual environment of wild monkeys. We have been able
to examine a large group of monkeys which had just been imported from
India into the United States as well as a group of Japanese Macaques. The
latter had lived in an open area in Japan and were captured as a group and
were transfered to Portland, Oregon, where they were again kept in very
large open pens which permitted visual distances of more than 300 ft.

We have not been able to generate comparable data on human populations
since all of the human groups we have studied such as the Eskimos in Barrow,

Alaska, and the Warm Springs, Oregon Native American (Indian) children have been characterized by a lack of random selection.

A recent publication by the National Center for Health Statistics of the U.S. Public Health Service, U.S. Department of Health, Education and Welfare, entitled 'Refraction Status and Motility Defects of Persons 4—74 Years — United States, 1971—1972' provides the type of random data which are necessary for 20 years and older; and examination of the pupil, lids, globes, conjunctiva, sclera, corneas, anterior chamber, irides and lenses.

The pupils were dilated in most instances for the spherical refraction and retinoscopy and for the examination of the vitreous and retina. Thus, while not all individuals had an actual retinoscopy, an approximately accurate determination of refractive error was made based upon a subjective trial lens determination of visual acuity and the use of glasses prescription for those who had normal 20/20 acuity through the glasses. Most determinations of those individuals with refractive errors were made under a cycloplegic.

DETERMINATION OF MONKEY VISUAL CHARACTERISTICS

All of the monkeys were refracted under Cyclogyl cycloplegia given in the sequence of one drop of 2% in each eye followed at 10 min intervals by an additional one drop of 1% in each eye for a total of three drops of 1% in addition to the one drop of 2%. Refractions were done between an hour and two hours after instillation of the drops. To facilitate the application of drops, adult animals were anesthetized with Sernylan for both the application of the drops and the refraction.

Since younger monkeys do not respond as well to Sernylan as do adult monkeys the procedure was varied in the younger animals such that the application of the drops was done in the alert monkey by capturing and holding the monkey while the drops were given and Sernylan was not administered until the refraction was to begin. It takes approximately 5—8 min for Anesthesia to Sernylan in the dosage level of 1 mg/lb of body weight. All of the monkey refractions except for the wild monkeys were done by the same investigator. The wild monkey refractions were done by a second investigator who had demonstrated consistent refractions to same criteria. All refractive errors were translated into spherical equivalents by algebraically adding half of the astigmatic correction to the spherical correction.

The refraction data presented by the National Center for Health Statistics were grouped under the following categories: 0.0 refractive error or no correction worn; a correction of 0.1—0.5 D either plus or minus; 0.6—1.0 D of plus or minus; 1.1—1.5 D plus or minus; 1.6—2.0 D plus or minus; 2.1—3.0 D plus or minus; 3.1—4.0 D plus or minus; 4.1—5.0 D plus or minus; 5.1 or more plus; 5.1—7.5 D minus; 7.6—10.0 minus; and 10.1 D or more minus. While the data available on the monkeys are available in actual refractive errors, for comparability the data were fit into the categories used by the National Center investigators for the human subjects. The information actually used for comparative purposes with the monkeys consisted of that obtained on 18 to 44 year old adults since these individuals showed the highest amount of myopia in the total population thereby representing the maximum amount of myopia which could be obtained in the human population in 1971–1972. These individuals totaled 3844 subjects.

The monkeys consisted of three groups, all of which were sexually mature and most of which were over six years of age which would be comparable to 18 year old humans. The wild monkeys consisted of 299 rhesus monkeys which had just been imported into the United States within a week of refraction and thus for practical purposes had never been caged except for the air transportation. To this group were added a group of 92 Japanese Macaque monkeys which again had not been exposed to a near-point environment other than the duration of the flight from Japan to the United States. These animals were housed in very large outdoor compounds which were approximately 200 ft by 600 ft enclosures with climbing towers for the animals which allowed them unrestricted distance vision.

The 174 caged laboratory monkeys were monkeys which were housed in standard laboratory cages in a number of Primate Centers. The near visual monkeys consisted of animals which had been placed in the near-visual situation in which the animals were housed, either in restraining chairs or in near point visual cages. The restraining chair animals were placed in the chair and the chair was enclosed within a translucent hood which restricted the visual distance to an average of 14 in. with a maximum of 20 in. Some of the animals were also housed in near-point visual cages which were approximately cubes of 24 in. with a translucent side. An adult mother and her infant were placed in these cages. After the mother had been in the cage situation for one to three years the mother was removed, and the infants were paired in a cage situation for another two or three years. After the infants had reached adulthood, they were refracted and their refraction data are included in the group of animals which were kept under the near visual situation which thus included all animals which had been in the situation for a year or more. There were a total of 186 animals which were exposed to this near visual situation.

In the case of the monkeys right eye refractions were used unless right eye refractions were not available, in which case left eye refractions were substituted. In the case of the human subjects it is not certain which eyes or whether both eyes were actually used. The distributions of refractive characteristics were translated into percentages. The monkey data were translated into the same categories and into percentages for comparison with the human data.

RESULTS

The means, medians and range of refractive characteristics for the four populations are presented in Table 1. The means given for the human subjects in Table 1 are somewhat biased since the actual values for the 1.43% of cases with more than 5 D Hyperopia and the 0.4% with 10.1 D or more myopia were not actually provided and there is no way of determining the exact means. However, in terms of the small number (less than 2% of the

Table 1. Comparison of human and monkey refraction distributions in terms of Number, means, medians and range of refractive errors.

Group	Number	Mean (D)	Median (D)	Range (D)
Adult humans	3844	− 0.04	+ 0.53	+ 5.0 to − 12.0
Children	1829	+ 0.64	+ 0.71	+ 4.0 to − 4.0
Wild monkeys	391	+ 0.64	+ 0.61	+ 4.0 to − 4.0
Caged lab monkeys	174	+ 0.16	+ 0.73	+ 7.5 to − 6.0
Near visual monkeys	186	− 0.71	+ 0.18	+ 7.0 to − 7.5

total population) the stability of the mean should be very high. Since the median in this situation does not depend upon the actual value of the individual marginal scores, the median is not affected by the missing data. The ranges are approximations for the human study subjects but are actual for the monkey groups.

Because of the number of distribution curves, the curves are presented two at a time in Figures 1−3. Figure 1 demonstrates the relationship between the wild and distance-space monkeys compared with a population of 1829 white children ranging in age from six to 12 years and older with a majority of the children (1001) being in the 12 years and older group. These children were given a cycloplegic retinoscopy examination in 1926−1927. (Kempf, *et al.* 1928).

Figure 2 shows the distribution of 3844 humans, ages 18 to 44 and 174 laboratory caged monkeys housed in ordinary sized laboratory vivaria rooms in standard monkey cages.

Figure 3 shows the distribution of the same human subjects compared with 186 experimental monkeys who had at some time or other been exposed to the near visual-space situation for at least one year.

DISCUSSION

Since the children in Washington, D.C. studies ranged in age from six to 12 and over with no breakdown of the age levels above 12, it was rather difficult to exactly specify the characteristics of the particular group of children. However, since the median age of the children was at least 12 since 55% of the children are in the 12 and over, the children would very likely have been born sometime around 1914. If so, they could be compared with the 55−64 year old age group of randomly selected adults in the population gathered by Roberts and Rolland in 1971−72 in the United States. This particular group of individuals showed a prevalence rate for myopia of 13.5%. This level is quite comparable again to the current European level and represents what maybe estimated to be the normal level of myopia for the U.S. population at earlier times. Quite clearly, the wild and distance visual situation monkeys are very similar not only in the shape of the distribution but in the means (+ 0.64 D in both groups) and in the medians (+ 0.61 in the monkeys and + 0.71 D in the humans).

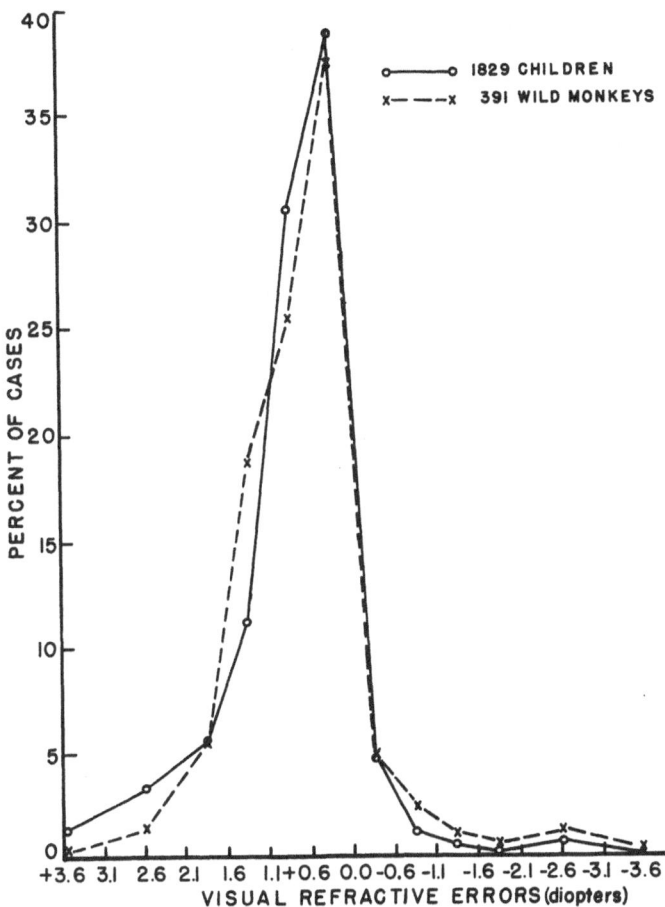

Fig. 1. Refractive distribution curve of the wild and distance-space monkeys of the present material (broken line) compared with a cycloplegic distribution curve of US children (Kempf *et al.* 1928, solid line).

When one compares the distribution of myopia in the 18—44 year old age human group with the distribution of myopia in animals which were raised or kept in the laboratory cage situation, there is also a fairly close approximation of these two distributions with respect to refractive errors. The caged laboratory animals have more hypermetropia than is found in the human population, and more low level myopia, but not as great a range of myopia as is found in the human population. When means and medians are compared, the human median is + 0.53 whereas the caged monkeys' is + 0.73, and the human mean is − 0.04 D where the animal mean is + 0.16 diopters. While these means are significantly different from each other (0.05 level), both are significantly different from those of the wild animals.

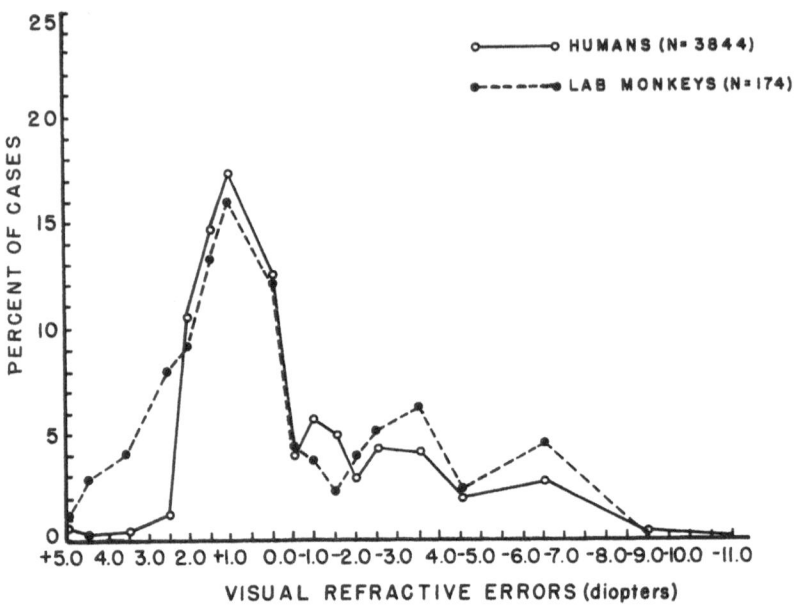

Fig. 2. Refractive distribution of laboratory monkeys housed in standard cages and ordinary rooms (broken line) compared with the distribution of humans aged 18 to 44 (cf. text, solid line).

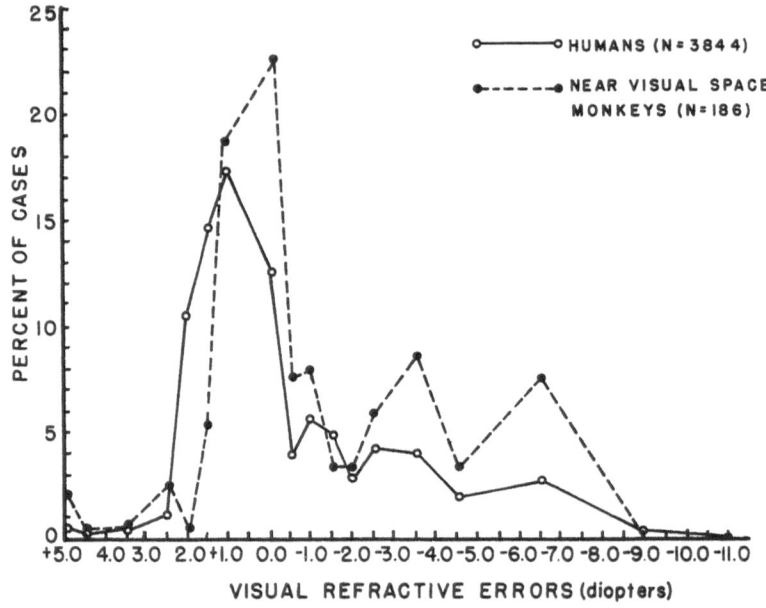

Fig. 3. Refractive distribution of near-visual-space experimental monkeys (broken line) compared with the same human sample as in Fig. 2.

10

Figure 3 shows the distributions for the humans and the experimental near-visual space monkeys. It is clear that there is considerable difference between the distributions in terms of the skewedness of the experimental monkeys toward myopia and in terms of the medians and means. While the median of the human distribution is $+ 0.53$ D, the median of the monkey distribution is $+ 0.18$ D. The mean difference is even greater since the monkeys have a mean refractive error of $- 0.71$ D compared with the human $- 0.04$. A t-test of the differences between the group means indicate that the near-visual space monkeys are significantly different from the means of the humans, the laboratory caged animals, or the wild animals, at the 0.01 level or higher.

A comparison of these distributions in terms of a Chi-square test of goodness of fit supports the mean and median differences. The wild monkeys and the Washington, D.C. children are not significantly different whereas the wild monkeys are significantly different from any of the other distributions. The near-visual space experimental animals are significantly more myopic than the human or caged laboratory animal monkeys which are not significantly different from each other.

The comparison of the wild monkey and Washington D.C. children, many of whom dropped out of school at the end of the eighth grade at a time when the total amount of myopia in the population was relatively low (13.5%), suggests that the type of visual environment which these individuals were exposed to was not greatly different from that to which the wild and distance vision animals were exposed. Comparably, the fact that animals are taken from the wild and put into the laboratory cage seems to have an effect upon the development of myopia in these caged animals, which develop a refraction distribution quite comparable to the general distribution of refractive characteristics of younger adults in our present human population of the United States. Placing animals in a near visual space situation is capable of developing amounts of myopia which are greater than those normally found in the human population. Thus it appears possible that the development of myopia in the human could easily be explained on the basis of exposure to a near visual space over a considerable time period.

REFERENCES

Kempf, G.A., et al., Refractive errors in the eyes of children as determined by retinoscopic examination with a cycloplegic. Public Health Bulletin (No. 182). US Government Printing Office Washington (1928).

Roberts, J. and Rowland, M. National Center for Health Statistics: Refraction Status and Motility Defects of Persons 4–74 Years – United States, 1971–1972. Vital and Health Statistics. Series 11-Number 206. DHEW Pub. No. (PHS) 78–1654. Health Resources Administration. US Government Printing Office (1978).

Author's address:
Professor F.A. Young, Ph.D.
Primate Research Center
Washington State University
Pullman, Washington 99164
U.S.A.

STUDY OF THE VISUAL ACUITY AND REFRACTION OF THE YAMI ON BOTEL TOBAGO ISLAND (LAN–YU)

R. YAMAJI, S. YOSHIDA, H. UCHIDA AND T. HIRANO

(Osaka, Japan)

ABSTRACT

Measurements of visual acuity of the Yami on Botel Tobago Island (Lan–Yu) were performed in July, 1971. The Yami have become completely isolated because of no chance to marry outsiders.
The results were as follows:
   (1) The visual acuity of the Yami ranged from 0.3 to 3.7.
   (2) The eyes with visual acuity from 1.2 to 2.0 accounted for 73.9% of the sample and eyes with visual acuity beyond 2.0, 19.9%. Visual acuity from 3.0 to 3.7 was found in 3.7%.
   (3) The number of eyes with visual acuity poorer than 1.0 accounted for 4%. Regarding visual disturbances, 2/3 had slight myopia and 1/3 astigmatismus myopicus inversus.
   (4) It is supposed that the excellent visual acuity of the Yami is attributable to their living circumstances with clear air at the blue sea and housing without artificial light.

INTRODUCTION

Measurements of visual acuity and refraction of the Yami living in Botel Tobago Island (Lan–Yu) were performed on the 12th–14th July, 1971. The Botel Tobago Island is located 80 km far east from the southern end of Taiwan and it is not so far from the Philippines. The Yami moved from the Philippines more than 1000 years ago. The Yami became completely isolated because of no chance to marry outsiders through 1000 years. Therefore, the Yami have been a pure tribe for at least 1000 years.

The map of Botel Tobago Island is shown in Figure 1.

METHOD

   (1) Objects of measurement were the Yami at school age (six to 18 years). The total number of objects were 202 persons and 403 eyes. The age distribution appears from Table 1.

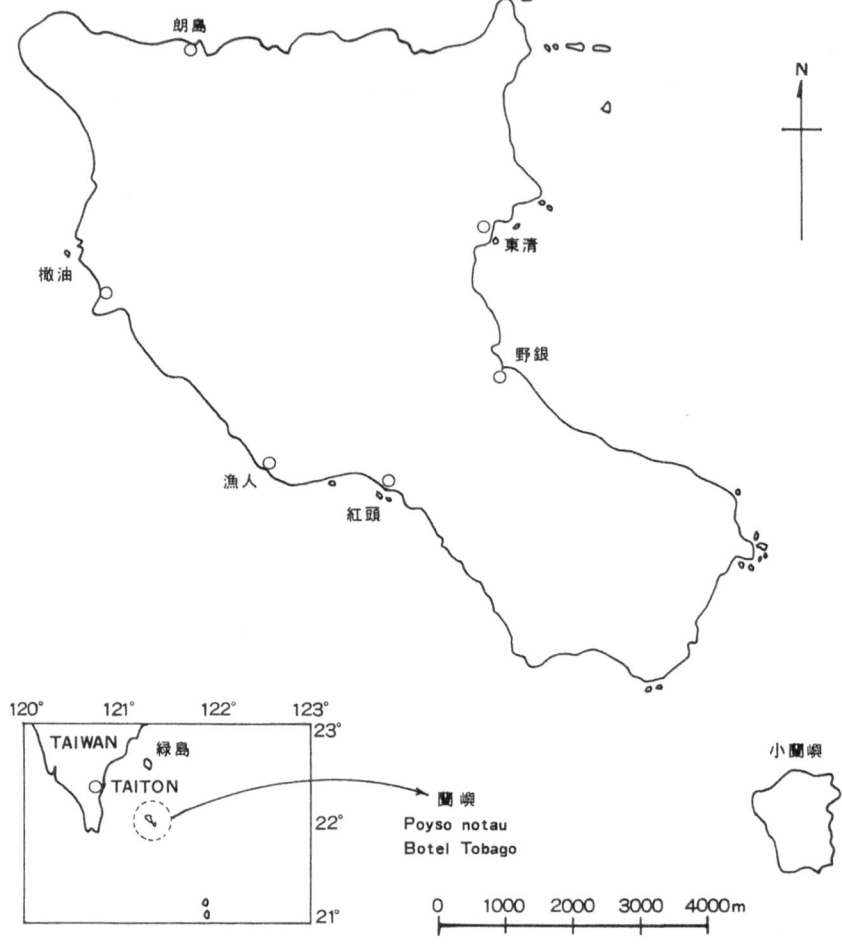

Fig. 1. Botel Tobago Island.

(2) Landolt rings, printed on paper, were used for the measurement of (uncorrected) visual acuity, at a distance of 5 m (or longer at high acuities).

(3) Skiascopy without cycloplegia was used for the measurement of refraction.

RESULTS

The visual acuity of the whole sample is shown in Table 1, subdivided according to age.

The visual acuity ranged from 0.3 to 3.7. The eyes with visual acuity from 1.2 to 2.0 accounted for 73.9% of the whole sample. Thus the eyes with visual acuity 1.2 made up 18.5%, those of 1.5—36.0% and those of

14

Table 1. The visual acuity of all eyes, according to age.

Age \ Visual acuity	0.3	0.4	0.5	0.6	0.7	0.8	0.9	1.0	1.2	1.5	2.0	2.2	2.4	2.6	2.8	3.0	3.2	3.4	3.4 over	3.6	3.7	Total
6									2	2												4
7						1		3	9	6	1											20
8					1	1	2	2	15	14	5	1	1	1	1				1			45
9						2	1	1	10	20	7	4	1	1	3	1		2				53
10			1		1				8	15	8	4	2	1								40
11			1			2		1	15	29	19	6	2		1	1			1	1		79
12	1	1						2	3	19	8	2	6	2	1	3	2		1		1	52
13			1						7	14	10	1	5	1								39
14									1	8	4		3		1		1					18
15									2	4	7	2		1								16
16									2	8	7	5										22
17										1	2	1	2	1	1							8
18									1	5	1											7
Total	1	1	3		2	4	5	9	75	145	78	27	22	8	8	5	3	2	3	1	1	403

% — 4.0 — ; 2.2 18.5 36.0 19.4 — ; 3.7 — ; 19.9

Table 2. The refraction of the eyes with visual acuity below or equal to 0.9.

| Degree of Refraction \ Age | S | | | C | S ⌢ C | Total |
	− 0.5 D	− 1.0 D	− 1.75 D	90° − 1.0 D ↑	S − 0.5 D 90° ⌢ C − 0.5 D ↑	
7	1					1
8	1	2			1	4
9	3					3
10				2		2
11		2			1	3
12			2			2
13					1	1
Total	5	4	2	2	3	16

2.0–19.4% respectively. A visual acuity beyond 2.0 was found in 19.9% of the eyes and a visual acuity from 3.0 to 3.7 in 3.7%.

As to the refraction of the eyes emmetropia accounted for 92% and hypermetropia for 4% of the eyes. All had visual acuity from 1.0 to 3.7. The degree of hypermetropia was + 0.5 D in all cases. The remaining 4% of the eyes were myopic (cf. Table 2).

The distribution of visual acuity of the primary school pupils aged from six to 12 years is shown in Figure 2. This group accounted for most of the eyes with visual acuity beyond 3.0, and for most of those below 0.9. This fact is very interesting. The refraction of the eyes with visual acuity ≤ 0.9 in this group showed slight myopia and astigmatismus myopicus inversus as shown in Table 2. It is assumed that their astigmatismus is due to heredity.

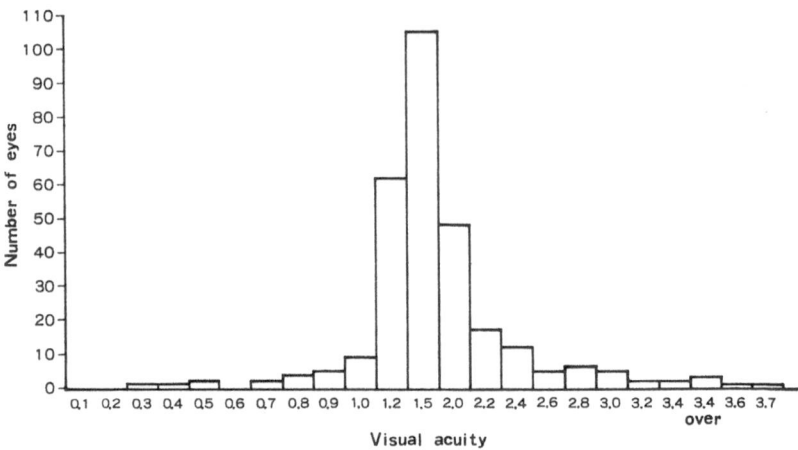

Fig. 2. Distribution of visual acuity of the primary school pupils aged from six to 12 years.

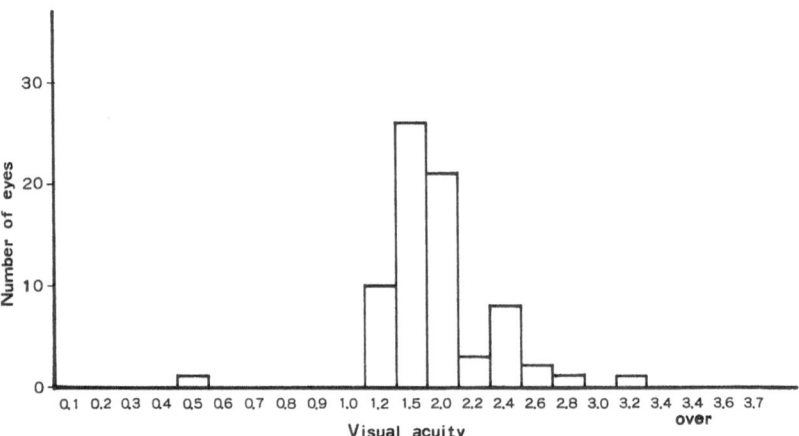

Fig. 3. Distribution of visual acuity of the middle school pupils aged from 13 to 15 years.

The distribution of visual acuity of the middle school pupils aged from 13 to 15 years is shown in Figure 3. Only one eye in this group showed the visual acuity 0.5 and its refraction is astigmatismus myopicus compositus inversus. The other eyes showed visual acuity beyond 1.0. The best visual acuity in this group was 3.2, in only one eye.

The distribution of visual acuity of objects aged from 16 to 18 years is shown in Figure 4. In this group, the visual acuity ranged from 1.2 to 2.8 and all showed emmetropia.

Thus, each group had different features. In spite of the difference, their visual acuity and refraction were excellent.

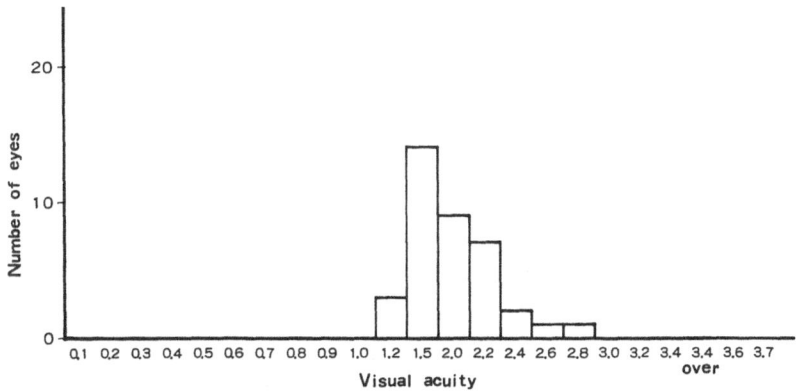

Fig. 4. Distribution of visual acuity of objects aged from 16 to 18 years.

Table 3. Visual acuity of various tribes in Taiwan.

Reporter	Tribe	Age	Total number of eyes	Visual acuity above 2.0		Best visual acuity
				n	%	
MOTEGI	Taiyal	~20	987	53	5.4	2.8
&						
KUNITOMO	Ami	~20	950	28	2.9	3.2
(1944)						
	Saishat		678	38	5.6	3.2
YAMAJI (1972)	Yami	6~18	403	80	19.9	3.7

DISCUSSION

As the reason of these results, it is considered that the living circumstances are of primary importance. The Yamis' houses have no electric equipment and artificial light is not usually used. They get up with sunrise and go to sleep with sunsink. Men take fishes in the sea and women cultivate the field. The air is clear and the sea is blue. This island is a completely unpolluted area. The dust of industry and disturbances by the medicaments of farmacy are unknown here.

The Yami have three tabus. The first is cutting the tree of the mountain. The second is walking at the night. The third is the prohibition of marriage within three degrees of relationships. The first is for the rain. The second is for the snake. The third is for the prevention of abnormal heredity.

Presumably therefore, they have escaped the hereditary factor of high myopia and astigmatismus rectus or obliquus.

It may be assumed that the life under these circumstances during 1000 years has brought an increase in the transparency of eye media, an activation of the accommodation and an increase in cone distribution of the retina and, consequently, a very good visual acuity.

The visual acuity of other tribes in Taiwan was measured by Motegi and Kunitomo in 1944. The results are shown in Table 3.

In the Saishat, the eyes with visual acuity from 2.2 to 3.2 accounted for 5.6%. In the Taiyal, eyes from 2.2 to 2.8 were found to make up 5.4% and in the Ami, those from 2.2 to 3.2 accounted for 2.9%. In the Yami, the eyes with visual acuity from 2.2 to 3.7 made up 19.9%. Therefore, the visual acuity of the Yami was the most excellent in these tribes. The Saishat and the Taiyal live in the mountains of Taiwan and the Ami lives at the seaside of Taiwan island. It is assumed that the difference in living circumstances has influenced these results.

REFERENCES

Kao, T., A human genetic study of an isolated group, the Yami. The public health institute of the medical department of Taiwan University, (1965).

Motegi, S., Kunitomo, N. et al. Ophthalmological research of the Takasago, part 1, the Saishat, Med J Taiwan 43: 778 (1944).

Motegi, S., Kunitomo, N. et al., Ophthalmological research of the Takasago, part 2, the Taiyal, Med J Taiwan 43: 826 (1944).

Motegi, S., Kunitomo, N. et al., Ophthalmological research of the Takasago, part 4, the Ami, Med J Taiwan 44: 71 (1946).

Yamaji, R., Yoshida, S. et al., Study of the visual acuity of the Yami on Botel Tobago Island (Lan–Yu), Folia Ophthalmol Jap., 23: 267 (1972).

Senior author's address:
R. Yamaji, M.D.
Eye Clinic
Osaka Otemae Hospital
Osaka, Japan

REFRACTION IN HUMANS FROM BIRTH TO FIVE YEARS

I. MOHINDRA and R. HELD

(Cambridge, Massachusetts, U.S.A.)

ABSTRACT

The results of refraction of 400 human infants from birth to five years of age are reported. In contrast to the traditional view that spherical equivalent refraction (SER) is hyperopic at birth, our results indicate that newborns are relatively myopic. With increasing age there is a decline in the myopic SER, becoming emmetropic around 6 months of age and hyperopic thereafter. Our results also show that the SER distribution is bell shaped at birth with a large variance. The degree of variance decreases with age and approaches the adult value close to one year of age. Incidence of astigmatism ($\geqslant 1$ D) is high in neonates, peaks around two to three months, and thereafter decreases slowly. The incidence is 35% for the age groups 129–256 weeks, which is still higher than 10% found in adults. Incidence of myopia ($\geqslant 1$ D) on the other hand decreases from 35% in the neonates to about 5% for the oldest age group (129–256 weeks). Incidence of hyperopia remains constant at 35% throughout the first five years of life. The lability of refraction during the first few years of life accompanies the fast rate of growth of the eye.

INTRODUCTION

Early visual deprivation can lead to deleterious and often irreversible effects as demonstrated by psychophysical, electrophysiological, and anatomical studies of animals, including primates (Hubel, *et al.* 1977; Mitchell 1978; Stone, *et al.* 1979). The refractive state of the eye is one of the factors that influences the quality of the visual input. In humans except for a few studies in the newborn (Banks 1979), very little is understood about the post-natal course of development of refraction. The spherical-equivalent refractive errors of newborns and neonates appear to be normally distributed (bell-shaped) with a mean of about $+2.0$ D and a standard deviation of 2.0 D as shown by several studies (Cook and Glasscock 1951; Goldschmidt 1969; Howland *et al.* 1978; Mehra *et al.* 1965). The refractive errors of adults, on the other hand, appear to have a leptokurtic distribution with a mean refraction between $+0.5$ and $+1.0$ D, generally considered to be emmetropic, and a standard deviation of about 1.0 D (Sorsby *et al.* 1960). The change in refractive error, showing that the variable and hypermetropic refraction of the neonate becomes emmetropic and less variable, has been called emmetropization (Sorsby 1960). Establishing the developmental course of emmetropization is important for assessing the role of refraction in early deprivation and in taking preventive measures.

The gap in our understanding of the development of refraction in human infants can be attributed to the difficulties of evaluating refractions in neonates, infants, and children. During early infancy, an infant is asleep nearly 80% of the time. During waking periods there is always an uncertainty of fixation either in distance or direction which raises questions about the state of the infant's accommodation. The common method of controlling accommodation in infants and young children is the use of cycloplegic drugs. Very little, however, is known regarding the action of these drugs on the developing ciliary musculature. In addition, there are no practical procedures to determine precisely the degree of residual ciliary muscle action in infants, i.e., the residual accommodation. Several systemic and local adverse side effects of cycloplegics are well established in the literature. Thus, use of cycloplegics for the young population becomes impractical and questionable.

In light of the above it becomes quite clear that there is definitely a need for procedures for refracting infants and young children, which do not require the use of cycloplegics and yet control the level of the infant's accommodation. Recently, we have developed the procedure of near-retinoscopy (Mohindra 1977). The purpose of this study is to assess refractions of infants from birth to five years of age by utilizing this non-cycloplegic procedure and formulating normative refractive data. The manner in which accommodation is controlled by near retinoscopy is shown by Owens et al. (1980).

SUBJECTS

A sample of 400 full-term healthy infants and children, of ages between birth and five years of age, from Cambridge and Boston, Massachusetts, was collected through letters promising tests of vision. The responders made up 15% of those invited. The older children were from local nursery schools and day care centers. The ages of 312 infants ranged from birth to approximately two years of age. The remaining 88 children were between two and five years of age. The mean birth weight was 3404 g with a standard deviation of 573 g.

PROCEDURE

For the purpose of this study only the refractions from the first visit of each infant were used. All refractions were obtained by using the near retinoscopy procedure. During this procedure retinoscopy is performed at a fixed distance of 50 cm on a non-cyclopleged eye, in an otherwise dark room. An adjustment factor of -1.25 D was added to the spherical component at neutrality to obtain the static distance refraction of the eye. The infants were divided into seven different age groups starting from the neonate group (0–4 weeks) and continuing in seven equal logarithmic steps.

The spherical equivalent refractions (SERs) were calculated by adding one-half the amount of the cylinder to the spherical component, for both the right and left eyes. For each age group percentages of hyperopic, myopic and emmetropic SERs were ascertained. The amount of astigmatism was classified in one diopter steps for each age group. Frequency of these classifications of astigmatism for each of the seven different age groups was also calculated. Distribution of anisometropia for the SERs was also determined.

RESULTS

Spherical Equivalent Refraction (SER)

Distribution curves for the SERs of the right eye of infants in each of the seven age groups are shown in Figure 1. The mean ($\bar{x}$), standard deviation (SD), standard error of the mean, kurtosis, and skewness of the SERs for the right eyes and the numbers of infants in each group are presented in Table 1.

Comparison of the SER of the neonates (0–4 weeks) obtained from the present study by near retinoscopy with those obtained from the cycloplegic refractions by Cook and Glasscock are presented in Figure 1. The percentage distributions of emmetropia and myopia, based on the SERs of infants in each of the seven age groups are presented in Figure 2. The means of the SERs for each age group are presented in Figure 3. Comparison of the SERs of children in the present study with those of adults obtained by Sorsby (Sorsby *et al.* 1960) from recruits of military services in the United Kingdom is shown in Figure 1.

Astigmatism

Incidence of astigmatism ($\geqslant 1.0$ D) from birth to five years of life is presented in Figure 2. The distribution of the mean amount of astigmatism for the right and left eyes of the infants with astigmatism equal to or exceeding 1 D in each of the seven age groups is presented in Figure 3.

DISCUSSION

Spherical Equivalent Refraction (SER)

The refractive distribution curves for SER of infants and children in each of the seven age groups of our sample, as shown in Figure 1, are in agreement with the traditional view that refractive distribution during infancy is bell shaped (Cook and Glasscock 1951; Goldschmidt 1969; Akiba 1969), with

21

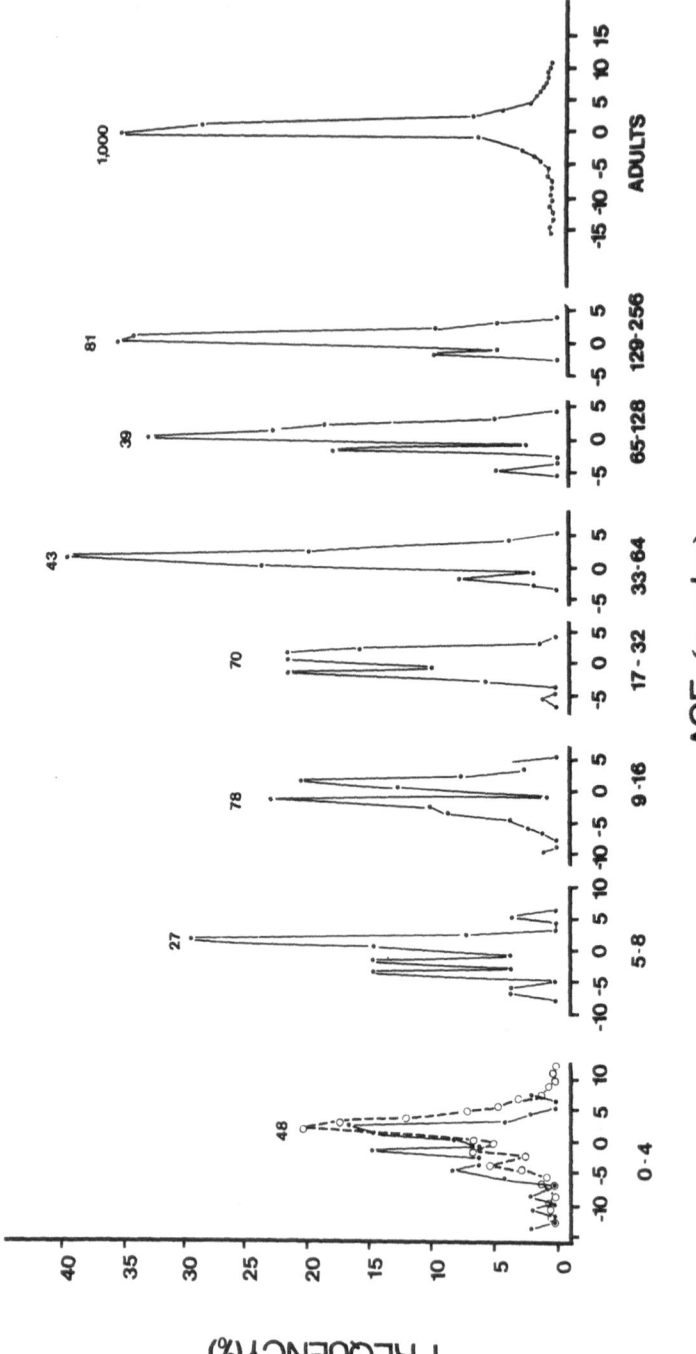

Fig. 1. Spherical Equivalent Refraction with increasing age groups. In group 0—4 the material of Cook & Glasscock (1951) is included (broken line and circles). Adults from Sorsby *et al.* (1960).

22

Table 1. Spherical equivalent refraction (SER). Distribution in seven age groups from birth to five years' age.

Age Group (weeks)	N	Mean ($\bar{X}$) of SER (D)	SD of SER (D)	Skewness SER	Kurtosis SER	Std_Error of $\bar{X}$ SER
0–4	48	− 0.70	3.20	− 0.96	2.10	0.46
5–8	27	− 0.35	2.30	− 0.60	0.98	0.44
9–16	78	− 0.52	2.25	− 0.90	2.21	0.25
17–32	70	0.13	1.29	− 0.79	2.27	0.15
33–64	50	0.78	0.97	− 0.15	0.25	0.14
65–128	39	0.43	1.32	− 1.03	2.70	0.21
129–256	81	0.59	0.85	0.97	1.05	0.09

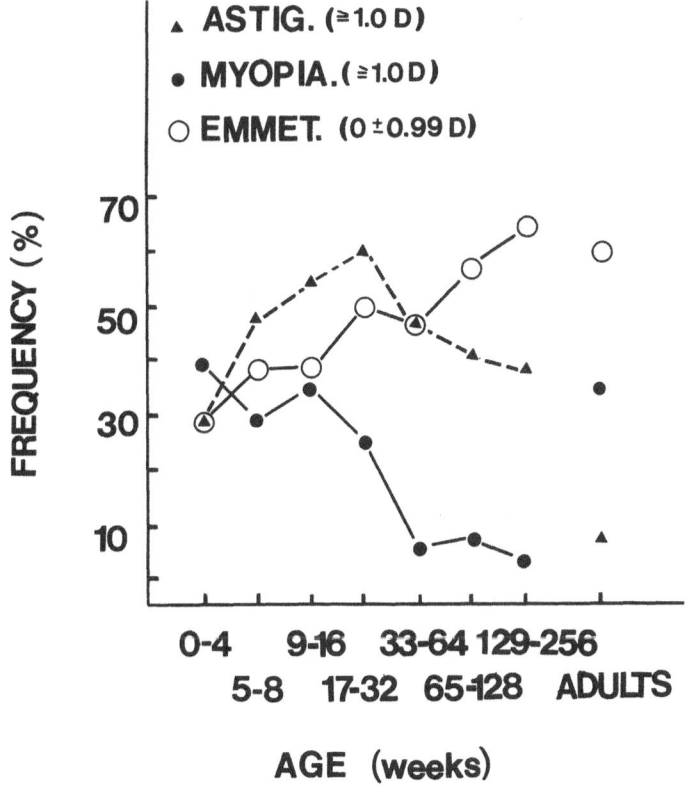

Fig. 2. Incidence of myopia, emmetropia, and astigmatism with increasing age groups.

a large variance. The mean of the SER for our age group of 0–4 weeks is − 0.69 D with a standard deviation of 3.21 and standard error of the mean of 0.46. Statistically, therefore, this − 0.69 D value for the mean of the SER is not significantly different than zero.

The mean of the SER determined by Cook and Glasscock using cyclo-plegia and confirmed by various other investigators (Goldschmidt 1969;

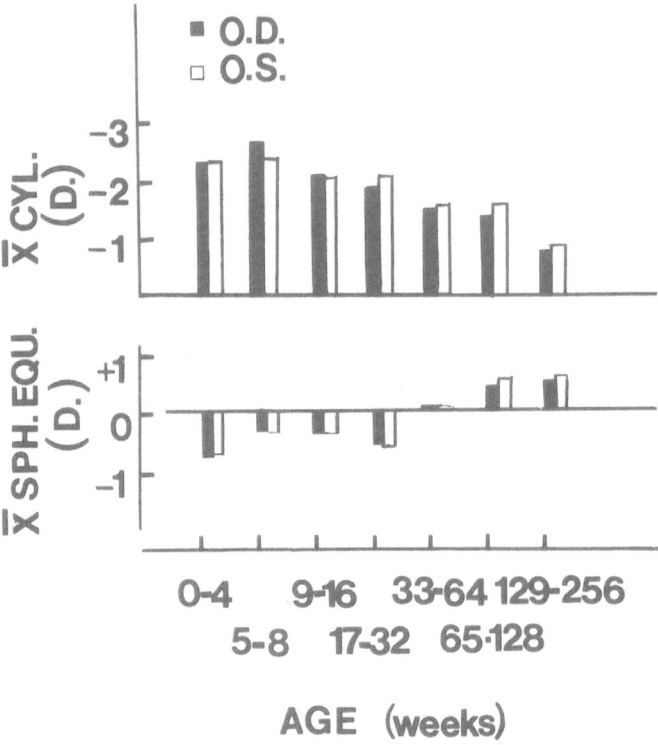

Fig. 3. Distribution of mean spherical equivalent refraction and cylinder for increasing age groups.

Zonis and Miller 1974) is + 2.0 D with a standard deviation of 2.0 D. Cook and Glasscock's sample consisted of 1000 newborns. Thus their mean of 2.0 D for SER becomes significantly different from zero, with a standard error of the mean of 0.06. These results are in contrast to the results obtained from our present study. We suspect that the differences in results can be accounted for by the fact that neither Cook and Glasscock nor any other investigators who used cycloplegia adjusted for loss of ciliary muscle tonus which occurs as a result of the actions of the cycloplegic agents. Tait (1975) extrapolated to 1.75 D the ciliary muscle tonus for infants and children under three years of age. Adjusting the + 2.0 D mean of the SER for the newborns, as determined by Cook and Glasscock (1951), by − 1.75 D yields the resultant mean of only + 0.25 D. This adjusted mean value for the SER is not significantly different from zero and does not disagree with our results.

The degree and incidence of myopia for the SER of the neonates as revealed by results of our study changes with age, as shown in Figure 2 and 3. During the first year SER begins to develop toward increasing hypermetropia. The histogram of Figure 3 shows the mean of the SER for all seven age groups from birth to five years of age. The regression line was

24

calculated by doing a linear regression of the mean of the SER on log age. The intersection of the regression line with the Y-axis predicts the average refraction at birth to be about -1.0 D, changing to emmetropia by about six months and becoming increasingly hypermetropic thereafter. Strömberg (1936), after examining eyes of 5000 adults, reported a mean and standard deviation for the SER of $+0.5$ D and 1.1 D respectively. Similarly Sorsby found a mean of $+0.50$ D with a standard deviation of 1.0 D after examining 2000 eyes of young British army recruits. These values compare favorably with the values obtained from our sample beyond the age group of 16–32 weeks. The myopic trend as shown by the means for the SER found in our younger age groups is also shown by the incidence of myopic, emmetropic, and hyperopic SER as shown in Figure 2. Incidence of myopia ($\geqslant 1.00$ D) reduces from 38% for the age group 0–4 weeks, to 3.7% for the age group 129–256 weeks. In contrast the incidence of emmetropia ($0 + 0.99$ D) increases from 29% for the youngest age group to 65% for the oldest age group. Incidence of hyperopia ($\geqslant 1.0$ D) on the other hand remains fairly stable for all age groups at around 35%. The incidence of myopia, emmetropia, and hyperopia in the adult population as cited in a US survey report of 1978 is 35%, 60%, and 5% respectively. The increased incidence of myopia in our younger infants agrees with that reported by Goldschmidt (1969) in his newborn population. The incidence of anisometropia based on the SER is around 22% in younger age groups and reduces to about 5% after $2\frac{1}{2}$ years of age.

Astigmatism

Recent reports by Howland *et al.* (1978) and Mohindra *et al.* (Mohindra 1978) have shown that there is a high incidence of astigmatism during infancy and early childhood. As reported by Mohindra *et al.* (1978), the incidence of astigmatism ($\geqslant 1$ D) is about 30% at birth rising to a peak of 51% between nine and 32 weeks. These results are confirmed by the results of our present study. As shown in Figure 2, the peak incidence of astigmatism of 59% occurs in the age group ranging from 17 to 32 weeks. It gradually decreases with increasing age and even for the oldest age group (129–256 weeks) the incidence remains at 39% which is higher than the 10% level found in adults (Sorsby *et al.* 1960; Sorsby 1979). The amount of astigmatism as determined by the mean of the cylinder values for each age group, and shown for both the right and left eyes in Figure 3, also declines with age. For instance, the linear regression for the amount of cylinder on log age predicts the cylinder to be 2.98 D at birth, and decreasing to about 1.0 D for the oldest age group (129–256 weeks). The mean cylinder amount of 1 D found in our oldest age group (129–256 weeks) is similar to the amount found in adults by Sorsby (Sorsby *et al.* 1960; Sorsby 1979), although the incidence of astigmatism is higher than that found in adults.

The etiology of this infantile astigmatism is not clear. All refractions were obtained by the near retinoscopy procedure. During this procedure the retinoscopy is performed as close to the visual axis of the infant's eye as possible as noted by the corneal reflex. Thus the measures of astigmatism due to oblique refraction (with respect to the visual axis) cannot account for this astigmatism. Observation of the reflections of a placido disc from the front surface of the cornea in several infants and keratometer measurements of several toddlers showed a good correlation between corneal astigmatism and that measured by near retinoscopy. It is possible that growth of the eye from birth, when the eye is two thirds of its adult weight and volume (Duke Elder 1963), influences the shape and size of the cornea. This change in shape is accompanied by a change in astigmatism. Because of some combination of the high lability of astigmatism, the low levels of visual resolution, and possible lack of neural susceptibility during the first year of the infant's life, the high amount of astigmatism does not appear to cause any deprivational neurological disorders, such as the meridional amblyopia found in adults. Thus far the earliest age at which we have found meridional amblyopia was two years and ten months. This toddler had had oblique anisometropic astigmatism of 2 D from eight months of life. However, after receiving his spectacle correction at two years and 10 months of age, the meridional amblyopia disappeared within a couple of months (by $3\frac{1}{2}$ years of age) (Held 1978).

SUMMARY

The concluding remarks are condensed in the abstract.

ACKNOWLEDGEMENT

This research was supported in part by grants from the National Institutes of Health (2RO1 EY-01191, 5 P30 EY-02621, and 3 MO1 RR 00088–17S1).

REFERENCES

Akiba, M., The studies on the refractive status of the normal infant. Acta Soc. Ophthalmol. Jap. 73, Tokyo Nippon Ganka Zasshi (March 1969).

Banks, M.S., Infants ocular refraction and accommodation, Int Ophthalmol Clin (1979).

Cook, R.G. & Glasscock, R.E., Refractive and ocular findings in the newborn. Am. J. Ophthalmol. 34: 1407–1413 (1951).

Duke Elder, Sir Stewart, Normal and abnormal development. 3(1) Embryology. pp. 310–311 (1963).

Goldschmidt, E., Refraction in the newborn. Acta Ophthalmol 47: 570–578 (1969).

Held, R., New methods of refracting infants and testing the visual resolution of infants. Symp Appl Psychophys Clin Probl Conf Behavioral and Social Sci. National Research Council, National Academy of Sciences, San Francisco, California (Oct. 30, 1978).

Howland, H.D., et al., Astigmatism measured by photorefraction. Science, 202: 900–902 (1978).

Hubel, D.H., et al., Plasticity of ocular dominance columns in monkey striate cortex. Phil. Trans. R. Soc. London, B-278: 377–409 (1977).

Mehra, K.S., et al., Refraction in full term babies. Br J. Ophthalmol. 49: 276–277 (1965).

Mitchell, D.E., Effect of early visual experience on the development of certain perceptual abilities in animals and man. In: Perception and Experience Eds. Walk R.D. Plenum Publishing Corp. New York pp. 37–75 (1978).

Mohindra, I., A non-cycloplegic refraction technique for infants and young children. J. of Am. Optom. Assoc. 48: 518–523 (1977).

Mohindra, I., et al., Astigmatism in infants. Science. 202: 329–331 (1978).

Owens, D. Alfred, Mohindra, I. Held, R., The effectiveness of a retinoscope beam as an accommodative stimulus. Invest. Ophthalmology and Visual Science., 19: 942–949 (1980).

Sorsby, A., et al., Visual acuity and ocular refraction of young men. Br. Med. J 1:1394 (1960).

Sorsby, A., Biology of the eye as an optical system. In: J.D. Duane (ed.): Clinical Ophthalmol. Vol. 1 (34). Harper & Row, New York (1976).

Stone, J., et al., Hierarchical and parallel mechanisms in the organization of visual cortex. Brain Res Rev 1: 345–394 (1979).

Stromberg, E., Uber Refraktion and Achsenlange des menschlichen Auges. Acta Ophthalmol. Kbh. 14: 281. 1936.

Tait, E.C., In: Pediatric Ophthalmology Ed. Harley Saunders Philadelphia pp. 113–131 (1975).

Zonis, S., and Miller, B., Refractions in the Israeli newborn. J. of Pediat Ophthal. 2: 77–81 (1974).

Authors' address:
Massachusetts Institute of Technology
Department of Psychology
Cambridge, Massachusetts 02139
U.S.A.

LONG-TERM FOLLOW-UP STUDIES OF MYOPIA

B. LECAILLON-THIBON

(*Perpignan, France*)

ABSTRACT

Results are given from long-term follow-up studies of myopic children and adolescents in two French province areas. Out of more than 600 cases under study, a scant hundred were followed regularly (twice a year) for more than eight years.

Atropine and contact lenses could arrest progression in some cases.

Cases with an early onset of myopia usually progress most. Most cases become stable at, or after the age of 20 years. The variability of progression is however stressed.

All considered, the present results are in accord with those of other myopia follow-up studies.

INTRODUCTION

Longitudinal studies with long-term follow-up were programmed at the First International Conference on Myopia (New York 1964), and several studies have been carried out since then, especially in Japan.

In Europe such studies are not possible in the big centers, due to changing examiners and due to the fact that patients often move. I therefore find it of interest to publish my own results, from French provincial areas, and to compare them with those obtained in other countries with different environmental factors. It will appear, that the conclusions are pretty similar.

In Yokohama, at the Second International Conference on Myopia, the effects of various treatments of myopia were emphasized. At the *present* conference we aim at getting further information about long-term progression and clinical types.

MATERIAL

In Normandy (North-western France), from 1954 to 1970, we observed more than 500 cases of acquired (= non-congenital) progressive myopia in children and adolescents. Eighty had been examined regularly, twice a year, for more than eight years.

Doc. Ophthal. Proc. Series, Vol. 28,
ed. by H.C. Fledelius, P.H. Alsbirk and E. Goldschmidt
© *1981 Dr W. Junk Publishers, The Hague*

In Perpignan (Southern France) we examined 100 similar cases, from 1970 to 1980. Sixteen had regular follow-ups for more than eight years.

METHODS

Circumstances of examination were kept identical, and the same examiner saw all cases (double blind examination is not possible in private practice):

(1) *Objective examination,* by streak retinoscopy (with cylinders).

(2) *Subjective examination,* binocular fogging method without cycloplegia, and monocular fogging method using atropine cycloplegia at first examination; on following occasions at least Mydrium M (Mydriaticum, Chibret) or cyclopentolate (Skiakol, P.O.S. Lab.) for cycloplegia.

Concerning the accuracy in single cases, we are without illusions, but we consider it possible to give refractive value by steps of 1/8 D. This is based on the *subjective* examination, through the influence on visual acuity of weak plus glasses during the fogging procedure, at a distance of 5 m (or ten, by mirror reading), according to this tabulation:

If correction to 'emmetropia' gives visual acuity $\geqslant 10/10$,

0.12 D fogging gives visual acuity	0.9,
0.25 D fogging gives visual acuity	0.7,
0.37 D fogging gives visual acuity	0.6,
0.50 D fogging gives visual acuity	0.5,
0.62 D fogging gives visual acuity	0.4,
0.75 D fogging gives visual acuity	0.3, and
1.00 D fogging gives about	0.2 in v.a..

The precision is good only in the upper part of the Table. When performed at 5 m, we have added 0.2 D to the refractive value, to obtain refraction at infinity (a fact often forgotten in optical corrections or in refraction recordings).

Conformity of results with and without cycloplegia demonstrates absence of accomodative spasm and signify a position of accommodative rest. When the patient is wearing a correct optical correction, the difference in refraction as related to ± cycloplegia seldom exceeds 0.25 D.

RESULTS, IN GENERAL

In the presentation given at the conference, evolution of single cases was shown by slides, with age on abscissa, and refraction, as spherical equivalent, on y-axis.

In some cases *treatment* had been given, to arrest myopia, for example with Mydrium M, Neosynephrine and Difrarel E. Occasionally there was a slight short-term effect of this treatment, but the long-term evolution was almost never modified.

Similarly, when treatment with the Diasonic of Yamamoto caused evident reduction in myopia (usually 0.25 D), the effect was not lasting, nor was the long-term result influenced.

Contrarily, stabilization of myopia appeared to be effective after treatment with atropine and treatment with contact lenses, and the natural evolution of the single case seemed entirely changed.

RESULTS, IN REFRACTIVE SUBGROUPS

Before analysing patterns of evolution in myopes, we may look at patterns of evolution in other refractive groups (apparent from statistical studies, which are not the direct subject of the present paper).

Hypermetropia usually decreases slowly with age, but in a few cases there is an increase, especially in cases of early and high hypermetropia. Such cases illustrate another way of missing emmetropisation.

Astigmatism, per se, is more stable than myopia is. We have, however, observed important long-term variations and modifications in a few cases. Axis and level change with age. Usually there is an amelioration of astigmatism with the rule and aggravation of against-rule astigmatism.

Astigmatism is more pronounced in high myopia. Rapidly progressing myopia is often associated with significant astigmatism, especially if uncorrected. Congenital myopia is less stable if astigmatism is associated as well. These facts support the theories of Otsuka.

Myopia progression: It may be difficult to establish the exact time of onset of acquired myopia. Usually it is discovered between the fourth and eighth school grade, but it may begin even earlier.

High myopia at a rather early age is probably *congenital,* especially if it is stable, because (conversely) it is well known that high congential myopia *is* usually stable. Often it is unilateral (confirming the importance of genetic factors in congenital myopia). In our material, we have observed a few congenital myopia cases with progression – *degenerative* myopia always begins before puberty.

The majority of *acquired* myopia cases show the more progression, the earlier they start. Thus:
(a) Most cases starting before the age of seven years are between − 3 and − 7 D eight years later, and are still progressing after 12 years observation.
(b) Those starting between the age of nine and 12 reach 2–5 D of myopia eight years later and still show progress after another eight years.
(c) With onset after the age of 14 years, myopia will increase to 1–3 D, and may show progress even after five years observation.

Myopia usually becomes stable after the age of 20, some earlier, while others are not stabilized before 30.

Deviations from the above rules do exist. Some precocious myopias remain of low order, and some late cases may show a rapid progression.

Comparison between right and left eye: If similar at onset, myopia progression is usually parallel. If one of the eyes is markedly more myopic at onset, the side difference usually increases with evolution.

31

DISCUSSION

It is not possible to generalize, and we must stress that myopia frequency and pattern of evolution vary with ethnic factors and environmental conditions.

Our results are valid only for the regions under study. We noticed that myopia is less frequent and progressive in Perpignan (Southern France) than in Evreux, in the Normandy. Possible factors may be discussed: Alcoholism in Normandy (in adults and babies?); a relative preponderance of blue eyes in Normandy and brown eyes in the south; living in the open air in the South, in-doors in Normandy; content of atmospheric carbon dioxide higher in Normandy, etc.

CONCLUDING REMARK

Definite associations exist between: time of onset, speed of initial progression, fundus changes, final progression, and final level of myopia. However, the variability and irregularity of myopia development make it difficult to give an exact prediction of the course in the individual patient.

Author's address:
B. Lecaillon-Thibon, M.D.
4 Rue des Jokglars
6600 Perpignan, France

THE ONSET AND PROGRESSION OF MYOPIA IN DANISH SCHOOL CHILDREN

T. ROSENBERG and E. GOLDSCHMIDT

(Svendborg and Odense, Denmark)

ABSTRACT

An analysis of a myopia material from a private practice, consisting of 122 boys and 158 girls, shows that myopia develops in all ages with a maximum around puberty. No major sex differences were observed. The progression during the first years varies with a tendency to a stronger yearly increase, if myopia develops before puberty. The great variation in yearly increase is demonstrated. The findings are in agreement with previous studies and do not indicate an increase in the progression of myopia in Danish school children.

INTRODUCTION

Few reports exist showing the variation in myopia progression or the importance of time of onset for the future development. In Denmark, a study by Blegvad 1918 illustrates the natural history of myopia in the beginning of the century and the present study gives a picture of the development of myopia in recent years.

MATERIAL AND METHODS

The material was selected from the files (1974–1979) of an ophthalmological practice in a Danish provincial town. All patients born 1958 or later (i.e. aged 20 or less at the time of the investigation) and seen in the office twice or more with a minimum observation time of 12 months were selected. In this way a material of 280 myopia cases were collected.

The routine procedure included the following measurements: refractometry (Rodenstock), subjective refraction (AO-phoropter, 6 m), heterophoria with correction (Maddox rod 6 m, 40 cm), near vision, binocular balance and stereopsis.

When the subjective refraction, esophoria or other observations gave suspicion of hyperactive accommodation a control examination in cycloplegia (cyclopentolate, Cyclogyl[(R)] 1%) was made.

Prescription of glasses in general was made according to the subjective value of the lowest myopia in duochrome test. Only monofocals were prescribed. The wearing instructions were liberal.

The age of onset of myopia was defined as the age at the first examination revealing myopia. In cases where glasses already were used the age at onset was defined from information on the age when glasses were first prescribed.

In astigmatism the degree of myopia was listed as the equivalent sphere.

As the majority of the children were still in the myopic progression phase, no data on the final degree of myopia can be derived from this material.

RESULTS

In Table 1 the age of onset is listed according to sex. The table indicates a slight tendency to earlier onset of myopia among girls.

The preschool-group consists of nine boys and seven girls. Apart from two girls being only ten years old at latest examination all have reached a myopia of at least 4 D.

Table 2 demonstrates the results from that part of the children where the initial two years' progression could be estimated. 252 children fulfilled this criterium. The mean progression of the two eyes was chosen as parameter.

Table 1. Age at onset in 280 myopia cases.

Age	Boys	Girls
< 7	9	7
7–8	16	19
9–10	21	42
11–12	40	43
13–14	24	33
15–16	11	13
⩾ 17	1	1
Total	122	158

Table 2. First two years' increase in school myopia.

Age at onset	Boys (n = 108)			Girls (n = 144)		
	⩽ 1 D	1.25–2 D	2.25–3 D	⩽ 1 D	1.25–2 D	2.25–3 D
7–8	7	6	2	7	9	2
9–10	9	9	2	15	19	4
11–12	18	19	1	26	10	6
13–14	14	10	–	23	8	2
15–16	11	–	–	12	1	–

34

Table 3. Annual increase in myopia.

Age at onset		No.	Observation (Months)	Mean (Dioptres)	SD
Girls	9–10	30	42.0	0.47	0.28
	11–12	36	37.8	0.37	0.42
Boys	11–12	37	40.1	0.40	0.22

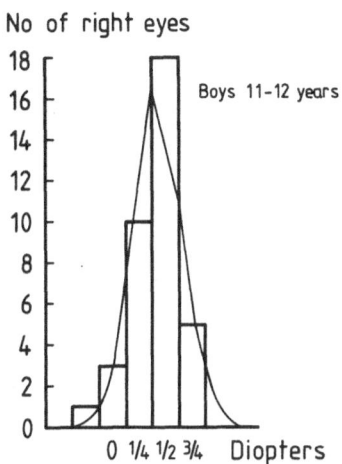

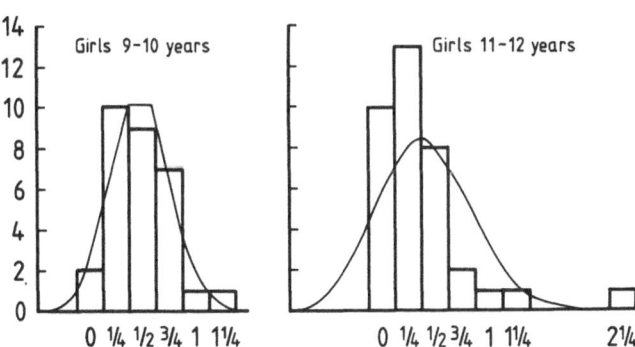

Fig. 1. Annual increase in myopia.

About 60% have a progression under 1 D. As the other extreme, only about 5% of the boys and about 10% of the girls increase more than 2 D during the first two years. There is a weak tendency that myopia starting before puberty exhibits a stronger progression than myopia starting in puberty, and the progression is particularly slight in late-onset myopia.

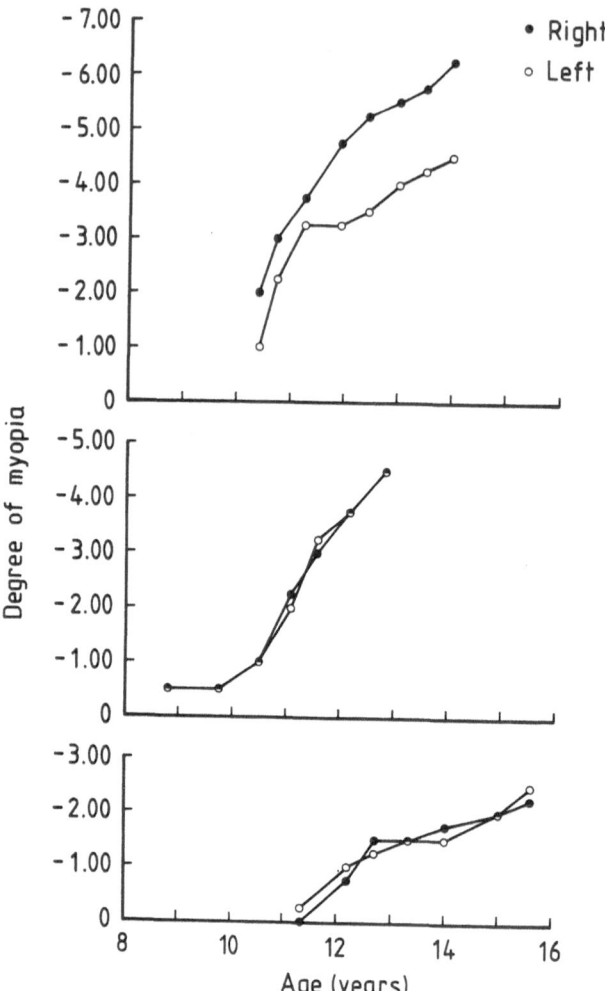

Fig. 2. Progression curves in myopia.

In order to minimize the effect of variation due to different age at onset, three numerically well-represented onset-age groups were selected (Table 3 and Figure 1). In these children the progression of the right eye was chosen (given as the difference between the myopia at the most recent examination and the initial value), using the mean annual progression during the whole observation period as parameter. With this technique a period with rapid progression could be 'hidden' by a long observation period after the myopia became stationary. This error was reduced by excluding end-periods of observation where no progression in an otherwise progressive myopia could be ascertained.

The annual progression rate is moderate, but the variations are rather

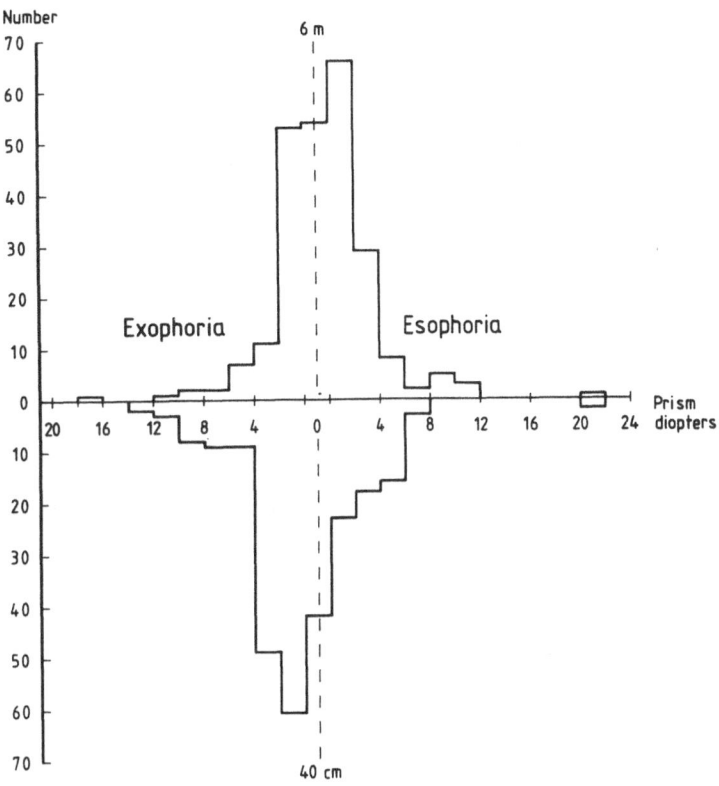

Fig. 3. Heterophoria measurements in 245 myopia cases.

great. Of particular interest is the group of girls in the onset-age group 11–12, which shows a greater variation than the other groups. In Figure 2 examples of the great variation in progression is demonstrated. Roughly speaking, the curves demonstrate three different types of progression: the hyperbolic, the logarithmic (or S-shaped) and the arithmetic or straight-line type. In addition the progression curves show the problems in using one eye as a control of the fellow-eye.

Periods without progression alternate with periods with progression and although the main type of progression is the same in the two eyes, the differences are striking. Despite the variation demonstrated, it seems justified to conclude that the progression of myopia among Danish school children in the late 1970s was in the range of 1/3 to 1/2 D per year.

The result of heterophoria measurements in 245 cases are shown in Figure 3.

As in other groups of 'normals', eso-deviations prevail when measured at 6 m, while exophorias dominate at near distance – in the individual cases, changes were observed in both directions. Thus 50 children had a

37

higher eso- or a lower exo-deviation at near when re-tested (range 1–17 PD, mean 3,5 PD), while 171 changed in the opposite direction (range 1–16 PD, mean 3,3 PD). Twenty-four children showed no change. All considered, changes towards exo (and away from eso, the deviation-type usually connected with accommodation) prevailed. Keeping in mind the fluctuations of repeated individual heterophoria measurement values, far-reached conclusions should not be drawn. Indirectly, the results may, however, suggest, that a hyper-accommodative state is not common in young myopes.

DISCUSSION

The age at onset of myopia is not a well defined parameter. In typical cases the first examination was preceded by six months to a year with complaints of reduced distant vision. Undoubtedly marked differences exist in children's adaptation to reduced distant vision. Some children have complaints when only 0.5 D of myopia or less can be found. In contrast, astonishingly often 1–2 D of myopia are measured during the first examination of children without any complaints. The pre-myopic period and the initial phase of myopia development seems so variable in respect to duration, symptomatology, and progression that retrograde extrapolation from the first examination is not justified in order to define the exact onset of myopia.

The material in average exhibits a moderate rate of progression. Compared with the findings by Blegvad 1918 (Table 4) there is no evidence of major changes in myopia progression during this century in Danish school children. Similar results were obtained by Fletcher 1964 in American school children, while Oakley and Young 1975 found higher rates of annual increase in American Caucasian groups.

A well-functioning school screening could be the explanation of a rather great proportion of low myopes with a low progression rate. It is also worth to mention the altered attitude among school children to spectacles. Modern spectacles are quite different from those 30 years ago. In fact, spectacles at some ages – especially among girls – are desired, independent of visual symptoms. In a material as the present this will induce a bias in favour of low, non-progressive myopia.

Another factor is that many low-myopes without progression omit controls or go to opticians when new glasses are needed. This will tend to bias the ophthalmologist's material in direction of the heavier cases.

Finally, the spectacle regime in the clinic was rather liberal. On this background adherents to theories of accommodation mechanisms in the etiology of myopia could use the rather low progression of the present material as an argument for their view.

The study emphasizes all the classical difficulties in handling a retrospectively collected, clinical material on myopia. The methodological problems that arise in the statistical treatise of these materials are well known. This implies that any study that claims a beneficial effect of any treatment must take into consideration that enormous materials have to be collected. This demand is so much the greater as double-blind techniques cannot be adapted to this field of clinical research.

Table 4. Average annual progression in 87 myopic children seen in a Copenhagen private practice 1905–1916 and re-examined 1917 (Blegvad 1918).

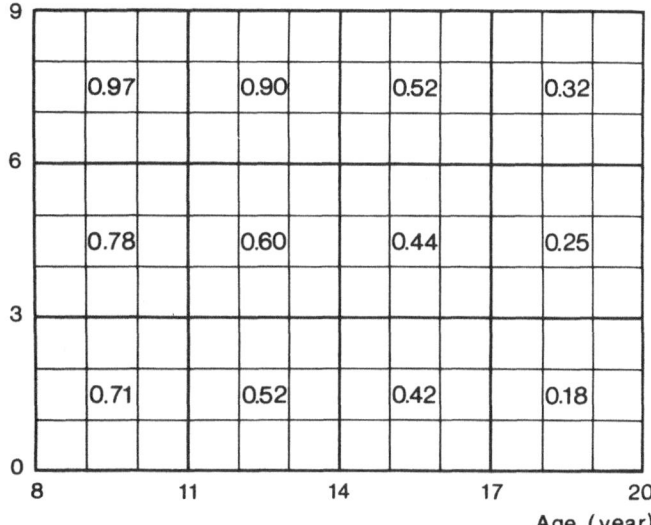

Average annual progression

Degree of myopia

0.97	0.90	0.52	0.32
0.78	0.60	0.44	0.25
0.71	0.52	0.42	0.18

Age (year)

It is not to be expected that the present rather small material can throw light upon the complex problem of the etiology of school myopia, but the heterophoria-measurements indicate no significant anomaly of the convergence-accommodation relation among myopes in general.

It seems medically and scientifically unsupported to define school myopia as a major threat to population health, at least in Denmark.

REFERENCES

Blegvad, O. Om myopiens Progression. Ugeskr. Laeger, 80 (1918).

Fletcher, M.C. Effect Of Contact Lens On School Myopia. Lecture delivered at First Int Conf Myopia, New York, N.Y., 10–13 September (1964).

Oakley, K.H. & F.A. Young. Bifocal Control Of Myopia. Am. J. Optom. & Physiol. Optics. 52 (1975).

Senior author's address:
T. Rosenberg, M.D.
Statens Øjenklinik Rymarksvej
Rymarksvej 1
DK-2900 Hellerup

NEARWORK AND FAMILIAL RESEMBLANCES IN OCULAR REFRACTION: A POPULATION STUDY IN NEWFOUNDLAND

A. RICHLER and J.C. BEAR

(St. John's, Newfoundland, Canada)

ABSTRACT

There is evidence that nearwork influences population variation in ocular refraction, and evidence of familial resemblances for this trait. The potential for nearwork, as an   aspect of common familial environment, to inflate correlations for ocular refraction among nuclear family members was therefore investigated in a sample of 957 persons aged five years and over (approximately 80% of the population above that age) in three communities on the west coast of Newfoundland.

Refraction was evaluated using standard optometric methods, nearwork measured as h/day as reported by the subject, education measured as last completed grade in years.

It was reasoned that the education and nearwork measures combined, rather than that of nearwork alone, best indicated lifetime nearwork levels. The effect of nearwork on refraction resemblances was therefore evaluated by calculating correlations or regressions among relatives before and after removing the effects of nearwork and education on refraction by linear regression. Reductions in sib-sib correlations and offspring-parent regressions were achieved, but patterns of resemblances among relatives after adjustment suggest nearwork effects on refraction resemblances were not completely removed.

Appropriate evaluation of the nearwork-refraction relationship, and its effects on familial resemblances, will require population-based longitudinal data. It is reasonable to suspect that the extent to which effects of common familial environment are confounded with genetically determined variation in ocular refraction differs from population to population, and over time within populations.

INTRODUCTION

The influences of nearwork and educational level on familial resemblances in ocular refraction have been investigated as part of a more extensive study (Richler and Bear 1980a) of ocular refraction variation in a rural Newfoundland population.

Doc. Ophthal. Proc. Series, Vol. 28,
ed. by H.C. Fledelius, P.H. Alsbirk and E. Goldschmidt
© 1981 Dr W. Junk Publishers, The Hague

Extensive epidemiological observation implicates nearwork, primarily the reading associated with formal education, as contributing to the prevalence of myopia (Richler and Bear 1980b). The few previous studies of the resemblances of nuclear family members in ocular refraction (Sorsby et al. 1966; Young et al. 1969; Hegmann et al. 1974; Alsbirk 1979) concur in reporting modest resemblances, with correlations between spouses being negligible and resemblances among sibs exceeding those of offspring to their parents. Greater sib-sib than offspring-parent resemblances in refraction may be attributed to the influences of dominant genes (Hegmann et al. 1974), common familial environment (Young et al. 1969), or both (Alsbirk 1979), increasing the resemblances of sibs to one another. Variance from these two sources cannot be partitioned using only data from first degree relatives (see for instance Li 1977). Whether nearwork, as an aspect of common familial environment, can inflate resemblances between relatives in ocular refraction, can however be evaluated by comparing resemblances with and without adjustment for the influences of nearwork.

SUBJECTS AND METHODS

The subjects of this investigation reside in three communities situated within 24 km of one another on the west coast of the Great Northern Peninsula of Newfoundland. Data were collected in 1974. All refractions were measured by one observer (AR) using standard, non-cycloplegic optometric methods. For analysis, any required cylindrical correction was converted to spherical power in the vertical meridian. Because right and left eye refractions are highly correlated ($R = 0.936$ in this series, $p < 10^{-5}$) only right eye refractions were analyzed.

Nine hundred and seventy-one (971) persons aged five years or over were refracted, about 80% of the total population above that age. Everyone attending for examination was refracted; subjects were not selected on visual grounds. Eleven persons with myopia greater than $-6D$ were, however, excluded from further analysis because of the considerable probability that their myopia was pathological, and three persons with right eye amblyopia were also excluded.

Nearwork was measured in h/day, as reported by the subject, spent in any task such as reading, sewing or knitting which required focusing of the eyes at a distance of 20 in. (50 cm) or less. This measure is approximate, depending upon accuracy of recall and the habitual attentiveness of subjects to nearwork tasks. Few subjects were engaged in occupations requiring even moderate amounts of nearwork or reading. Education was measured in years as last completed grade.

In view of age trends in refraction and the introduction of compulsory education in 1949, the association of refraction with other variables was considered in five age intervals: 5–14, 15–29, 30–44, 45–59, and 60 years and up (Richler and Bear 1980b). It was reasoned that the combined values of nearwork measured at the time of the investigation, and education as an indicator of nearwork in earlier life, provided the best measure possible in the data of the potential influence of nearwork on refraction. For each age interval a multiple linear regression of refraction on age, sex, education and nearwork was therefore calculated and deviations of individual refractions from regression predictions used as measures, first of refraction adjusted for age and sex (hereafter R1), and second of refraction adjusted for age, sex, education and nearwork (hereafter R2).

For R1 and R2 values, intraclass correlations of sibs, and regressions of offspring on parents, were calculated allowing for unequal sibship size (Falconer 1963). For spouses the intraclass correlation coefficient was found (Fisher 1967). Resemblances were considered separately for the age intervals 5–14 years and 15–29 years; pairs of relatives aged over 45 were few, and were combined for analysis with persons aged 30–44.

Table 1. Intraclass correlations of father-mother pairs.

Age of offspring	Pairs	R1	R2
5–14	95	0.06	− 0.02
15–29	62	− 0.05	− 0.06
30–	21	0.06	0.01
All	123*	0.04	− 0.03

*Some parents have offspring in more than one age interval.

Table 2. Intraclass correlation of sibs.

Age	Sibships	Subjects	R1	R2
5–14	87	242	0.29	0.25
15–29	56	158	0.26	0.16
30–	76	232	0.39	0.36
All	215	714	0.29	0.24

RESULTS

Intraclass correlations of spouses (Table 1), overall and grouped by virtue of having a child in a particular age interval, are consistently small or negative, giving no indication of assortative mating for refraction in this population.

Intraclass correlations of sibs (Table 2) are substantially larger than those between spouses; R2 correlations are consistently less than R1. Correlations among sibs tend to increase with age, perhaps because the linear regression adjustment employed does not completely remove age variation in refraction at younger ages.

Among offspring-parent regressions, (Table 3) different sex and age comparisons vary considerably. Again R2 values are less than R1, with two minor exceptions. Again there are indications that age adjustment may be incomplete. In particular, offspring-parent similarities are consistently greatest for the 15–29 year age interval, perhaps because these persons and their parents are of ages at which refraction is relatively stable. Resemblances for the 5–14 year group may be relatively low because these children's refractions are changing relatively rapidly. The relatively slight

Table 3. Offspring-parent regressions. Weighted by the number of parent-offspring pairs in each category, overall values are R1 = 0.23 and R2 = 0.15.

Son-father					Son-mother			
Age of sons	Sibships	Sons	R1	R2	Sibships	Sons	R1	R2
5–14	75	107	0.36	0.19	112	167	0.03	−0.02
15–29	43	62	0.40	0.20	49	70	0.30	0.27
30–	18	22	−0.06	−0.11	32	43	0.08	0.09
All	111	191	0.33	0.15	161	280	0.10	0.06

Daughter-mother					Daughter-father			
Age of daughters	Sibships	Daughters	R1	R2	Sibships	Daughters	R1	R2
5–14	94	131	0.22	0.12	60	85	0.08	0.03
15–29	71	111	0.46	0.51	56	85	0.31	0.21
30–	31	55	0.18	0.13	21	36	0.26	0.18
All	164	297	0.28	0.25	106	206	0.22	0.15

resemblance of persons aged 30 and over to their parents is based on small numbers of observations, but may indicate the influence of presbyopic changes in older subjects.

DISCUSSION

In this population, as in others investigated, resemblances of nuclear family members in ocular refraction are modest, sib-sib resemblance exceeds offspring-parent, and there is no indication of correlation of spouses in this trait. For numerous comparisons drawn, over a wide range of ages, statistical adjustment of refraction for nearwork and education very generally reduces resemblance. This suggests that nearwork, as a feature of common familial environment, can inflate estimates of the genetic component in refraction variation if not taken into account. The overall reduction of sib-sib correlation achieved by adjustment is 20%, the overall reduction of offspring-parent regression is 35%. Inflation of familial resemblances by the effects of common familial environment could be larger in populations in which nearwork levels are high.

Statistical adjustments used probably did not completely remove bio-logical nearwork effects on refraction resemblances. Among persons aged less than 30, like-sex offspring-parent resemblances are generally greater than unlike-sex resemblances. This is not explicable on any simple genetic hypothesis but could result if refraction were influenced by sex-specific aspects of familial environment. Nearwork habits, on the reasonable assumption that they were acquired preferentially from the parent of the same sex, would fill this role. Offspring-parent regressions are relatively small for persons aged 30 years and up, and sib-sib correlations in R2 are generally somewhat greater than offspring-parent regressions. This mirrors population similarities and differences in educational level.

Present findings indicate a contribution of common environment to resemblances among close relatives in ocular refraction, but the contribution of genetic dominance to sib-sib correlations remains unassessed. In the 15−29 year age interval, comparisons are of refractions measured at ages when they are changing little, and sib-sib resemblances adjusted for near-work and education are in fact lower than offspring-parent resemblances. Outside this age interval, however, the greater resemblances of sibs to one another than to their parents remain even after adjustment for nearwork and education. Inadequate adjustment, dominance effects, or both, may contribute to this greater resemblance. The influence of dominant alleles on refraction variation in this population has been investigated by examination of the relationship between refraction and homozygosity as measured in pedigree data (Bear and Richler, this Conference).

Observed resemblances among relatives in refraction after adjustment for education and nearwork (R2) remain large by comparison with reductions achieved by such adjustment and comparable in magnitude to those observed in other studies. This indicates a substantial genetic influence in the development of refraction, as must be expected from the complexity and organization of the eye.

REFERENCES

Alsbirk, P.H. Refraction in adult West Greenland Eskimos. Acta Ophthalmol. 57: 84−95 (1979).

Bear, J.C. et al. Nearwork and familial resemblances in ocular refraction: A population study in Newfoundland. Clinical Genetics (in press).

Falconer, D.S. Introduction to Quantitative Genetics. Oliver and Boyd, Edinburgh (1960).

Falconer, D.S. Quantitative inheritance. In: Methodology in Mammalian Genetics, Ed. W.J. Burdette, P. 193−216. Holden-Day, San Francisco (1963).

Fisher, R.A. Statistical Methods for Research Workers, 13th edition, Hafner Publishing Company Inc., New York (1967).

Hegmann, J.P., et al., Genetic analysis of human visual parameters in populations with varying incidences of strabismus. Am. J. Hum. Genet. 26: 549−562 (1974).

Li, C.C. Separation of common environment and dominance effects with classic kinship correlation models. Social Biol 24: 259−266 (1977).

Miller, R.W. Distant visual acuity loss among Japanese grammar school children: the roles of heredity and the environment. J. Chron. Dis. 16: 31−54 (1963).

Neel, J.V., et al., The effect of parental consanguinity and inbreeding in Hirado, Japan. III. Vision and hearing. Hum. Hered. 20: 129−155 (1970).

Richler, A. & Bear, J.C. The distribution of refraction in three isolated communities in Western Newfoundland. Am. J. Optom. & Physiol. Optics, 57:861−871 (1980a).

Richler, A. & Bear, J.C. Refraction, nearwork and education: a population study in Newfoundland. Acta Ophthalmol 58: 468−477 (1980b).

Salmon, D., et al., A familial aggregate of common variable immunodeficiency, Hodgkin disease and other malignancies in Newfoundland − II. Genealogical analysis and conclusions regarding hereditary determinants. Clin. & Investig. Med. 2: 175−181 (1980).

Sorsby, A., et al., Family studies on ocular refraction and its components. J. Med. Genet. 3: 269−273 (1966).

Wright, S. Coefficients of inbreeding and relationship. Am. Naturalist 56: 330–338 (1922).

Young, F.A., et al., The transmission of refractive errors within Eskimo families. Am. J. Optom. and Arch. Am. Acad. Optom. 46: 676–685 (1969).

Authors' address:
Division of Community Medicine
Faculty of Medicine
Health Sciences Centre
Memorial University of Newfoundland
St. John's
Newfoundland
Canada A1B 3V6

INBREEDING EFFECTS ON OCULAR REFRACTION:
FINDINGS FROM WESTERN NEWFOUNDLAND

J.C. BEAR and A. RICHLER

(St. John's, Newfoundland, Canada)

ABSTRACT

It has been generally observed that resemblances between sibs in ocular refraction are greater than those of offspring to parents. Influences of common environment, of genetic dominance, or some combination of these factors may increase the resemblance of sibs. A companion paper presents evidence that environmental factors increase both sib-sib and offspring-parent resemblances, but that statistical correction for common environment does not equalize these measures. This leaves open the question of the influence of genetic dominance, which cannot be distinguished from that of the common environment using only the available data on first degree relatives.

As an alternative approach, the relationship between ocular refraction and consanguinity (Wright's coefficient of inbreeding, f) has been evaluated in the western Newfoundland data. f could be calculated for 926 subjects. Subjects were grouped in age intervals 5–14, 15–29, 30–44, 45–59, and 60 years and up. In each age interval, vertical ocular refraction (right eye) was regressed on f, adjusting both for age, sex, education and nearwork, and for age and sex only. After adjustment for age, sex, education and nearwork, a small negative regression of refraction on f was found at ages 5–14 years. A marked negative regression was found at ages 60 years and up. Regressions for the intermediate age groups were small and not significantly different from zero. Without adjustment for education and nearwork, regressions were slightly less negative (more positive). Inspection of scatter-plots of refraction against f suggests that with increasing consanguinity, subjects are less often highly hyperopic and more often moderately myopic.

Findings in the young indicate a contribution of genetic dominance to population variation in refraction, dominance being in the direction of hyperopia, and are in agreement with findings of Japanese investigations in this age group, of a decline in visual acuity with consanguinity. There are no other studies with which to compare the findings in subjects aged 60 years and over; the striking negative relationship of refraction to consanguinity at this age remains unexplained.

Doc. Ophthal. Proc. Series, Vol. 28,
ed. by H.C. Fledelius, P.H. Alsbirk and E. Goldschmidt
© 1981 Dr W. Junk Publishers, The Hague

INTRODUCTION

Resemblances between sibs in ocular refraction are consistently observed to be greater than those of offspring to their parents (Sorsby, *et al.* 1966; Young *et al.* 1969; Hegmann, *et al.* 1974; Alsbirk 1979; Richler and Bear, this Conference). This may indicate the influence of common family environment increasing the resemblance of sibs to one another, or a contribution of genetic dominance to refraction variance, or both. These possibilities cannot be distinguished using only data from first degree relatives (Li 1977).

If there is a dominance component in refraction variance, the mean of refraction should change with inbreeding. The reason is as follows. If alleles at loci contributing to variation in a metric trait are purely additive in their effects, heterozygotes will be phenotypically intermediate, compared to homozygotes. If however, some relevant alleles are partially or completely dominant in their effects, phenotypes will deviate toward one or other homozygote value. Since inbreeding increases the population frequency of homozygotes and decreases that of heterozygotes, the mean value of a metric trait for an inbred population will be different from that in a comparable non-inbred population, if dominant alleles influence the trait (Falconer 1960).

Changes in refractive error with inbreeding have been evaluated in a western Newfoundland population as part of a more general investigation of the genetics and epidemiology of ocular refraction (Richler and Bear 1980a). Such inbreeding effects are of interest both in themselves and, as indicated, as a measure of the contribution of dominant alleles to population variation in refraction.

SUBJECTS AND METHODS

The subjects of this investigation reside in three small communities, located within 24 km of one another, on the west coast of the Great Northern Peninsula of Newfoundland.

Extensive *pedigree data* for the communities were compiled from parish and other historical records, in connection with the investigation of a familial aggregation of Hodgkin's disease in the area (Salmon *et al.* (1980). From this data, Wright's (1922) coefficient of inbreeding f was calculated for each subject for whom both parents were recorded (926 subjects in all).

Refraction data were collected in 1974, following standard, non-cycloplegic optometric techniques. Vertical ocular refraction, the combined power of the spherical and cylindrical corrections in the vertical meridian, was used as the basic measure of refractive error; only right eye refractions were analyzed. Subjects were not visually selected (Richler and Bear, this Conference). Subjects were considered in five age intervals: 5–14, 15–29, 30–44, 45–59, and 60 years and up.

The *nearwork* activity of subjects was measured in h/day, self-reported, spent in any task such as reading, sewing or knitting, requiring focusing of the eyes at a distance of 20 in. (50 cm) or less. Aside from children and adolescents attending school, few subjects were engaged in occupations requiring even moderate amounts of nearwork activity. *Education* was measured in years as last completed grade.

To allow for influences of education and nearwork on refraction (Richler and Bear 1980b) the relationship between refraction and f was analyzed twice, once using refraction values adjusted by linear regression (in each age interval) for age and sex (designated R1), and again using refraction values similarly adjusted for education and nearwork as well as age and sex (hereafter R2). Linear regressions of R1 and R2 on f were calculated, including and excluding subjects whose f coefficient was zero.

Table 1. Regression of R1 on f (see text).

Age interval (yr)	N	Regression coefficient	SE	Intercept
5–14	322	− 3.2964	3.4796	0.0620
15–29	264	6.9901	5.4194	− 0.1049
30–44	154	3.8659	4.2572	− 0.0612
45–59	122	− 2.4982	4.5349	0.0505
60–	64	− 20.1560**	7.3916	0.2789
All ages	926	− 1.2473	2.1486	0.0223
		Excluding persons with $f = 0$:		
5–14	187	− 4.3385	3.9442	0.1008
15–29	168	5.1376	6.1180	− 0.0374
30–44	96	1.6814	4.4441	0.0375
45–59	69	− 7.7669	5.0918	0.3008
60–	22	− 35.4953**	10.3565	1.1392
All ages	542	− 3.5113	2.4079	0.1163

**p < 0.01

Table 2. Regression of R2 on f (see text).

Age interval (yr)	N	Regression coefficient	SE	Intercept
5–14	322	− 5.4699	3.2279	0.0808
15–29	264	4.1766	5.1072	− 0.0672
30–44	154	0.3075	3.6675	− 0.0113
45–59	122	− 2.5789	4.3856	0.0522
60–	64	− 20.6425**	7.3257	0.2886
All ages	926	− 3.2574	2.0094	0.0468
		Excluding persons with $f = 0$:		
5–14	187	− 6.1330	3.7851	0.1054
15–29	168	5.1392	5.6410	− 0.1022
30–44	96	0.0884	3.6149	− 0.0014
45–59	69	− 8.0985	4.9401	0.3144
60–	22	− 36.8830**	9.9530	1.1995
All ages	542	− 4.3212	2.2326	0.0909

**p < 0.01

49

RESULTS AND DISCUSSION

Regressions of R1 on f (Table 1) and R2 on f (Table 2) are not significantly different from zero, except for those for the age interval 60 years and up. Consistent with previous observations for Japanese populations (Miller 1963; Neel *et al.* 1970), regressions are negative in the 5—14 year age interval, but not in general at higher ages. The significant negative regression for persons aged 60 years and over is a unique observation; subjects of these ages were excluded in Japanese studies. Adjustment for education and near-work (Table 2) had little effect on the standard error or intercept of regressions, but rendered regression slopes somewhat more negative, particularly for the 5—14 year group, suggesting variation from these sources could obscure the relationship between refraction and f if not taken into account. Exclusion of apparently non-inbred subjects gave more negative regressions, possibly because for some of these subjects inbreeding was not ascertained.

These findings, for subjects aged less than 60 years, parallel those of earlier Japanese investigations, indicating reduction in visual acuity consequent upon inbreeding, if any, appears generally negligible.

A contribution from dominant genes of large effect to population variation in refraction cannot be ruled out; such genes would however appear rare. Greater sib-sib than offspring-parent resemblances for refraction in this population probably result from imperfect statistical adjustment for environment common to sibs. Such imperfection will not be remedied without extensive normative data to allow appropriate comparison of refractions of persons of different ages. Better quantification of the susceptibility of refraction to environmental influences is also necessary; it is of particular interest whether or not nearwork influences the refraction of all persons equally.

REFERENCES

Alsbirk, P.H. Refraction in adult West Greenland Eskimos. Acta Ophthalmol 57: 84—95 (1979).

Bear, J.C. & Richler, A. Ocular refraction and inbreeding: A population study in Newfoundland. J. biosoc. Sci. 13: in press (1981).

Falconer, D.S. Introduction ot Quantitative Genetics. Oliver and Boyd, Edinburgh (1960).

Falconer, D.S. Quantitative inheritance. In: Methodology in Mammalian Genetics, Ed W.J. Burdette, P. 193—216. Holden-Day, San Francisco (1963).

Fisher, R.A. Statistical Methods for Research Workers, 13th edition, Hafner Publishing Company Inc., New York (1967).

Hegmann, J.P., et al., Genetic analysis of human visual parameters in populations with varying incidences of strabismus. Am. J. Hum. Genet. 26: 549—562 (1974).

Li, C.C. Separation of common environment and dominance effects with classic kinship correlation models. Social Biology 24: 259—266 (1977).

Miller, R.W. Distant visual acuity loss among Japanese grammar school children: the roles of heredity and the environment. J. Chron. Dis. 16: 31—54 (1963).

Neel, J.V., et al., The effect of parental consanguinity and inbreeding in Hirado, Japan. III. Vision and hearing. Hum. Hered. 20: 129—155 (1970).

Richler, A. & Bear, J.C. The distribution of refraction in three isolated communities in Western Newfoundland. Am. J. Optom. & Physiol. Optics, 57: 861–871 (1980a).

Richler, A. & Bear, J.C. Refraction, nearwork and education: a population study in Newfoundland. Acta Ophthalmol., 58: 468–477 (1980b).

Salmon, D., et al., A familial aggregate of common variable immunodeficiency, Hodgkin disease and other malignancies in Newfoundland – II. Genealogical analysis and conclusions regarding hereditary determinants. Clin. & Investig. Med. 2: 175–181 (1980).

Sorsby, A., et al., Family studies on ocular refraction and its components. J. Med. Genet. 3: 269–273 (1966).

Wright, S. Coefficients of inbreeding and relationship. Am. Naturalist 56: 330–338 (1922).

Young, F.A., et al., The transmission of refractive errors within Eskimo families. Am. J. Optom. and Arch. Am. Acad. Optom. 46: 676–685 (1969).

Authors' address:
Division of Community Medicine
Faculty of Medicine
Memorial University of Newfoundland
St. John's
Newfoundland
Canada A1B 3V6

SECULAR CHANGE IN ANTERIOR CHAMBER DEPTH, A REFRACTIVE COMPONENT OF HIGH HERITABILITY

P.H. ALSBIRK

(Copenhagen and Odense, Denmark)

ABSTRACT

Axial anterior chamber depth (ACD) – a refractive component of admittedly minor optical importance – has been extensively studied in Greenland Eskimos due to frequent angle-closure glaucoma. In this population ACD showed a high heritability, $h^2 \pm SE = 0.71 \pm 0.08$. Thus about 70% of age- and sex-independent ACD variations seemed to be genetically determined. Corresponding h^2 estimates were found in axial length and corneal curvature radius while refractive error showed a low heritability: $h^2 = 0.14 \pm 0.12$ in this as in other recent surveys.

On this background two studies have now been performed: (1) An ACD and refractive error estimation of 63 Greenland Eskimo women more than 40 years old, who had lived in Denmark for at least 25 years. (2) A ten-year follow-up study of about 550 Eskimos in Greenland. ACD was re-measured optically, using Haag Streit equipment as in 1969 at the first population survey. Both studies showed a significant secular change, the chambers being less shallow than the basic cross-sectional study had suggested. The refractive errors of Eskimo immigrants in Denmark did not differ from the level in Greenland.

Thus a mainly genetically determined ocular parameter has been found to show a secular change due to environmental influence, cf. anthropometric traits like human height and cephalic index. Heritability estimates are not hard facts. In ocular and other quantitative variations conspicuous plasticity is to be anticipated, not least in low heritability characters like human refraction.

INTRODUCTION

The relative importance of genes and environment is one of the basic questions in all biological sciences, and so it is in the field of myopia research. The additive genetic variance, taken as a proportion of the total phenotypic variance of a trait may be one answer to this question. The *heritability*, h^2, of a quantitative trait is estimated statistically through familial resemblance studies. However, interpretation of the results thus obtained is never straightforward.

Doc. Ophthal. Proc. Series, Vol. 28,
ed. by H.C. Fledelius, P.H. Alsbirk and E. Goldschmidt
© *1981 Dr W. Junk Publishers, The Hague*

Table 1. Heritability (h^2) of ocular dimensions and refraction.

	No. of child-parent pairs	Heritability h^2	Standard error of h^2
Anterior chamber depth*	564	0.71	0.08
Corneal thickness*	452	0.61	0.08
Corneal diameter*	138	0.80	0.14
Corneal curvature radius	159	0.64	0.14
Axial length	159	0.76	0.18
Refractive error	159	0.14	0.12

*h^2 estimates based on child on midparent regression coefficients. (Data collected from Alsbirk 1975a, b; 1978; 1979).

The heritability of ocular dimensions and refraction had been studied in a series of population surveys among Greenland Eskimos. Table 1 gives a brief summary. Frequent angle-closure glaucoma motivated the surveys. As the Table shows, heritability was found to be high, about 60—80% for all anatomical parameters, indicating a major genetic determination. On this background I was initially surprised to find a much lower heritability of refractive error in the population, indicating environmental factors as more important than genes. However, this result agreed with other recent studies, cf. Spivey (1976). Furthermore, it appeared on the remarkable background of the Eskimoan 'epidemic of myopia', observed among adolescents in Alaska and Canada, cf. Young *et al.* (1969), Morgan *et al.* (1975), Johnson *et al.* (1979). In Greenland, no similar myopic change was found. The relatively stable West Greenland community, where all have learned to read, had fairly frequent myopia in all age groups (Alsbirk 1979).

So far all findings have been based on cross-sectional studies. Quantitative geneticists stress that in principle heritability studies are valid only in the population studied, at the time of the survey. Even in highly heritable anthropometric traits like human height, secular trends or changes have frequently been disclosed which are unexplainable by genetic factors, cf. e.g. Cavalli-Sforza and Bodmer (1971).

In the following a secular change in anterior chamber depth will be reported, based on two sources: (1) an investigation of Eskimoan immigrants in Copenhagen and (2) a ten-year follow-up study of my original sample in Greenland. Although the main purpose of both studies was angle-closure glaucoma risk estimation, some aspects are relevant to ophthalmo-genetics and to human refraction due to its foundation in ocular anatomy.

MATERIAL

The samples were collected from two sources: (1) A census register collection of all women aged 40 years or more, who were born in Greenland and lived in Major Copenhagen (n = 171). Through interviews the subsample of Eskimo women who had lived more than 25 years in Denmark was selected (n = 71). Of these a total of 64 (90%) were examined at the University Eye Clinic,

Rigshospitalet, Copenhagen (one was excluded due to bilateral aphakia, i.e. n = 63). (2) A ten-year follow-up sample of Greenland Eskimos (in the district of Umanaq, n.l. 71°) originally examined in 1969 (Alsbirk 1974). Out of this sample of 928 persons 541 were reexamined (58.3%) while 387 were either dead (127), moved (218) or disabled (15). Only 22 did not attend or overtly refused to come (5), and thus only 5% (27/568) of available persons were not seen. Statistically, the original ACD distribution of non-examined as well as examined persons could not be shown to differ from the basic population, i.e. a representative subsample with respect to ACD was at hand.

METHODS

In Copenhagen as well as in Greenland *Haag Streit pachymetry* was used at the optical ACD measurements, subtracting the corneal thickness measure from the distance between front of cornea and lens. *Statistically,* age- and sex-variability of ACD had been outlined in the primary population study. An age- and sex- independent *deviation score* was used again, taking the standard deviation about the linear regression $(s_{y.x})$ as a unit of measurement (Alsbirk 1975b). *Subjective refraction* in front of Snellen's chart at 6 m was used, following Javal-Schiøtz keratometry. Refractive errors were transformed to spherical equivalents

RESULTS

(1) *Anterior chamber depth in Copenhagen immigrants compared with a background population in Greenland*

Figure 1 illustrates the individual ACD results in 63 women of Eskimoan descent who had lived for at least 25 years in Denmark. The usual wide dispersion is illustrated by the scattergram, the standard deviation about the regression line $(s_{y.x})$ being: 0.32 mm. The mean level of immigrants was significantly higher than the level of their background population, $P < 0.001$ by a t-test.

Caucasian admixture was estimated by interviewing the women examined and was found to be higher in the immigrant sample than in the native Umanaq group. Figure 1 shows that 14% (9/63) of the immigrants had $\geq 50\%$ Caucasian admixture (against 3% in Umanaq, 5/160). In Figure 2 persons without known admixture are indicated as 'pure' and persons with known, even remote, admixture as 'mixed', in Copenhagen as in Greenland. *Within* these locations mixed groups had deeper chambers than groups of pure Eskimos, significantly so in Greenland. This relationship indicated a *genetic influence.* However, when comparing groups of ethnically pure with pure and mixed with mixed persons *between* the locations a significant difference was found in both comparisons. Thus a deeper chamber *was* found in Copenhagen Eskimos in pure as well as in mixed Eskimos. This finding

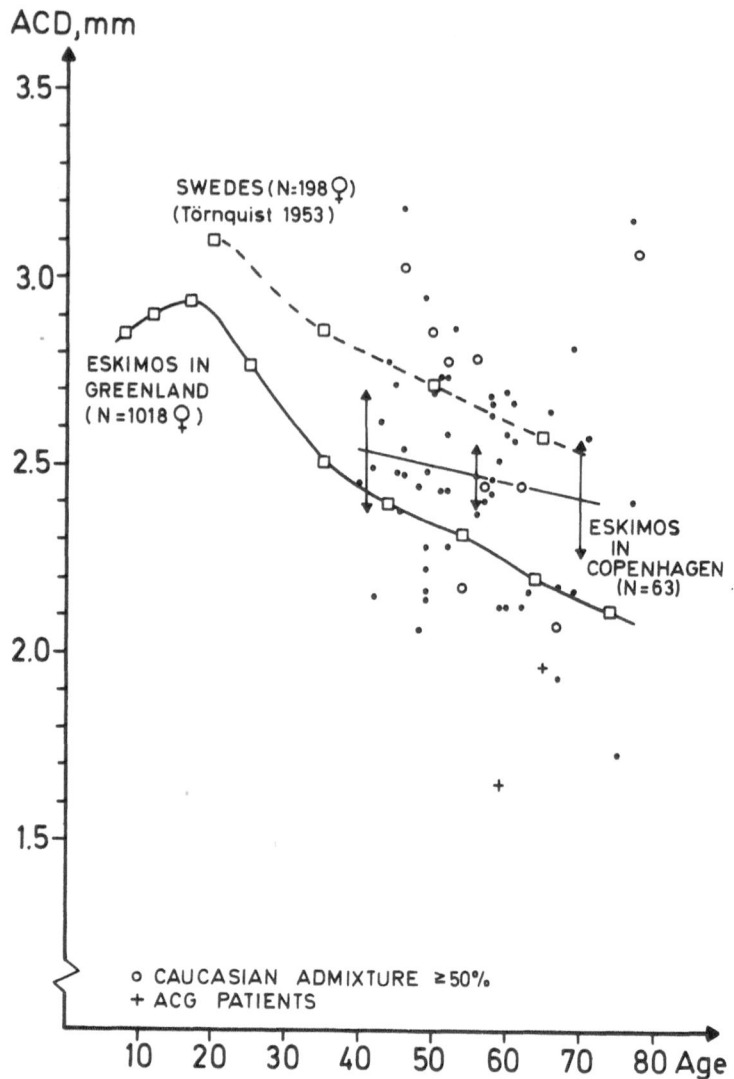

Fig. 1. Anterior chamber depth (ACD) and age, given as curves through a number of mean values, in women from Sweden and Greenland, cf. Alsbirk 1974. Eskimo immigrants in Copenhagen are shown as a scattergram and a linear regression line with 95% confidence limits at mean age (⊕) and arbitrary extreme ages (⊕). ACG indicates primary angle-closure glaucoma patients of the sample.

strongly suggested an influence of *environmental* factors overlying genetic variability.

Evidently the study could not disclose which type of environmental influence was of special importance. As apparent from Figure 3 the distribution

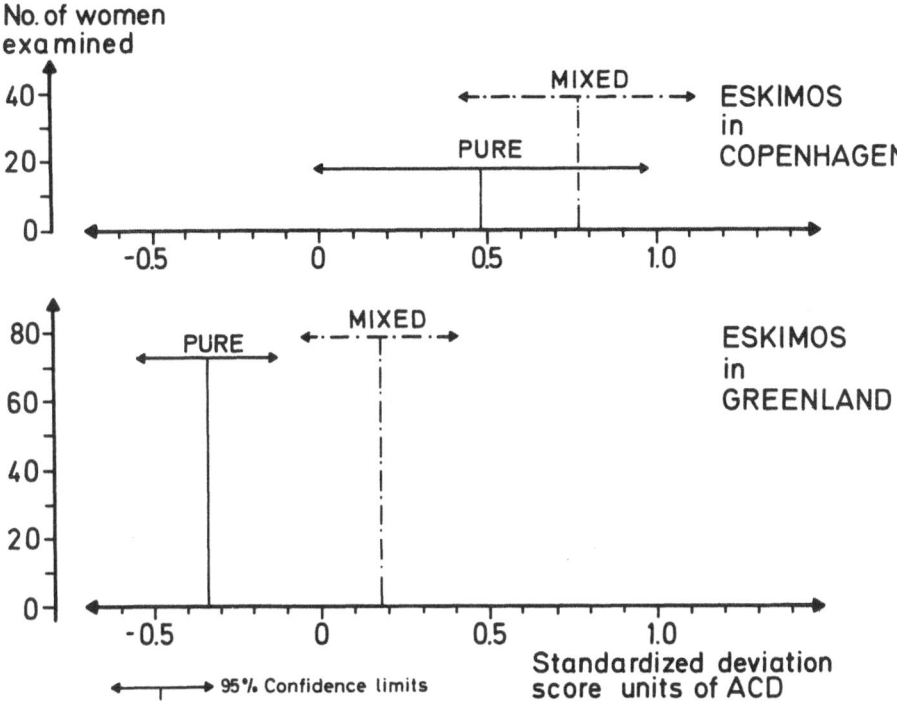

No. of women
examined

Fig. 2. ACD in Copenhagen Eskimo immigrants versus Eskimos in Greenland. The samples are subdivided in 'pure' and 'mixed' groups according to the pedigrees obtained, 'mixed' indicating persons with well-known Caucasian admixture (down to 12.5% or less).

of *refractive errors* showed range and mean value very close to the level known from the same age groups in Greenland. No significant excess of myopes in Copenhagen Eskimos was fond. Thus the well-known correlation between low-grade myopia and chamber depth could not explain the deeper chambers in Copenhagen.

(2) *Change of ACD in ten years. A longitudinal investigation*

In Figure 4 the change of ACD is analysed in eight age groups. The increase in the child group, originally aged 7–9 years, the plateau around puberty and the shallowing of ACD through all adult age groups corresponded largely to the cross-sectional curve in Figure 1. However, most of the adult groups had decreased less than expected from the cross-sectional study. Table 2 gives some details of an analysis of these data, which as an overall result showed a highly significant (positive) difference between observation and expectation. Thus in both sexes the chambers in 1979 were found to be

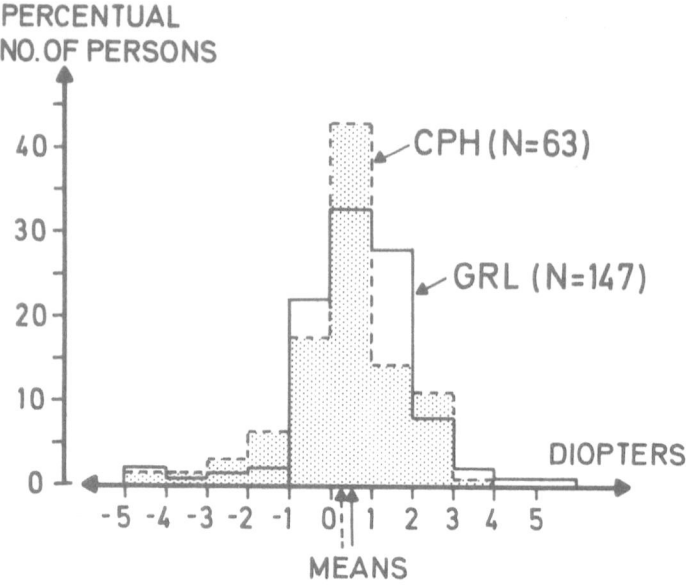

Fig. 3. Refraction (in averaged spherical equivalents of both eyes) of Eskimo women, aged ≧ 40 years, in Greenland (GRL) and Copenhagen immigrants (CPH).

slightly deeper than the regressions of ACD on age from the 1969 study had predicted. The Table also shows a remarkable age effect. In the group of younger adults (15–39 years old) the secular trend was highly significant, while elderly persons showed an ACD shallowing closely agreeing with expectation.

DISCUSSION

The present study has focused on a refractive component of admittedly minor optical importance. However, as an example of a highly heritable ocular parameter it was interesting to look at the stability of anterior chamber depth variations. This possibility occurred for reasons inherent in the remarkable angle-closure glaucoma morbidity of Eskimos.

Studies of *immigrants* and comparison with their background populations have been of great importance in human anthropology, cf. the classical study of Shapiro (1939) and e.g. Froehlich (1970) who demonstrated remarkable changes, mainly due to environment, in numerous physical characteristics of Japanese immigrants to Hawaii. The present study of Greenland Eskimo women who had lived in Denmark for at least 25 years, showed less shallow chambers than their background population which had been extensively studied a few years earlier. However, the possibility

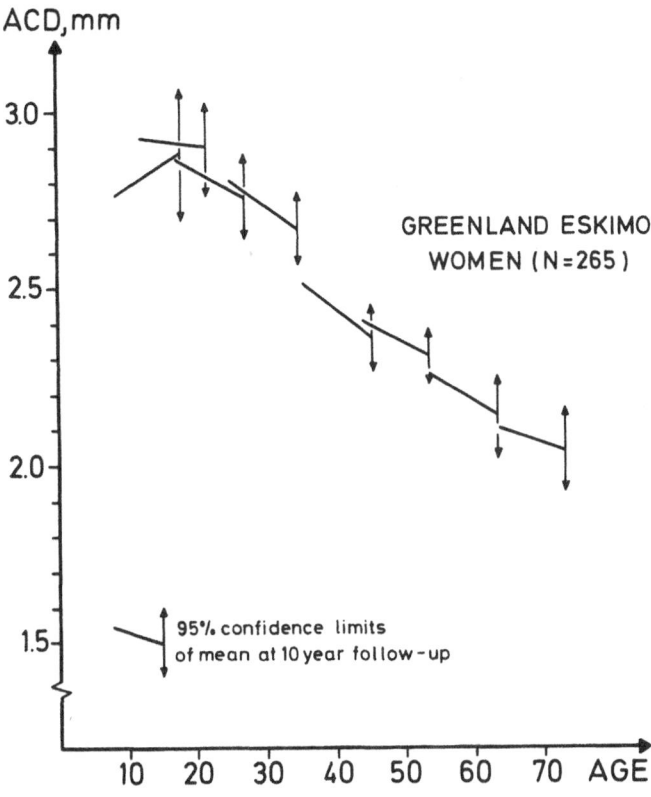

Fig. 4. Change of anterior chamber depth (ACD) in 10 years. The eight oblique lines are drawn between mean values in 1969 and in 1979 of the same persons (as average of both eyes). The vertical double arrows indicate 95% confidence limits of the latter mean value in each age group.

Table 2. Ten-year change ($\bar{\Delta}$) of anterior chamber depth, analysed as individual age and sex independent deviation scores, 1979 minus 1969 values.

Age groups in 1969	Men n	$\bar{\Delta}$	SD	Women n	$\bar{\Delta}$	SD	All n	$\bar{\Delta}$	SD
7–14	56	0.03	0.38	26	0.17[a]	0.39	82	0.07	0.39
15–39	90	0.16[c]	0.36	108	0.16[c]	0.39	198	0.16[c]	0.37
40 +	128	−0.01	0.31	131	0.02	0.35	259	0.00	0.33
Total	274	0.05[b]	0.35	265	0.09[c]	0.37	539	0.07[c]	0.36

Significance of mean changes ($\bar{\Delta}$, by t-tests): [a] $p < 0.05$, [b] $p < 0.02$ and [c] $p < 0.001$; other $\bar{\Delta}$ values not significant. One deviation score unit = 0.28 mm ACD below and 0.31 mm above age 40.

59

of a (self-) selective process, making the individual an atypical representative of her background population also with respect to a trait like ACD, clearly may exist. In this context it was convincing that the 'immigration effect' was obvious in 'pure' as well as 'mixed' Eskimos, cf. Figure 2.

The results of the *longitudinal,* ten-year *follow-up study* gave further support to the results of the immigrant study. The Greenland communities have experienced large socio-cultural changes through the last 30 years. However, living circumstances are still — and will always be — different from those of Copenhagen for evident geographical reasons.

The confounding of age effects and secular trends in cross-sectional studies is a well-known difficulty in anthropometry. cf. Damon 1965. Also in the present study this problem was apparent. It became clear that several age groups had not followed the cross-sectional age curve but taken a slightly higher course. Especially younger adults of both sexes showed a trend towards chambers which were less shallow than predicted. These results will be documented in further detail elsewhere. In principle, they are in good agreement with several anthropometric studies in other isolated and homo-geneous populations in which secular trends have been convincingly demonstrated, due to changing environmental conditions, cf. e.g. Lewin *et al.* (1973). Anterior chamber depth is a measure, dependent on lens position and thickness which continue to change throughout life. Although genetic influence is certainly demonstrable in family resemblance studies, plasticity due to environmental influence does also exist as long as ocular structures are not definitively stabilized.

Remarkable myopic changes have been demonstrated in several recent population studies of refraction, cf. the introduction and e.g. Richler and Bear 1980. These results strongly indicate an often dramatic secular change in human refraction and, consequently, the static genetic concept of refraction prevailing in Euro-American ophthalmology through most of this century has to be abandoned. The present study confirms that the human eye and its natural growth and development is not fully determined at conception by the genetic complements of the sperm and the egg cell. It is further modulated throughout life by environmental factors. Future research has much to do in disclosing the nature of this environmental variability or plasticity of the human eye and its refraction.

REFERENCES

Alsbirk, P.H., Anterior chamber depth in Greenland Eskimos. I. A population study of variation with age and sex. Acta ophthalmol. (Kbh.) 52: 551 (1974).
Alsbirk, P.H., Corneal diameter in Greenland Eskimos. Anthropometric and genetic studies with special reference to primary angle-closure glaucoma. Acta ophthalmol. (Kbh.) 53: 635 (1975a).
Alsbirk, P.H., Anterior chamber of the eye. A genetic and anthropological study in Greenland Eskimos. Human Heredity 25: 418 (1975b).
Alsbirk, P.H., Corneal thickness. II. Environmental and genetic factors. Acta ophthalmol. (Kbh.) 56: 105 (1978).
Alsbirk, P.H., Refraction in adult West Greenland Eskimos. A population study of spherical refractive errors, including oculometric and familial correlations. Acta

ophthalmol. (Kbh.) 57: 84 (1979).

Cavalli-Sforza L.L. & Bodmer W., The genetics of human populations, Freeman, San Francisco pp. 597–602 (1971).

Damon, A., Discrepancies between findings of longitudinal and cross-sectional studies in adult life: Physique and Physiology. Human Devel. 8: 16 (1965).

Froehlich, J.W., Migration and the plasticity of physique in the Japanese-Americans of Hawaii. Am. J. phys. Anthrop. 32: 429 (1970).

Johnson, G.J., et al., Survey of ophthalmic conditions in a Labrador community. I. Refractive errors. Br. J. Ophthalmol. 63: 440 (1979).

Lewin, T., et al., Secular changes in craniofacial dimensions in a homogeneous population. Acta morphol. Neerl. -Scand. 11: 289 (1973).

Morgan, R.W., et al., Inuit myopia: An environmentally-induced epidemic? Can. Med. Assoc. J. 112: 575 (1975).

Richler, A. & Bear, J.C., Refraction, nearwork and education. A population study in Newfoundland, Acta ophthalmol. (Kbh.) 58: 468 (1979).

Shapiro, H.L., Migration and environment. A study of the physical characteristics of the Japanese immigrants to Hawaii and the effects of environment on their descendants. Oxford University Press/London, New York, Toronto (1939).

Spivey, B.E., Quantitative genetics and clinical medicin. Trans. Am. ophthalmol. Soc. 74: 661 (1976).

Törnquist, R., Shallow anterior chamber in acute glaucoma. A clinical and genetic study, Acta ophthalmol. (Kbh.) Suppl. 39 (1953).

Young, F.A., et al., The transmission of refractive errors within Eskimo families. Am. J. Optom. 43: 676 (1969).

Author's address:
P.H. Alsbirk, M.D.
University Eye Clinic,
Rigshospitalet,
DK-2100 Copenhagen Ø,
Denmark

CHANGES IN REFRACTION AND EYE SIZE DURING ADOLESCENCE

With special reference to the influence of low birth weight

H.C. FLEDELIUS

(Copenhagen, Denmark)

ABSTRACT

Ophthalmic follow-up has been performed in 137 18-year-old Danes. Being part of a previous (larger) study on ophthalmic sequelae to low birth weight, 70 have a low birth weight (< 2000 g), while 67 are full-term controls.

Longitudinal data are given concerning three major items:
    (a) Changes in refraction from age of ten to 18 years,
    (b) Changes in eye size from age of ten to 18, and
    (c) The influence of low birth weight on ocular development.

The *myopes* show the most marked refractive change (up to 6.25 D, median value 1.75 D) during adolescence. The *population* norm of refractive change is estimated to be in the area 0.5–0.7 D.

There is a *basic* eye growth of 0.4–0.5 mm around puberty (at variance with previous statements by Sorsby *et al.*).

Low birth weight leaves (1) a (minor) group of pathological myopia ('of prematurity'), and (2) a permanent LBW size deficit, *also* including eyes that otherwise appear and function as normal.

INTRODUCTION

From available refractive curves in literature it may be deduced, that the marked *changes* are confined to the first years of life. The refractive curve shows an early shift from the newborns' Gaussian curve to the established leptokurtotic distribution of later childhood and of adult life ('Emmetropization', Sato 1968; Gernet and Olbrich 1969).

From the age of ten years, refractive changes are usually of a low order, except for the *minor* part of the teenagers making up the 'myopic tail' of the refractive curve. Myopia is associated with an axial elongation of the eye. Otherwise eye size is regarded as pretty stable during adolescence (Sorsby *et al.* 1961–1973).

The present study is based on longitudinal ophthalmic data from the ages of 10 and of 18 years. It deals with *changes in refraction and eye size* between these age levels. According to the aims of the initial ten-year study (cf. Material), the influence of *low birth weight* (on changes during adolescence) will further be analysed.

MATERIAL AND METHODS

The present study, comprising 137 18-year-old Danes, is a longitudinal follow-up of children who were originally examined around the age of ten, as part of a larger-scale investigation (n = 539) into ophthalmic sequels to a low birth weight (Fledelius 1976; 1980).

In selection for follow-up, there is a deliberate refractive skewing, because it was attempted to re-examine all known cases of myopia (diagnosed *at* the 10-year assessment, *or* later developed, based on information achieved from school medical records). The present results concerning eye changes during adolescence will therefore be skewed, to some extent, *away* from the presumed rather static population norm, and *towards* the more progressing myopes.

Out of the 137 under study, 70 had a *low* birth weight (below 2000 g; mean BW 1561 g ± 249). The remaining 67 were full-term controls, with a presumed optimum weight at delivery (between 3000 and 4000 g; mean BW 3455 g ± 224).

On both occasions, cycloplegic refraction is given as spherical equivalent (in D), keratometry as corneal curvature radius (in mm), and axial ultrasound oculometry (Kretztechnik 7000, Ultrasonolux 12 or 10 MC transducers) also in mm.

RESULTS

Refraction at the age of 18 years

Assuming that not *all* myopic cases have been recorded (in school medical records or in my own files), an 18-year population *incidence of myopia* can be given only as a *minimum* figure: The incidence thus found is 13.1% in the original full-term sample (n = 237), and 17.6% in ex-prematures (n = 302). The difference between groups is due to the fraction with 'myopia of prematurity', which is considered a pathological sequel to the premature birth (Fledelius 1981). Concerning the incidence of ordinary *juvenile* myopia, birth weight has not shown any significant influence.

The skewing of the follow-up sample is given by the fact that 45% of the actually re-examined 137 are myopic (cf. Material).

Age at onset of myopia: According to the definition used, 'myopia of prematurity' is of a definite early onset, being diagnosed already in pre-school years (⩽ six years). Conversely, *juvenile* myopia occurred at so-called school age, that means from the age of seven. The median age at onset is 11 years, with 85% of all included juvenile cases being diagnosed before the age of 15.

A fair picture of the 18-year distribution within *emmetropes and hypermetropes* cannot be given, because so relatively few of these were invited for follow-up. (School medical records alone do not allow an estimate; refractive values are *not* assessed as routine in the *many,* who pass the customary visual tests without any trouble).

64

Refractive change (ΔR) is calculated as the ten-year value minus the 18-year value. A dioptric shift towards myopia (increase in refraction) is thus given a positive sign. This applied to 127 of the 137 re-examined. The remainder were static or showed a slight decrease in refraction.

Table 1 shows refractive change in the material subdivided by birth weight and sex, given by mean values and ranges. The subgroups do not differ significantly, and in the following they will be pooled on most occasions.

Table 1. Refractive change (ΔR) from the age of ten to 18 years in the present sample, divided by birth weight and sex. Low birth weight is abbreviated to LBW.

	Number and sex	ΔR, in D, mean and SD	ΔR, range, in D
LBW group	36 ♂	1.75 ± 1.66	0–6.3
	34 ♀	1.29 ± 1.03	0–4.0
Full-terms	36 ♂	1.26 ± 1.23	− 0.2–4.3
	31 ♀	1.07 ± 0.91	− 0.5–3.8

Usually only right eyes are entered into calculations (n = 137), but in assessing refractive *change* some left eyes (n = 20) are included too. They derive from cases of anisometropia (where the two eyes often develop quite differently).

Figure 1 shows refractive change as percentage distribution on four ΔR-classes, in myopia (left) compared with emmetropia + hypermetropia (right). The latter group is clearly the more static one, with a median ΔR-value of 0.7 D. Conversely, the myopes have undergone more marked changes: 54% have increased more than 1.5 D during adolescence, and the median value is 1.7 D.

Figure 1 further shows (at bottom) an estimated population 'norm' of refractive change during adolescence. The percentages are calculated from the above distributions (Figure 1, top), on the assumption of a 15% general incidence of myopia around the age of 18 years.

In juvenile myopia, the progression is usually considered more marked, the earlier the onset. In the present sample, this is confirmed by linear regression, with age at onset on abscissa and ΔR on the y-axis. The correlation is significant, but not strong. The regression line is given by: $\dot{y} = -0.164 x + 4.15$, and $r = -0.34$.

Birth weight showed no (significant) influence on the refractive change patterns.

Changes in eye size from age of ten to 18

An ocular growth *norm* of adolescence will not appear from the mean values and ranges of the present sample, due to its skewing towards myopic cases. Too high values will be obtained, because myopic eyes elongate not only

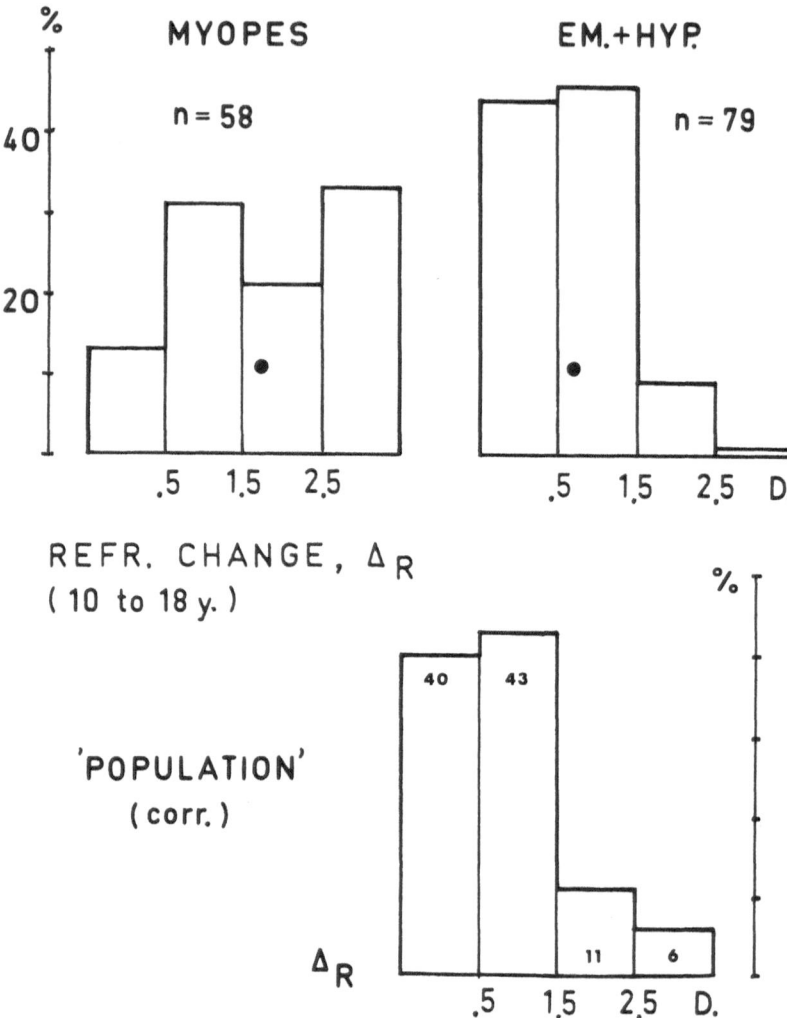

Fig. 1. Refractive change from the age of 10 to 18 years in myopes (top, left) and in emmetropes + hypermetropes (top, right). Percentage distribution on four refractive change groups (as divided by ΔR values of 0.5, 1.5 and 2.5 D). Black dot signifies median value. Below: a calculated population norm distribution (cf. text).

according to a possible 'basic growth', but also associated with the increase in refraction.

This additional influence of refractive change can be neutralized by dividing (once again) the sample according to degree of ΔR. Table 2 accordingly gives mean values in the four ΔR groups. The *static* eyes show an axial length increase of 0.4–0.5 mm, almost harmoniously divided on posterior and anterior eye segment (80%/20%). In eyes with *higher* degree

Table 2. Axial eye measurement changes from the age of ten to 18 years, given in four refractive change classes, by mean values. AL = axial length, VL = vitr. length, LT = lens thickness, ACD = ant. chamber depth; ΔVL/ΔAL = relative proportion of posterior eye segment increase of *total* axial increase, in per cent. 157 eyes are included, cf. text.

		ΔAL, in mm	ΔVL, in mm	$\dfrac{\Delta VL}{\Delta AL}$, in per cent	ΔLT, in mm	ΔACD, in mm
Static eyes	ΔR ⩽ 0.5 D (n = 49)	0.45	0.35		0	0.10
	ΔR 0.6–1.5 D (n = 61)	0.49	0.40	80%	0	0.09
Progressive eyes	ΔR 1.6–2.5 D (n = 24)	1.15	1.07		− 0.04	0.13
	ΔR > 2.5 D (n = 23)	1.61	1.44	91%	0.04	0.13

Table 3. Axial eye length and corneal curvature radius (given as mean values) at the age of ten (top) and 18 years (bottom), further divided by birth weight group. A LBW-deficit appears in the last column (right). The data are longitudinal only to some extent, cf. text.

		LBW group	Full-terms	Deficit due to LBW
Emmetropia at age of ten (n = 47)	axial length (mm)	23.0	23.47	0.47
	corn. curv. rad. (mm)	7.60	7.86	0.26
Emmetropia at age of 18 (n = 56)	axial length (mm)	23.29	23.76	0.47
	corn. curv. rad. (mm)	7.67	7.90	0.23

of refractive change, the increase in vitreous length (posterior eye segment) clearly predominates. This is in keeping with our common knowledge of axial elongation in relation to myopia. The correlation (by linear regression) between ΔR (y-axis) and Δ vitreous length (x), from age of ten to 18, is thus found to be high:

full terms: y = 1.60 x + 0.38;   r = 0.76.

LBW group: y = 1.39 x + 0.52;   r = 0.62.

The influence of *low birth weight* on eye dimensions is demonstrated in Table 3, which deals with the optically most 'normal' eyes, those with emmetropia. At the age of ten, it was obvious that ex-prematures had not (yet?) caught up. Their axial lengths were shorter and the corneae smaller and more curved (cf. also Fledelius 1976).

Being myopic today, some formerly emmetropic eyes are *not* included in the 18-year group of emmetropia, which has instead received some (relatively shorter) eyes from the previous hypermetropes. In spite of this deviating from the truly longitudinal set-up, the size differences between ex-prematures and full-terms appear amazingly similar at follow-up. Ex-prematures have *not* caught up, even at the age of 18 years.

DISCUSSION AND CONCLUDING REMARKS

Being the subject of more extended presentations elsewhere, only a brief account of the results is given here.

At the age of 18 years, the *incidence of juvenile myopia* is about 13%. This is probably a minimum figure (based as it is on *available* information about the full 10-year material (n = 539)). Most examined cases of juvenile myopia had their *onset* between the ages of seven and 14, with a median value of 11 years.

Concerning *refractive change* from the age of ten to 18 in those re-examined (n = 137), 93% showed an *increase* in refraction (change towards myopia), the remaining 7% being static. The latter percentage is probably somewhat higher in the population (which is not skewed towards myopia, as is the present follow-up sample).

The *median* refractive change is 1.75 D in myopes, 0.7 D. in emmetropes, and 0.5 D. in hypermetropes. Within the group of juvenile myopia, a usually accepted trend is confirmed: Cases of early clinical onset progress more than the late teenage cases.

Concerning *eye size*, the refractively most *static* eyes of the sample show an axial elongation of 0.4–0.5 mm during adolescence. This is regarded the *basic growth* that *has* to occur in relation to puberty. The result is at variance with classical statements by Sorsby and co-workers, who considered the eye to be fully grown already *before* puberty.

Finally a brief mention of two features associated with *low* birth weight. First, there is the subgroup of 'myopia of prematurity', which is regarded *pathological* (abortive retrolental fibroplasia?) with a clear relationship to the premature birth (Fledelius 1976, 1981).

Next, it is shown that the eyes of ex-prematures remain of smaller size than those of full-term controls. They appear dimensionally retarded at ten-year assessment, but do not catch up during adolescence either; the eye size deficit is permanent.

This is paralleled by similar growth deficits regarding *other* somatic parameters (body height, cranial circumference, interpupillary distance, Fledelius 1979).

REFERENCES

Fledelius, H.C. Prematurity and the Eye (thesis). Ophthalmic follow-up of children of low and normal birth weight. Acta Ophthalmol (Kbh.), suppl. 128 (1976).

Fledelius, H.C. Prematurity and the eye. Some results from two follow-up studies of children from the longitudinal Copenhagen University Project 1959—61, Paper read in Dan. Paed. Soc. (1979).

Fledelius, H.C. Ophthalmic changes from age of ten to 18 years. A longitudinal study of sequels to low birth weight. I., Refraction. Acta Ophthal. (Kbh.), 58: 889—898. (1980).

Fledelius, H.C. Myopia of prematurity, changes during adolescence. Paper read at SIDUO VIII Symposium Nijmegen, Sept. 1980, To appear in Conference Report (1981).

Gernet, H. & Olbrich, E. Excess of the human refractive curve and its cause. In, Ophthalmic Ultrasound. Eds. K.A. Gitter et al. pp. 142—148 Mosby, St Louis (1969).

Sato, T. Acquired myopia. J. Pediat. Ophthalmol. 5: 238—241 (1968).

Sorsby, A., Benjamin, B. & Sheridan, M. Refraction and its components during growth of the eye from the age of three. Medical Research Council SRS 301, London, H.M.S.O. (1961).

Sorsby, A. & Leary, G.A. A longitudinal study of refraction and its components during growth. Medical Research Council SRS 309. London, H.M.S.O. (1970).

Sorsby, A. Growth of the eye in relation to refraction. In, Modern Trends in Ophthalmology-5. Eds. A. Sorsby & S. Miller, pp. 100—108 Butterworth, London (1973).

Author's address:
H.C. Fledelius, M.D.
University Eye Clinic
Rigshospitalet
DK-2100 Copenhagen Ø
Denmark

OCULOMETRIC FINDINGS IN MYOPIA

H. GERNET

(Münster, Germany)

ABSTRACT

Measurements of more than 3000 emmetropic and ametropic eyes have shown that in medium and high myopia the lengthening of the vitreous is the refraction-determining factor.

In emmetropes and myopes the mean values of corneal curvature are equal (7.8 mm). Lenticular refractive power in myopia is distinctly diminished as compared with emmetropic eyes (process of emmetropization).

Assessment of intraocular optics by ultrasound echometry enables the ophthalmologist to prescribe contact lens – spectacle combinations or intraocular lens – spectacle combinations in unilateral aphakia or planned unilateral pseudophakia of myopes, in order to avoid the obstacles of aniseiconia.

INTRODUCTION

For more than 70 years our knowledge about the dimensions and optical components of living eyes was based on the ingenious work of Gullstrand, who developed his eye model, the schematic eye, based on findings in enucleated eyes. Theoretical calculations were necessary because before echography it was impossible to measure the vitreous length and the lens thickness in living eyes.

Oculometry by ultrasound (as we have performed it since 1963 in about 5000 emmetropic and ametropic eyes) together with other clinical measurements (refraction and keratometry) and appropriate formulas (Gernet, Osthold and Werner 1971), allows for the first time an exact analysis of all optical components of living emmetropic and ametropic eyes. Since 1969 we have used a high-precision ultrasonic equipment (with special calibration), the error of axial partial dimensions being only ± 0.05 mm and of the axial length measurement ± 0.15 mm.

OCULOMETRY IN MYOPIA

Figure 1 summarizes findings in myopia (Franceschetti and Gernet 1965, Gernet 1969). In myopia, the mean value of corneal curvature is almost

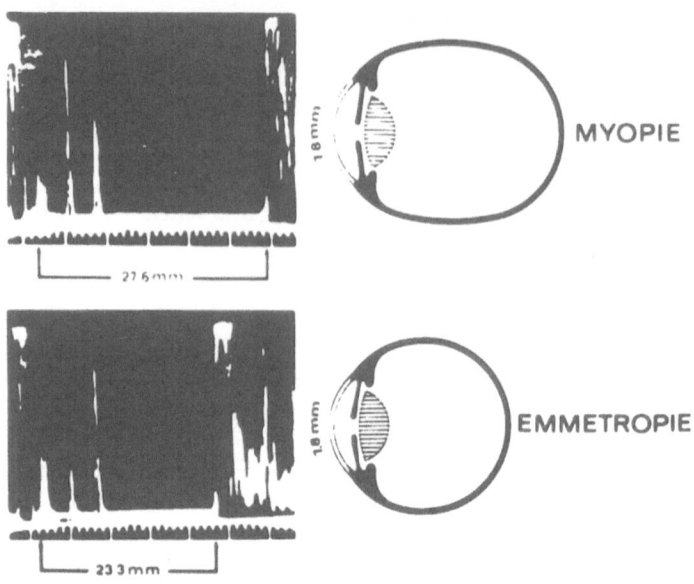

Fig. 1. Ultrasonic echograms and morphological findings in myopia and emmetropia.

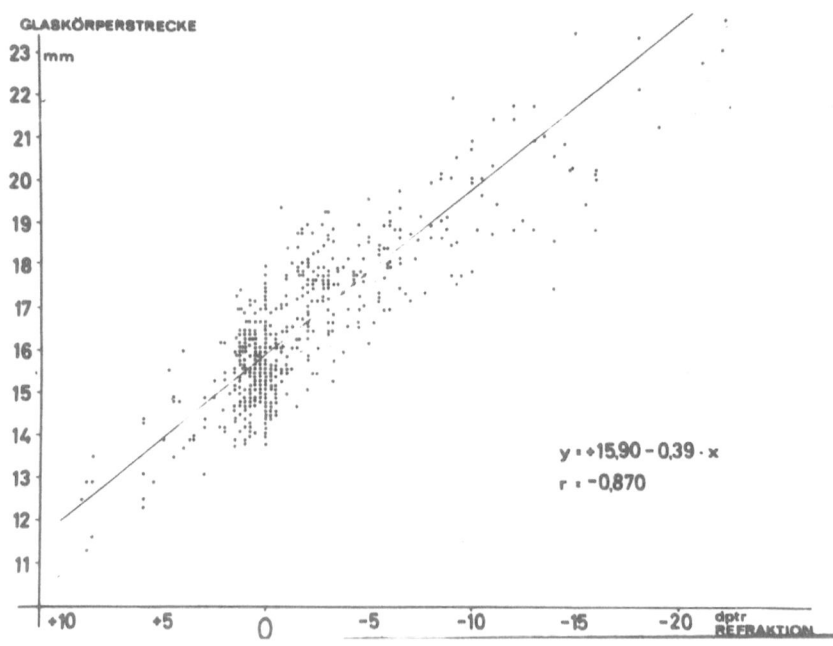

Fig. 2. Association between refractive value (abscissa) and vitreous length (ordinate) in 608 eyes.

the same as in emmetropia; in myopia higher than 2–2.5 D we find almost constantly a lengthening of the vitreous. Myopia exceeding 2.5 D, without pathological changes in cornea or lens, is thus usually caused by an augmented vitreous length. In low grade myopia (< 2.5 D) a marked curvature of the cornea *may* lead to myopia but only in a minority of cases.

Being based on 608 eyes, Figure 2 shows a very strong correlation between refraction and vitreous length (− 0.870); this is even a little stronger than that between refraction an axial length (− 0.845).

OCULOMETRY IN ANISOMETROPIA

Table 1 shows oculometric features of high anisometropia in 59 consecutive cases (Gernet 1979). Amblyopia being infrequent, aniseiconia is mostly overcome by microstrabismus and sensory anomalies. The table clearly shows that the refraction determining factor is the vitreous length (and the axial length) whereas corneal curvature, anterior chamber depth and lens thickness are almost equal. This allows a *rule of thumb* for the practitioner not using echometry:

In cases of high anisometropia with equal keratometer readings and no lens or fundus pathology, the anisometropia is an *axial* anisometropia.

Table 1. Optical components in high anisometropia.

Anisometropie (≥ 2,5 dptr)
(59 Fälle · 118 Augen)
Mittelwerte

	weniger ametr. oder emmetr. Auge	Differenz	stärker ametropes Auge
Achsenlänge (mm)	23,5 ± 1,4	2,5 ± 1,6	26,0 ± 2,1
		Korrelation	
		0,62	
Glaskörperstrecke (mm)	15,9 ± 1,2	Differenz	18,3 ± 1,9
		2,4 ± 1,6	
		Korrelation	
		0,54	
Refraktion (dptr)	-1,1 ± 2,6	Differenz	-8,4 ± 5,3
		7,2 ± 5,0	
		Korrelation	
		0,37	
Hornhautkrümmung (mm)	7,7 ± 0,27	Differenz	7,7 ± 0,28
		0,0 ± 0,1	
		Korrelation	
		0,93	
Vorderabschnitt (mm)	3,6 ± 0,34	Differenz	3,7 ± 0,34
		0,1 ± 0,14	
		Korrelation	
		0,92	
Linsendicke (mm)	3,8 ± 0,35	Differenz	3,8 ± 0,35
		0,0 ± 0,2	
		Korrelation	
		0,91	

Table 2. Optical components in myopia corrected by spectacles (Brille, left) and contact lenses (Haftschale).

Retinale Bildgrößen Achsenmyoper mit Brille und Haftschale

$D_C \cdot 7.8$ $d \cdot 5.8$ $D \cdot 10.0$

BRILLE				HAFTSCHALE			
L (mm)	Dptr	F (mm)	%	L (mm)	Dptr	F (mm)	%
24.2	- 1.0	22.2	103	24.2	- 1.0	22.4	104
24.6	- 2.0	22.3	103	24.6	- 2.0	22.8	106
25.0	- 3.0	22.4	104	25.0	- 3.0	23.2	107
25.4	- 4.0	22.5	104	25.4	- 4.0	23.6	109
25.8	- 5.0	22.6	105	25.8	- 5.0	23.9	110
26.2	- 6.0	22.7	105	26.2	- 6.0	24.2	112
26.5	- 7.0	22.7	105	26.5	- 6.5	24.6	113
26.8	- 8.0	22.7	105	26.8	- 7.5	24.8	115
27.1	- 9.0	22.6	105	27.1	- 8.0	25.0	116
27.4	-10.0	22.6	105	27.4	- 9.0	25.3	117
27.7	-11.0	22.6	105	27.7	-10.0	25.6	118
28.0	-12.0	22.5	104	28.0	-10.5	25.8	119
28.3	-13.0	22.5	104	28.3	-11.0	26.1	121
28.6	-14.0	22.5	104	28.6	-12.0	26.3	122
29.1	-15.0	22.6	105	29.1	-13.0	26.7	124
29.6	-16.0	22.7	105	29.6	-13.5	27.2	126
30.0	-17.0	22.8	105	30.0	-14.0	27.6	128
30.4	-18.0	22.9	106	30.4	-15.0	28.0	130
30.7	-19.0	22.9	106	30.7	-15.5	28.2	131
31.1	-20.0	22.9	106	31.1	-16.5	28.5	132
32.8	-25.0	22.8	105				

D_C · Hornhautkrummung (mm)

L · Achsenlange (mm)

F · Hintere Brennweite (mm)

F · Hintere Brennweite ( )

d · Hornhautscheitel · Linsenhauptebene

D · Abstand Brillenglas · Hornhautscheitel

INTRAOCULAR OPTICS AND ANISEICONIA, SPECTACLES VS. CONTACT LENSES

Table 2 shows mean refraction and axial length values in 235 myopic eyes; further posterior focal distances and retinal image-sizes are presented with spectacles and with contact lenses. The values are considered representative up to a refraction of -8 D. The number of cases with higher refraction is low and the values for axial length accordingly not as reliable as those of the more numerous low-grade myopes. Further, the difficulty regarding exact assessment of refractive value may play a role in high myopia. Nevertheless the table shows an interesting fact. In myopia – without taking in account the scarcely known changes in cone *density* in the macula of the elongated myopic eye – spectable-correction leads more or less to an equal retinal image-size all over the myopic range, because the lengthening of the axis is compensated for by a 'shortening' of the focal distance by the spectacles' minus lenses. On the contrary, contact lens correction leads to a gradual

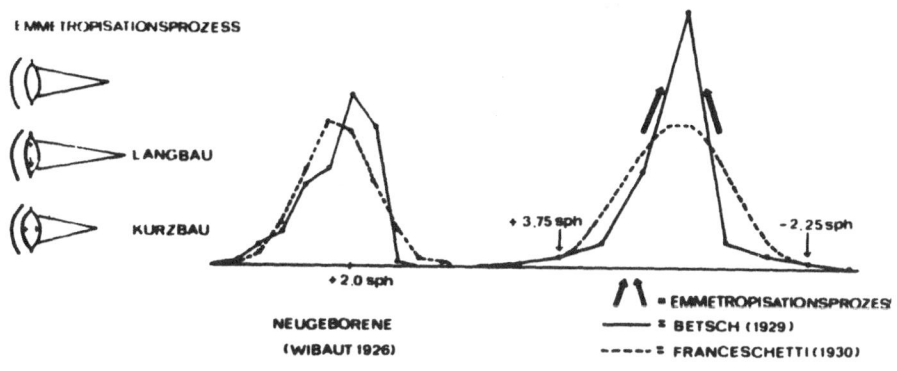

Myopia and Human Lens Refractive Powers

	Refraction Dptr.	Axial Length mm	Corneal Curvature mm	Distance Cornea- - Main Plane Human Lens mm	Human Lens Refractive Power Dptr.
Gullstrands Eye	± 0	24,0	7,8	6,0	+ 21,6
Normal Eye (Mean val. 446 emmetr. eyes)	± 0	23,5	7,8	6,0	+ 23,7
Myopia (235 myopic eyes)	- 3,0	25,0	7,8	6,0	+ 22,1
	- 7,0	26,5	7,8	6,0 6,2	+22,1 +22,5
	-12,0	28,0	7,8	6,0 6,2	+23,4 +23,8
	-17,0	30,0	7,8	6,0 6,2	+23,3 +23,9

Fig. 3. The process of ememtropization (above) and the decrease of human lens refractive power (below) in myopia.

magnification of the retinal image by increase of myopia, going from 104% in low to 130% in high myopia. This finding clearly applies to the wellknown clinical fact, that contact lens correction of myopia creates a magnification and thereby a better vision.

LENS AND EMMETROPIZATION

Previously we have demonstrated that the proces of emmetropization (Gernet and Olbrich 1968 and 1969) is mainly based on the adaptation of the refractive power of the human lens to the eye dimensions.

In myopes the emmetropization is due to the fact that refractive power of human lenses in *myopic* eyes is a little lower than in our *normal* eye, the features of the latter being based on oculometric findings in 446 emmetropic eyes of adults (Gernet and Ostholt 1973). We could prove these facts by our formulas, developed in 1971, concerning calculation of the lens refractive power in emmetropia and ametropia.

Figure 3 shows that in the normal eye the lens refractive power is + 23.7 D, whereas the corresponding value in Gullstrand's simplified schematic eye is + 21.6 D. In myopia up to 7 D we therefore find a decrease in human lens refractive power as compared with our normal eye. As mentioned already, the values for the higher myopic refractions are not regarded representative because of smallness of number and possible errors in the spectacle refraction. In high myopia this error-possibility plays an important role.

HOW TO AVOID ANISEICONIA

Ultrasound oculometry and appropriate formulas allow the ophthalmologist, for the first time, to assess very exactly the lens refractive power and the posterior focal distance and so also the optical aniseiconia in unilateral aphakia or in unilateral pseudophakia. Since 1973 we developed our database on Intraocular Optics in order to treat – after careful echometry – a) unilateral aphakia with individual contact lens-spectacle-combinations (Gernet 1973, 1976, 1977) and b) unilateral cataract by artificial lens-spectacle-combinations (Gernet, Osthold and Werner 1971, 1978). Thus we are able to provide our patients with nearly equal retinal images and comfortable binocular vision in unilateral aphakia and pseudophakia (clinical examples are demonstrated).

CONCLUDING REMARKS

In summary myopia is created by a lengthening of the axial vitreous. In myopia the corneal curvature is mostly identical to that of normal eyes and the lens refractive power is not augmented, but slightly diminished. That means that myopia is essentially *axial*, and not curvature or index myopia. The same is true for myopic anisometropia.

REFERENCES

Franceschetti, A. and Gernet, H. Über optische Größen bei leichter und hoher Myopie auf Grund echographischer Befunde, Graefe's Arch. Ophthalmol. 168: 1–16 (1965).

Gernet, H. Okulometrie-Daten bei Augengesunden 70. Tagung der Dtsch. Ophthalmol. Gesell. 597–599 (1969).

Gernet, H. Okulometrie zur Erkennung von Anomalien der Bulbusdimension Ultrasonographia Medica, Herausgeber: J. Böck u. K. Ossoinig, Verlag der Wiener Med. Akademie II, 455–466 (1969).

Gernet, H. Zur Behandlung der hochgradigen Anisometropie Sitzungsbericht der 126. Vers. d. Ver. rhein.-westf. Augenärzte, Verlag Zimmermann Balve, 46–50 (1973).

Gernet, H. Intraocular Optics, Aniseikonia and Combined Correction of Unilateral Aphakia. The Soft Contact Lenses. II. Intern. Symposium Tokyo, Ed S. Mishima 38–49 (1976).

Gernet, H. Posttraumatic unilateral aphakia. Results of combined correction. Metabolic Ophthalmology, Pergamon Press 2: 307–309 (1978).

Gernet, H. and Ostholt, H. Augenseitige Optik. Ein neues Gebiet der klinischen Okulometrie, Ophthalmologica 166: 120–143 (1973).

Gernet, H. and Olbrich, E. The excess of human refractive curve and its cause Ophthalmic Ultrasound, Ed. Gitter, et al. Mosby-Comp. St. Louis 142–148 (1969).

Gernet, H., Ostholt, H. and Werner, H. Neue klinische Grundlagen zur Binkhorst-Linseneinpflanzung bei Altersstar 123. Vers. d. Ver. rhein.-westf. Augenärzte, Verlag Zimmermann Balve 58–82 (1971).

Gernet, H., Ostholt, H. and Werner, H. Intraokulare Optik in Klinik und Praxis Rothacker, Buchhdlg. f. Medizin, Berlin Köln, München, Regensburg sowie Urban u. Schwarzenberg, 168 S Wien (1978).

Author's address:
Professor H. Gernet, M.D.
University Eye Clinic,
Westring 15
D-4400 Münster
West Germany

THE AETIOLOGY OF MYOPIA AS CONSIDERED FROM THE DIFFERENCES IN THE REFRACTIVE COMPONENTS OF THE RIGHT AND LEFT EYES

J. OTSUKA, T. SUGATA and M. ARAKI

(Tokyo, Japan)

J. Otsuka (1951) and T. Sugata (1958) measured the axial length of the eye with X-ray-vision and calculated the refractive power of the crystalline lens from the axial length and the degree of ametropia of the eye. M. Araki (1962) made ultrasonic measurements of the axial length, anterior chamber depth and lens thickness and calculated the refractive power of the crystalline lens using these values and the degree of ametropia of the eye. The authors discovered in 1979 that most of the age and sex differences in refraction can be eliminated by determining the differences in the mean values of the refractive components of the two eyes in each patient, which were classified into the eye with the higher degree of ametropia and the eye with the lower degree (Table 1). They then applied this method of calculation to their subject groups composed of bilateral emmetropes, isometropes and aniso-metropes, and obtained the following results:

Table 1. The statistical significance of the differences between the refractive components of the eyes with higher refraction and those of the corresponding other eyes with lower refraction in 42 low and high anisometropic subjects (Calculated from M. Araki's data).

	H or L	Mean	V.	S.D.	Max.	Min.	Skew	Krut.	Mean	V.	S.D.	t₀	d.f.	t	Significance
Age		20.35	37.69	6.13	34.00	9.00	0.39	2.78							
Refraction (D)	H	-4.61	20.56	4.53	1.50	-18.00	-1.37	4.43	-1.60	4.92	2.21	-4.69	41	2.03	Sig.
	L	-3.00	12.43	3.52	1.75	-12.00	-1.08	3.37							
Anterior chamber depth (mm)	H	3.74	0.10	0.32	4.80	3.08	0.29	4.61	0.08	0.08	0.29	1.89	41	2.03	Insig.
	L	3.66	0.12	0.35	4.46	2.82	0.00	2.89							
Lens thickness (mm)	H	3.79	0.10	0.32	4.37	3.18	-0.08	2.02	0.04	0.09	0.31	1.01	41	2.03	Insig.
	L	3.74	0.07	0.27	4.28	3.06	-0.02	2.65							
Vitreous chamber depth (mm)	H	18.15	3.62	1.90	22.97	15.04	0.86	3.18	0.43	1.45	1.20	2.34	41	2.03	Sig.
	L	17.72	2.77	1.66	22.68	14.05	0.83	4.38							
Axial length (mm)	H	25.71	3.70	1.92	30.49	22.45	0.75	2.96	0.58	1.42	1.19	3.15	41	2.03	Sig.
	L	25.13	2.54	1.59	29.57	22.32	0.78	3.62							
Corneal power (D)	H	43.46	2.08	1.44	46.53	40.57	-0.24	2.24	0.01	0.25	0.50	0.23	41	2.03	Insig.
	L	43.44	1.96	1.40	46.02	40.00	-0.44	2.30							
Lens power (D)	H	20.51	8.40	2.89	24.92	12.46	-0.73	3.22	0.55	3.61	1.90	1.87	41	2.03	Insig.
	L	19.96	7.15	2.67	13.39	12.65	-0.56	2.89							
Total refractive power (D)	H	60.01	6.05	2.46	64.12	54.70	-0.32	2.23	0.33	2.09	1.44	1.51	41	2.03	Insig.
	L	59.68	5.36	2.31	64.69	55.34	0.08	2.26							

Notes: Abbreviated words should be treated in the same sense as in the other table

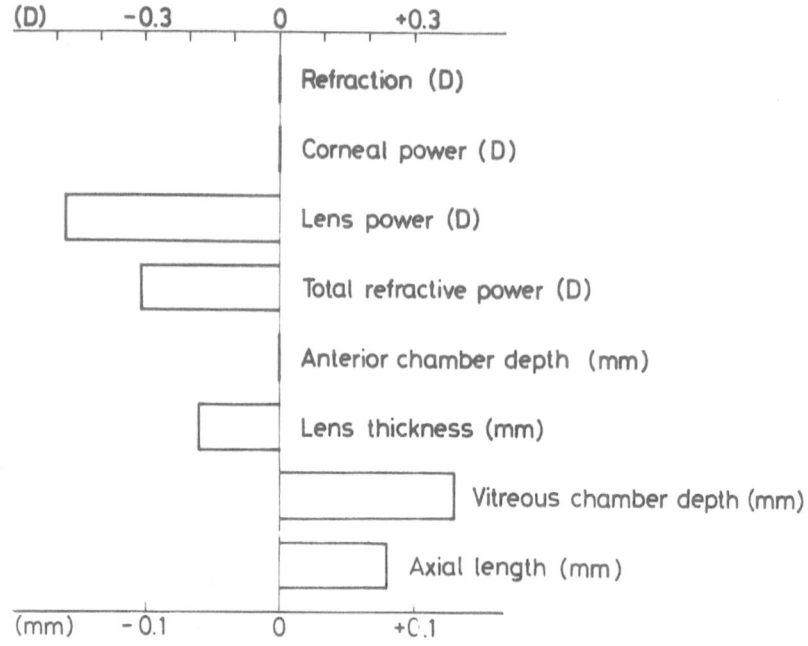

Fig. 1. The differences between the refractive components of the right eyes and those of the corresponding left eyes in 42 isometropic subjects. (Calculated from M. Araki's data).

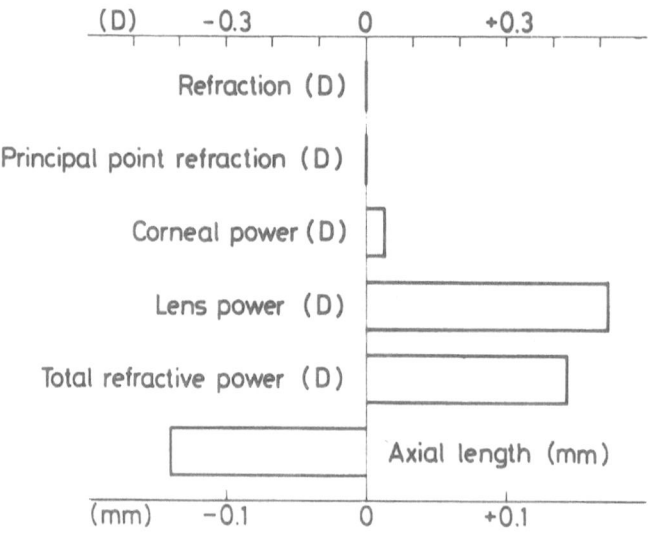

Fig. 2. The differences between the refractive components of right eyes and those of the corresponding left eyes in 21 isometropic subjects (Calculated from T. Sugata's data).

80

(1) In the groups with bilateral emmetropia or with isometropia of various degrees of ametropia, no statistically significant difference was found in any of the refractive components of either eye (Figure 1—Figure 2), except for 24 isometropic subjects of low hypermetropia.

(2) In the group with low anisometropia of less than 2D with low, medium

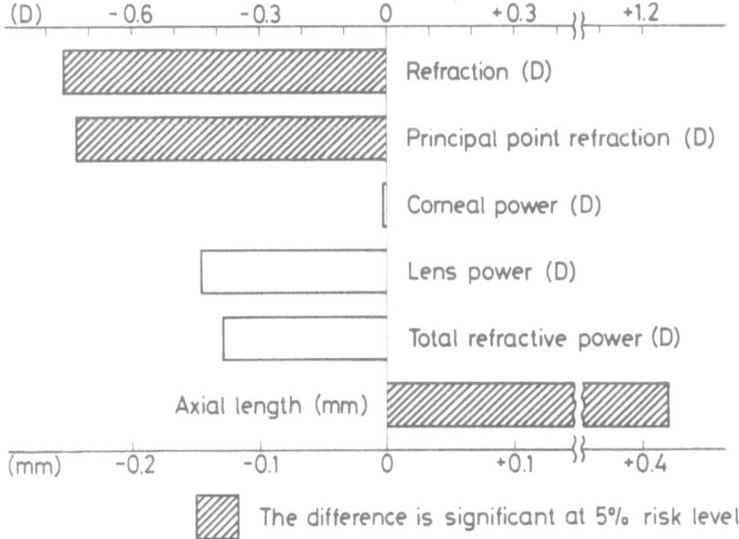

Fig. 3. The differences between the refractive components of the eyes with higher refraction and those of the corresponding other eyes with lower refraction in 49 low anisometropic subjects (Calculated from T. Sugata's data).

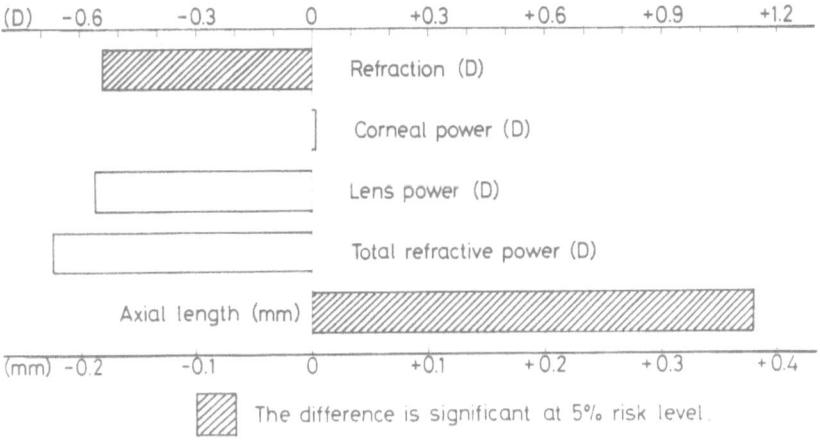

Fig. 4. The differences between the refractive components of the eyes with higher refraction and those of the corresponding other eyes with lower refraction in low anisometropia of 51 low myopic subjects. (Calculated from J. Otsuka's data).

81

or high myopia, a statistically significant difference was found only in the degree of ametropia and axial length with little or no difference in the corneal power, lenticular power or total refractive power of either eye (Figure 3—Figure 6).

(3) In the group with anisometropia of over 2D with medium or high

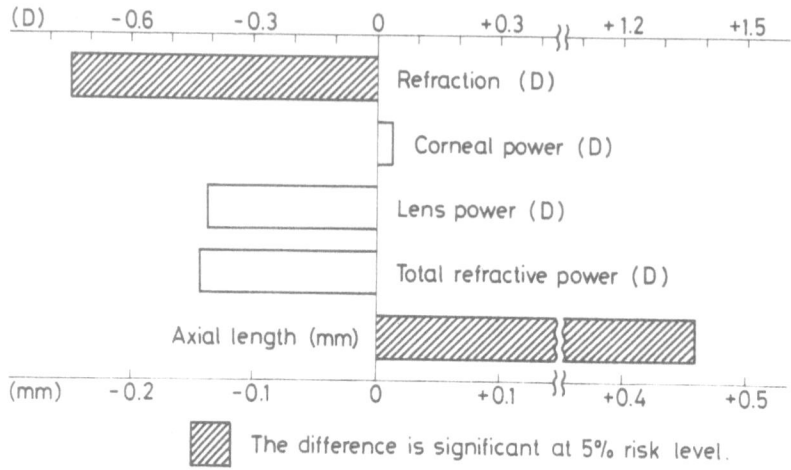

Fig. 5. The differences between the refractive components of the eyes with higher refraction and those of the corresponding other eyes with lower refraction in low anisometropia of 32 medium or high myopic subjects. (Calculated from J. Otsuka's data).

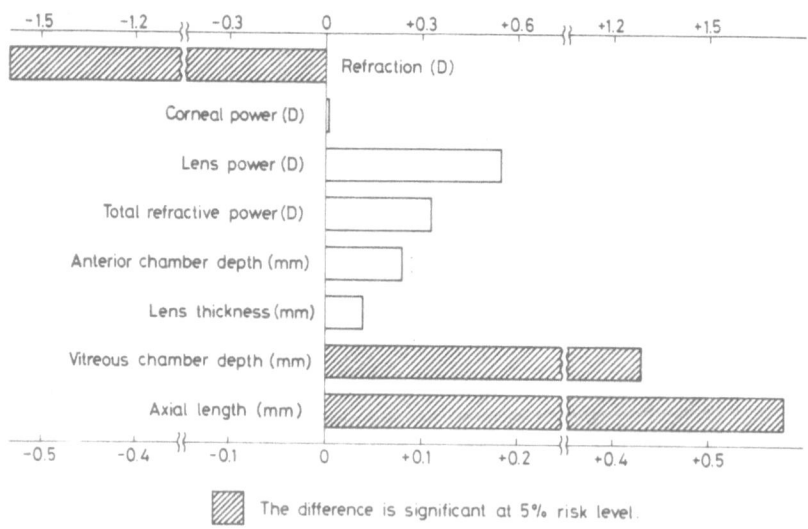

Fig. 6. The statistical significance of the differences between the refractive components of the eyes with higher refraction and those of the corresponding other eyes with lower refraction in 42 low and high anisometropic subjects (Calculated from M. Araki's data).

82

myopia again a statistically significant difference was only found in the degree of ametropia and axial length of the two eyes with little or no difference in the refractive power of the refractive components of either eye. (Figure 7).

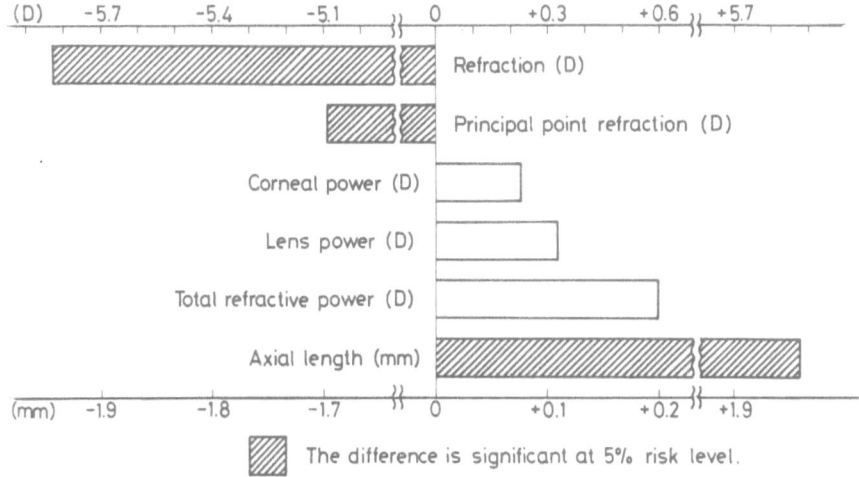

Fig. 7. The differences between the refractive components of the eyes with higher refraction and those of the corresponding other eyes with lower refraction in 23 anisometropic subjects. (Calculated from T. Sugata's data).

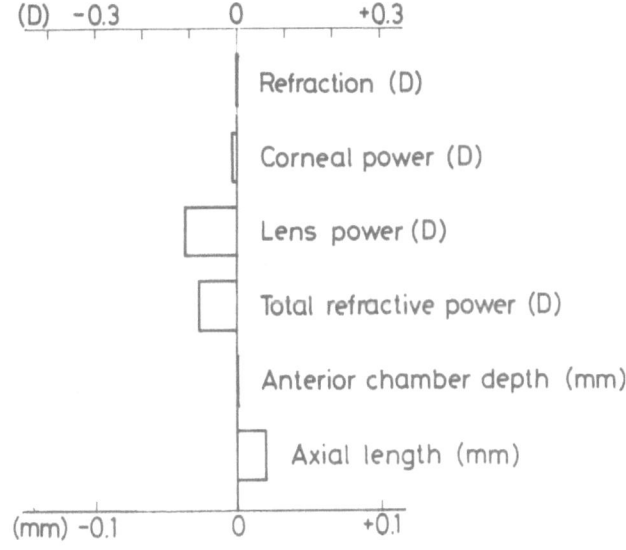

Fig. 8. The differences between the refractive components of the right eyes and those of the corresponding left eyes in 75 isometropic subjects with emmetropic, low or medium hyperopic refraction. (Calculated from A. Sorsby's paper on refraction in twins).

83

(4) Using the same statistical calculation method, we examined the findings covering the 447 subjects studied by Sorsby *et al.* (1956, 1961, 1962)
whose eyes were instilled with cycloplegics such as Homatropine, Atropine,
Hyoscine or Cyclopentolate. The results are as follows:

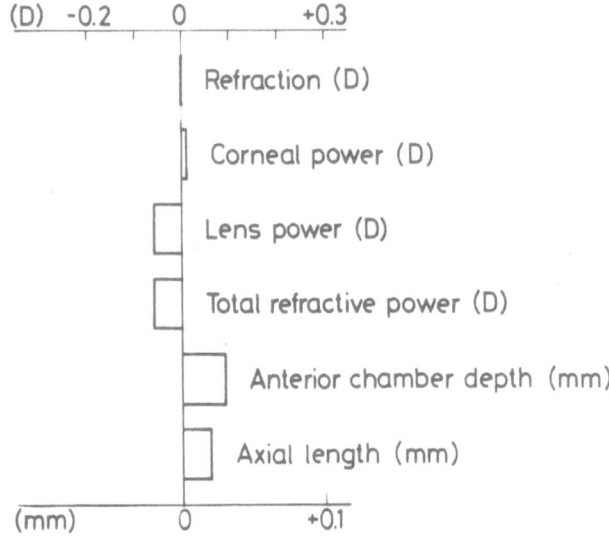

Fig. 9. The differences between the refractive components of the right eyes and those
of the corresponding left eyes in 15 isometropic subjects with low myopia. (Calculated
from A. Sorsby's paper on refraction in twins).

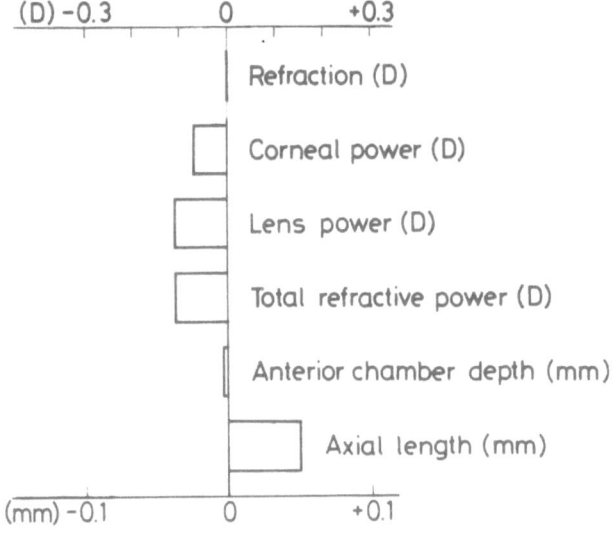

Fig. 10. The differences between the refractive components of the right eyes and those
of the corresponding left eyes in 41 hypermetropic or emmetropic cases of isometropia
aged 20–54 years. (Calculated from A. Sorsby's data).

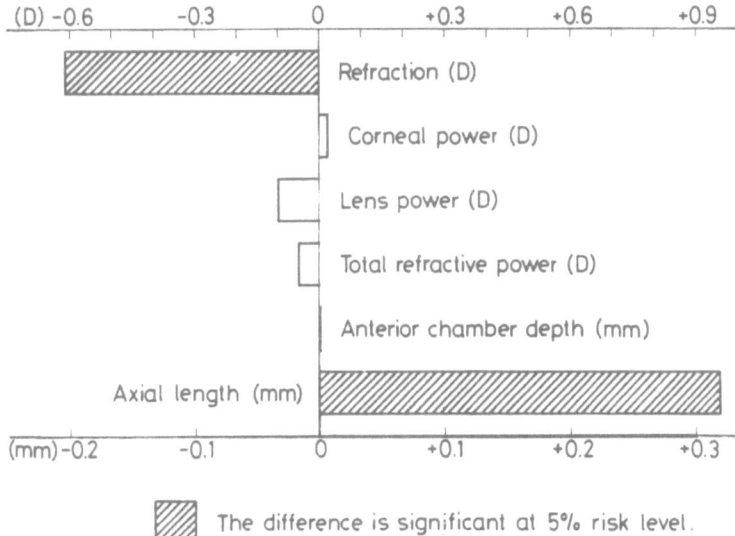

Fig. 11. The differences between the refractive components of the eyes with higher refraction and those of the corresponding other eyes with lower refraction in 43 low myopic anisometropic cases aged 20–58 years. (Calculated from A. Sorsby's data).

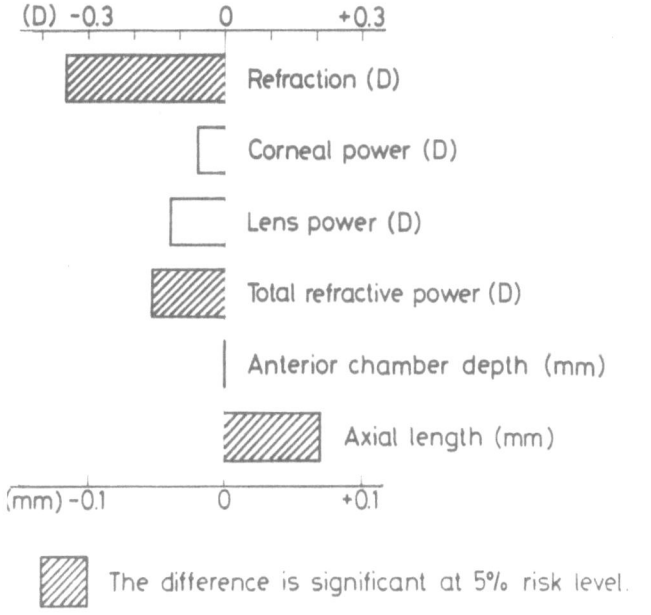

Fig. 12. The differences between the refractive components of the eyes with higher refraction and those of corresponding other eyes with lower refraction in 117 low anisometropic subjects with low hyperopia (Calculated from A. Sorsby's paper refraction in twins).

(a) Isometropes with various degrees of ametropia showed no significant differences between the corresponding refractive components of their eyes (Figure 8–Figure 10).

(b) Low anisometropes with low myopia, with medium and high hyperopia, and with medium myopia, showed a significant correlation between

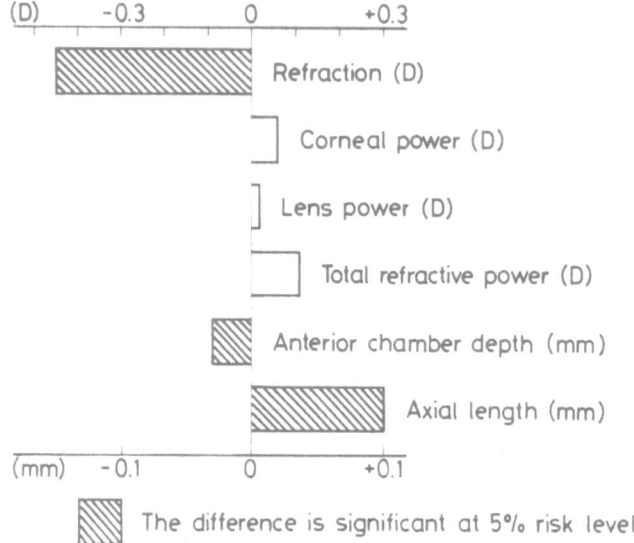

Fig. 13. The differences between the refractive components of the eyes with higher refraction and those of the corresponding other eyes with lower refraction in 53 low hyperopic anisometropes aged 20–60 years. (Calculated from A. Sorsby's data).

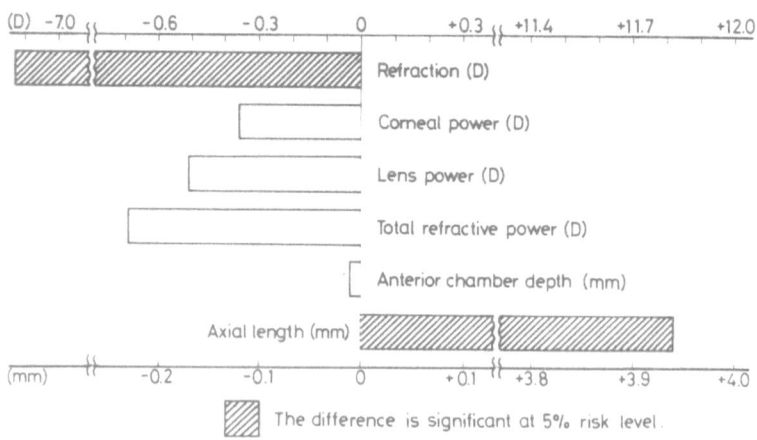

Fig. 14. The differences between the refractive components of the eyes with higher refraction and those of the corresponding other eyes with lower refraction in 13 anisometropic high myopic subjects aged 20–57 years. (Calculated from A. Sorsby's data).

the axial lengths and degrees of ametropia of their two eyes (Figure 11). Moreover, in low anisometropes with low hyperopia, a significant correlation was found between the total refractive powers and anterior chamber depths of their two eyes (Figure 12–Figure 13).

(c) Anisometropes with medium and high myopia also showed a significant correlation between the degrees of ametropia and axial lengths of their two eyes (Figure 14).

(5) The authors are therefore of the opinion that this statistical calculation method is not only simpler but decidedly superior to the method comparing correlation coefficients or distribution curves, as the differences due to age and sex can largely be eliminated. From the findings covering the subjects studied by Sorsby *et al.* the authors conclude that the aetiology of low and medium, as well as high myopia lies equally and principally in the elongation of the ocular axis.

REFERENCES

Araki, M., Studies on refractive components of human eye by means of ultrasonic echogram. Report III. The correlation of refractive components. Acta Soc. Ophthalmol. Jap. 66: 129 (1962).

Otsuka, J. et al., The axial length and the refractive power of the crystalline lens of the eye. Acta Soc. Ophthalmol. Jap. 55: 100 (1951).

Otsuka, J., Research on the etiology and treatment of myopia. Acta Soc. Ophthalmol. Jap. 71: Suppl. 1–212 (1967).

Otsuka, J., Supplementary studies to the genesis and treatment of myopia. Acta Soc. Ophthalmol. Jap. 72: 2012 (1968).

Sorsby, A. et al., Refraction and its components in twins. Medical research council. Special report series 303 (1962).

Sorsby, A. et al., Emmetropia and its aberrations. A study in the correlation of the optical components of the eye. Medical research council. Special report series 293 (1956).

Sorsby, A. et al., Refraction and its components during the growth of the eye from the age of three. Medical research council. Special report series 301 (1961).

Sugata, T., Studies on myopia by X-ray-vision. Acta Soc. Ophthalmol. Jap. 62: 1841 (1958).

Author's address:
T. Sugata, M.D.
Department of Ophthalmology
Tokyo Medical and Dental University School of Medicine
Tokyo
Japan

REFRACTIVE COMPONENTS IN ANISO- AND ISOMETROPIA

An oculometric study (by ultrasonography and keratometry)

H.C. FLEDELIUS

(*Copenhagen, Denmark*)

ABSTRACT

Side differences are assessed concerning axial eye dimensions (by ultrasound) and corneal refractive power (by keratometry) in cases of anisometropia (n = 28) and isometropia (n = 63).

Isometropia: Concerning refractive level, the cases cluster around the emmetropic population norm. With the measurement techniques employed, the optically important eye components of the two eyes are practically identical (as is refractive value).

Anisometropia: Most eyes being myopic, the cases are skewed away from the above emmetropic population norm. The correlation between side differences in refraction and axial length is high (r = 0.94). Anisometropic myopia in young Danes is of a clearly axial nature.

INTRODUCTION

Ophthalmology has – among other medical branches – benefitted from ultrasound examining techniques. Important diagnostic information is gained concerning eye pathology behind opaque media, and it is possible to measure eye distances by ultrasound. The latter has applied especially to studies of refractive components (as evident from a blooming literature, e.g. Delmarcelle *et al.* 1976), including the important field of myopia.

During ultrasound studies one decade ago, my routine was to measure axial length of *right* eyes (and not both). Only in cases of anisometropia the rule was deviated from.

For a period, however, I also measured *bilaterally* in so-called isometropia, partly to check my ultrasound measuring technique (Fledelius 1970; 1976). The other reason was, that such knowledge was not apparent from ophthalmic literature, probably because everyone 'just knows' that the two eyes usually *are* of equal size. More recently there has been a report by Karantinos *et al.* (1974) to cope with the subject.

The aim of the present paper is to report on axially measured right-left differences in isometropia and anisometropia. The latter group is included

Doc. Ophthal. Proc. Series, Vol. 28,
ed. by H.C. Fledelius, P.H. Alsbirk and E. Goldschmidt
© 1981 Dr W. Junk Publishers, The Hague

because there is still some controversy as to the role of the various eye components in myopia. Since anisometropia relates mainly to myopic eyes, some knowledge may be gained concerning myopia *in general*.

MATERIAL AND METHODS

The material comprised 28 persons with *anisometropia* (a cycloplegic side difference above one diopter) and 63 with *isometropia* (cycloplegic side difference $\leqslant 0.5$ D).

Table 1. Composition of the material, by sex and age (range 11–48 years).

		Anisometropia (n = 28)	Isometropia (n = 63)
Sex	male	18	33
	female	10	30
Age	10–19	19	56
	20–29	7	5
	30–49	2	2

Most persons were quite young (Table 1) due to the fact that they attended a larger scale ophthalmic investigation into sequelae to a low birth weight ($<$ 2000 g, Fledelius 1976). They were 10–12 years old at examination. The remainder were random cases from the University Eye Clinic, all being referred from other departments for routine examination, and *not* due to eye disease.

Refractive values were assessed by retinoscopy, in cycloplegia, with subjective confirmation whenever possible.

Anterior corneal curvature radius was measured by Javal-Schiøtz keratometry.

Axial eye distances were measured by ultrasound (Kretztechnik 7000, contact glass method with methylcellulose and Ultrasonolux 12 Mc transducer, cf. Fledelius 1976).

RESULTS

Table 2 gives refractive distribution in the two groups under study. Isometropic cases show the usual accumulation around emmetropia (with a median value of + 0.75 D), while anisometropic eye pairs are skewed away from this norm, towards myopia. Anisometropic median value is − 6 D of the stronger refracting eye and − 1 D of the fellow eye.

The individual eyes of the anisometropia group are shown graphically in Figure 1. They are scattered over the full refractive range. Isometropic cases (forming a cluster of dots between 0 and + 2 D) are not shown.

90

Table 2. Refractive distribution, in per cent, in the two refractive groups under study (top). *Median value* is given (bottom), in anisometropia for stronger and weaker refracting eye, in isometropia for right eyes.

	Anisometropia (n = 2 × 28 eyes)	Isometropia (n = 63 right eyes)
< − 6 D	29%	6%
− 6 to − 2.25	29%	8%
− 2 to − 0.25	16%	3%
0 to + 1.75	16%	75%
⩾ + 2 D	10%	8%
Median refractive value	− 6 and − 1 D	+ 0.75 D

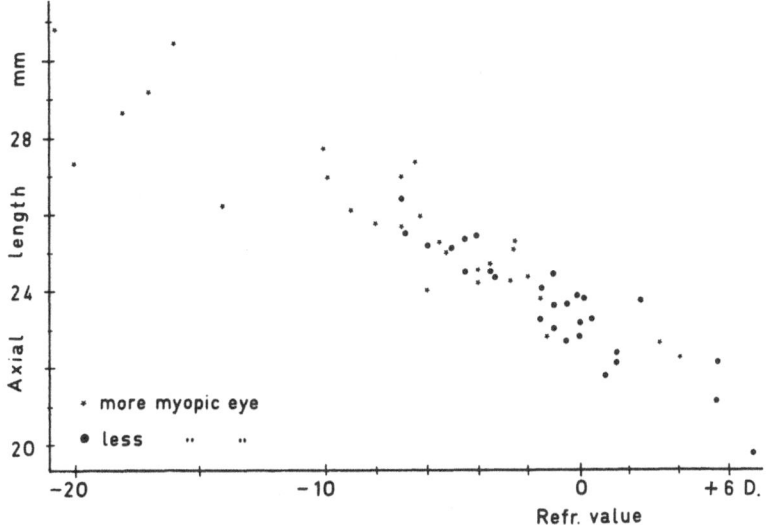

Fig. 1. The eyes of the anisometropic group shown graphically (refractive value on x-axis, axial length on y-axis). Linear regression: $y = -0.328x + 23.36$; $r = -0.93$, n = 56 eyes.

Table 3. Side differences (Δ) between so-called stronger refracting (more myopic/less hypermetropic) and weaker refracting eye in anisometropia (left) and isometropia (right). Mean values and SD.

	Anisometropia (28 eye pairs)	Isometropia (63 eye pairs)
Δ Refraction (D)	− 6.15 ± 6.24	− 0.12 ± 0.17
Δ Axial length (mm)	2.23 ± 2.15	0.13 ± 0.12
Δ Ant. chamber D (mm)	0.086 ± 0.14	− 0.002 ± 0.12
Δ Lens thickness (mm)	0.036 ± 0.19	0.004 ± 0.11
Δ Corneal power (D)	0.00 ± 0.29	0.01 ± 0.16

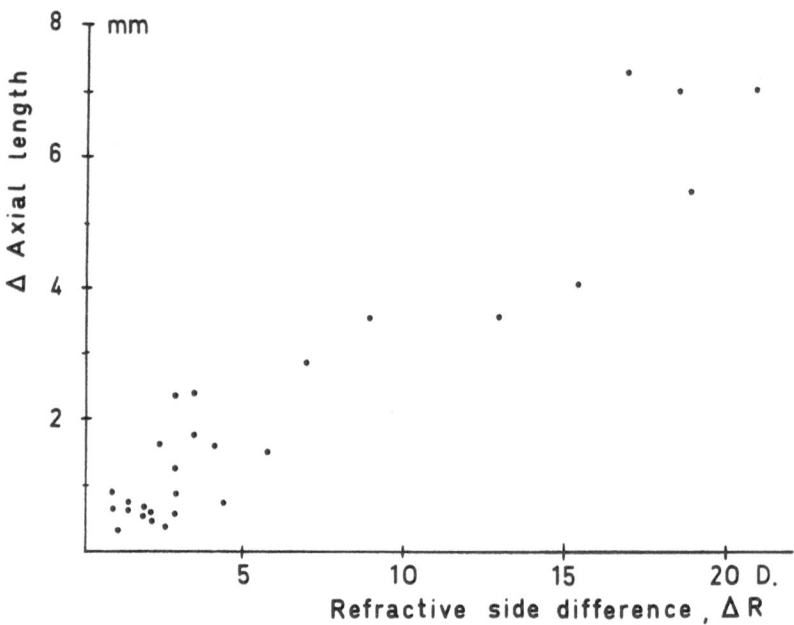

Fig. 2. Correlation between refractive side difference (on x-axis, given as *numerical value*), and axial length side difference (y-axis) in 28 cases of anisometropia, shown graphically. r = 0.94, cf. text.

Table 3 shows intra-individual side differences between the so-called 'stronger' and 'weaker' refracting eye in the two groups. According to tradition, 'stronger refractive' means the more myopic/or the less hypermetropic, of the two eyes. Side differences are shown concerning refraction, axial length, anterior chamber depth, lens thickness, and corneal refractive power.

The results of *isometropes* confirm our working hypothesis, that the two eyes are indeed very much alike, as regards the parameters of Table 3.

The average degree of *anisometropia* appears to be − 6.15 D. Correspondingly there is an axial elongation of the more myopic eye, with a mean side difference of 2.23 mm. The mean *side difference ratio* is − 2.7 D/1 mm axial length.

Further there is a slight, but significant side difference as concerns anterior chamber depth, with the deeper chamber occurring in the more myopic of the two eyes. Concerning lens thickness and corneal power, the differences between the two eyes are not significant.

It thus appears that only one of the four presented parameters, namely axial length, shows a *strong* correlation to refractive side difference in anisometropic eye-pairs. This association is obvious also from Figure 2, where side differences in refraction (in D, numerical values) and in axial length

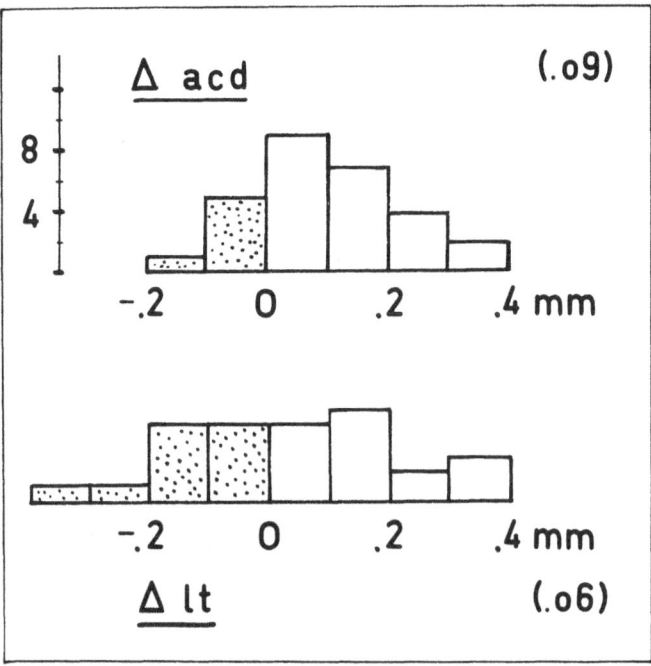

Fig. 3. Side differences in anisometropic eye-pairs (stronger minus weaker refracting eye's value) regarding anterior chamber depth (top) and lens thickness (bottom). The tendency towards a deeper chamber in the more myopic eye is apparent also from Table 3. Number of cases on ordinate, mean values (in mm) in parentheses.

(in mm) are on abscissa and ordinate. The 28 points lie close to a line, and by linear regression the equation is found:

$$y = 0.325 x + 0.234 \qquad (r = 0.94!)$$

Figure 3 shows, in column diagrams, anisometropic side differences regarding anterior chamber depth and lens thickness, again calculated as the value of the weaker refractive eye subtracted from that of the stronger (within the eye-pair). There is a certain scatter, which *may* however be related to the measuring error of the ultrasound method. At least, tendencies are not obvious, but it cannot be denied that a *thick* lens may occasionally contribute to the myopia.

In this context, it is to be kept in mind that only lens *thickness* is measured (even with a certain error due to the method), and not the *optical* properties of the lens (curvatures of refracting lens surfaces, refractive index).

DISCUSSION

A summary discussion of the results is already given above. Concerning refractive components in anisometropia, the present findings are in keeping with

93

those of previous authors (Sugata 1959; Sorsby *et al.* 1962; Franceschetti *et al.* 1968). They stress the *prime* importance of axial length (or vitreous length) as related to side difference in refraction. Lens factors seem to be of far less importance, a view which is, however, still questioned by Sato (1968, 1981).

Analysing anisometropic (*within*-eye-pair) differences, inter-individual variation is (to some extent) discarded. Theoretically such results concerning the dominant role of axial length therefore apply only to anisometropic myopia. The conditions are, however, considered valid also for myopia *in general*. This is evident from a large (and unanimous) number of cross-sectional studies in literature (Stenström 1946; Franken 1961; Jansson 1963; and many others). Thus, the association between refraction and axial length *is* indeed strong, and apparently not obscurred by the inter-individual variation.

Concerning *isometropia,* the trivial confirmation of equal eye dimensions cannot surprise. As compared with the oculometric study of isometropia by Karantinos *et al.* (1974), the right-left fluctuations of the present study are somewhat smaller. Karantinos et al. reported on intraindividual right-left side differences up to ± 0.75 mm, however, without a significant side difference when assessing statistically the *whole* sample. The high intra-individual differences reported are probably (mainly) due to the measuring error of the ultrasound method employed.

Refractive value made up the criterion for inclusion into the present study. Next, refractive components were analysed, and conclusions are drawn *from* refractive value *to* the latter parameters (among which is axial eye length).

The results seem to justify also the 'inverse' conclusions, namely from axial length (as measured by ultrasound) to refraction. In eyes with opaque media, equal axial lengths probably signify isometropia, and eyes with axial elongation are probably (more) myopic.

This has bearing on another paper given at this conference, on the distensability of the young eye (Fledelius 1981) based on eyes with opaque media due to trauma.

SUMMARY

Intraindividual side differences are reported concerning ocular refractive value, keratometry, and axial ultrasound oculometry in anisometropia (n = 28) and isometropia (n = 63).

The conclusions are, in brief:

(1) The more myopic eye of an anisometropic eye-pair invariably had the greater axial length. Corresponding *mean* differences were − 6.15 D and 2.33 mm axial length. The anterior chambers were also a little deeper, while significant side differences concerning lens thickness (and corneal power) did not appear. Myopia of young anisometropic Danes is thus clearly axial, and not lenticular.

(2) In *isometropia* there was an equal eye size of the two eyes. The

same applied to corneal power and the axial dimensions of the various eye segments.

(3) The ultrasound measuring method seems reliable as assessed with the best suited *in vivo* control for comparison, the fellow eye in individuals with equal refraction of the two eyes.

(4) Finally, the results imply that it is justified to conclude from axial elongation to refractive state (towards myopia), also in eyes where refractive value cannot be determined due to opaque media.

REFERENCES

Delmarcelle, Y., François, J., Goes, F., Collignon-Brach, J., Luyckx-Bacus, J. & Verbraeken, H. Biométrie oculaire clinique. Masson, Paris (1976).

Fledelius, H. Ultrasound (A-mode) in a case of nasal posterior scleral ectasy. Acta ophthalmol. (Kbh.) 48: 502–507 (1970).

Fledelius, H. Prematurity and the Eye. Thesis. Acta opthalmol. (Kbh.) Suppl. 128 (1976).

Fledelius, H. Distensability of the young eye. Docum. Ophthalmol. Proc. Series 28: 117–120 (1981).

Franceschetti, A.T., Linder, A. & Franceschetti, A. New results concerning the problem of axial lengths of the eye in anisometropia. In, Diagnostica Ultrasonica in Ophthalmologia, Ed. Vanysek J. pp. 235–238, Brno (1968).

Franken, S. Metingen aan het levende menselijke oog met behulp van ultrasone trillingen (Thesis), Utrecht (1961).

Jansson, F. Measurements of intraocular distances by ultrasound. Acta ophthalmol. (Kbh.) suppl. 74 (1963).

Karantinos, D., Papacharalampous, E., Theodossiadis, G. & Velissaropoulos, P. Biométrie oculaire par échographie A. Arch. Ophthalmol. 34: 581–586 (Paris 1974).

Sato, T. Acquired myopia. J. Ped. Ophthalmol. 5: 238–241 (1968).

Sato, T. Criticism of various accommodogeneous theories on school myopia. Paper read at III. Int. Conf. on Myopia, Copenhagen Aug. 1980. To appear in conf. report (1981).

Sorsby, A., Leary, G.A. & Richards, J. The optical components in anisometropia. Vision Res. 2: 43–51 (1962).

Stenström, S. Untersuchungen über die Variation und Kovariation der optischen Elemente des menschlichen Auges. Acta ophthalmol (Kbh.), suppl. 24 (1946).

Sugata, T. Studies on myopia by estimating aniseikonia and the refractive components of both eyes. Jap. J. Ophthalmol. 3: 142–148 (1959).

Author's address:
H.C. Fledelius, M.D.
University Eye Clinic
Rigshospitalet
DK-2100 Copenhagen Ø
Denmark

CRITICISM OF VARIOUS ACCOMMODOGENEOUS THEORIES ON SCHOOL MYOPIA

Judging from explanation on emmetropization

T. SATO

(*Yokohama, Japan*)

ABSTRACT

The importance of school myopia and its accommodogeneous cause are unquestionable. In order to know which theory is right with regard to school myopia, axial theories or Sato's theory, I took up, as a standard of estimation, 'emmetropization' (EM) which has a very close relationship with accommodation and school myopia. Sato's theory can rationally explain EM by the braking mechanism of tonus. On the contrary, none of the axial theories can explain EM as they cannot contain the braking mechanism. A theory which is a compromise between the refractive theory related to tonus and the axial theory has not received support by comparing bony arm length, corresponding to axial eye length, of the dominant arm with that of the other arm.

INTRODUCTION

At the international conference on myopia held in 1978, environmental myopia was selected as the main theme, and school myopia, making up the majority of cases of environmental myopia, was discussed in detail. The following points were ascertained, cf. Sato (1979):

Firstly, though many textbooks teach that school myopia does not exist, it really exists. Furthermore, it is no doubt increasing rapidly due to the spread of education and the increase of near work.

Secondly, the cause of school myopia was assumed epidemiologically to be excessive accommodation, and this assumption was supported by experiments on monkeys.

Thirdly, there are surely two fundamental mistakes in the logic of the traditional theory on school myopia. The traditional theory deduced the environmental axial elongation directly from an undoubted phenomenon that the myopic ocular axis is generally long or elongating. Next, the traditional theory denied the environmental lenticular role played in the case of school myopia, judging from an undoubted phenomenon that lens refractive power is generally small or becoming smaller. However, the traditional theory on school myopia ignored remarkable hereditary axial elongation when insisting on environmental axial elongation and on the other hand ignored a big environmental role of the crystalline lens in accomplishing emmetropization when denying environmental factors influencing the crystalline lens (Sato 1978). It is also possible to prove, mathematically, that the deduction by the traditional theory is surely wrong. In the case of emmetropization in teenagers, the absolute value of the lenticular power may decrease in myopes to accomplish emmetropization, but its relative value increases through excessive accommodation, resulting in development of school (weak) myopia. As hypermetropes accommodate more than myopes, the lenticular power of the latter is weaker than that of the former.

Fourthly, it is impossible to tell which is correct, the axial theory or Sato's theory from the facts based on which the traditional theory was formed. Sato's theory (1957, 1980) says that hereditary factors of refraction, including school myopia, are mainly determining the ocular axis, whereas environmental factors work through accommodative adaptation of the crystalline lens and the ciliary muscle. This theory is based upon many sound experiments, and is able to explain any phenomenon of school myopia. Furthermore, the theory gives a basis for prevention and cure of school myopia.

The remaining problems are: (1) will any of various accommodogeneous axial theories be established? (2) if so, how will it be? To answer these questions, each theory was estimated by judging whether it is able to explain emmetropization which is closely related to accommodation and school myopia.

METHODS, RESULTS AND DISCUSSION

1. The reason why 'emmetropization' was chosen as a standard of estimation of accommodogeneous theories

The refractive curve of newborn babies is similar to the normal curve following the biological law; however, when they start to see their surroundings, the refractive curve suddenly shows concentration approximately on emmetropia (Figure 1). Straub (1909) called this phenomenon 'Emmetropisation'. Erggelet (1932) assumed that this sudden change was caused by the start of accommodation in babies. To prove this assumption the other way round, I performed an experiment in which accommodation was paralyzed by atropine. Then it was found with certainty that the phenomenon of emmetropization became much less distinct, showing its very close relationship with accommodation (Figure 2).

Now, let's examine the relation between emmetropization and school myopia. School myopia was discovered by Cohn (1867), and was found by Tscherning (1883) to be weak myopia and not strong myopia. Observing the refractive curve, they found that school myopia is either contained in the part which is concentrated due to emmetropization, or adjacent to that part. This central region of the distribution decreases remarkably when atropine is applied, cf. Figure 1 and 2. However, strong myopia exists

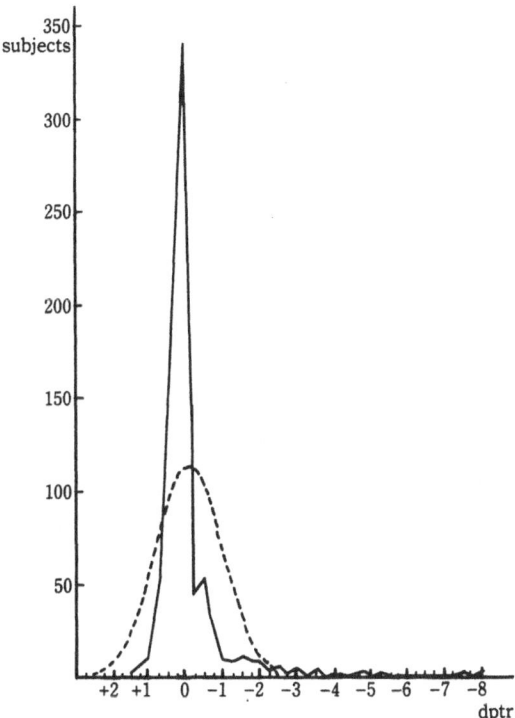

Fig. 1. The refractive curve of 1.034 children before the instillation of atropine, and the corresponding normal curve. This shows the remarkable emmetropization. (Sato 1941).

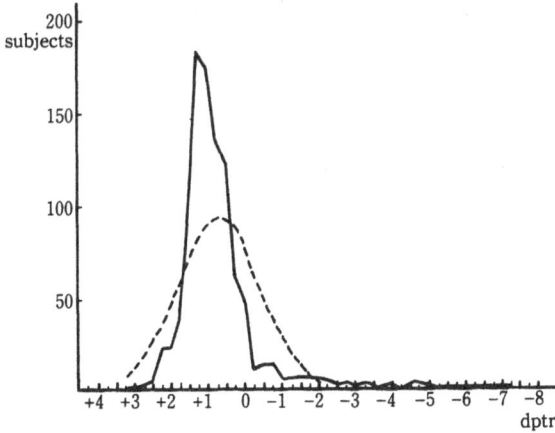

Fig. 2. The refractive curve of 1.034 atropinized children and the corresponding normal curve. By atropinization emmetropization decreased remarkably (Sato 1941).

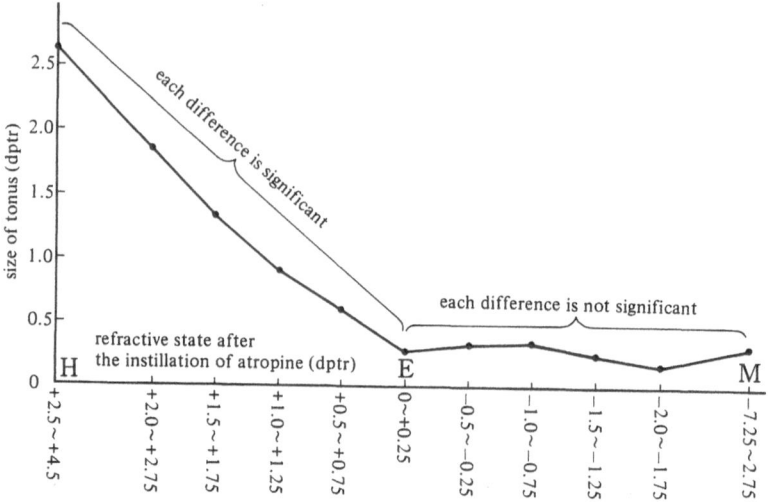

Fig. 3. The relation between the refraction without tonus (abscissa) and the average tonus (ordinate) (Sato 1942).

distant from the concentrated part; it is hardly influenced by atropine and seems to differ from school myopia in its nature. Therefore, in order to examine the various accommodogeneous theories on school myopia, it would be appropriate to choose, as the standard of estimation, the question whether each of the theories can explain emmetropization or not.

2. Examination of Sato's theory, with 'emmetropization' as a standard of estimation

Sato's theory explains emmetropization by tonus. Tonus is not a pathological spasm but a kind of physiological contraction, as explained in detail in my previous papers (Sato 1942, 1957). It is unconscious and static, thus differing from another physiological contraction (so-called tetanus). The degree of tonus of the ciliary muscle can be determined as the refractive change arising when tonus is paralyzed by atropine instillation.

In order to know how tonus of the ciliary muscle will influence refraction, I examined the relationship between the degree of tonus and the refractive state without tonus in a sample of 1034 primary school children (Figure 3). The graph obtained has a slope of 45° on the hypermetropic side and is almost horizontal on the myopic side, with the bend at emmetropia. On the hypermetropic side, tonus corresponds approximately to the degree of hypermetropia. As a result, hypermetropic eyes are emmetropized. The correlation in hypermetropes was statistically significant while it was insignificant in myopes (Sato 1942). Thus, on the myopic side emmetropization by tonus suddenly ceases at the point of emmetropia, as if braked.

Despite the continuous normal accommodation from the hypermetropic to the myopic end of the range, development of tonus caused by this accommodation is not continuous as it suddenly ceases at emmetropia

100

as if braked. This peculiarity of tonus is explained by the laws of physiology (cf. Bayliss 1927). When muscles contract consciously to various degrees (tetanus) for a long time, tonus develops to the minimum necessary degree of contraction. It is unconscious and stable, in contrast to tetanus which is conscious and labile, and development of tonus is inhibited when it exceeds the minimum necessary contraction, as if braked. For example, the shape of the body is controlled by tonus. If tonus were to develop continuously without such braking mechanism, its degree would continue to increase, resulting in a deformed body. In the case of refraction it can be said that if no brake was found, i.e. there was no restraining function to keep the refractive state emmetropic, the peak of the refractive curve would shift far to the myopic side, presenting not a concentrated distribution but a normal curve. Thus no emmetropization would occur and strong myopia would be more frequent.

As shown by the foregoing, Sato's theory, which bases the mechanism of school myopia on tonus, can explain emmetropization reasonably.

3. Examination of the axial theories, with 'emmetropization' as a standard of estimation.

The accommodogeneous axial theories on school myopia have been explained by many mechanisms like ocular hypertension, intoxication, spasm of the ciliary muscle, inflammation, hyperaemia, traction of the tensor muscle, etc., but none of them contained the braking phenomenon at emmetropia. According to them, the ocular axis will continue to elongate, and there will be no emmetropization. Therefore, it is concluded that these theories are unable to explain emmetropization, and thus they are feeble. We cannot expect that any axial theory, in the past or in the future, will be able reasonably to explain the braking mechanism at emmetropia. When the other six bases for non-establishment of the axial theory are also considered (cf. Sato 1979), it could be said that no axial theory will ever be established in the future, and even if an axial theory should exist, it would be feeble.

4. The axial theories regarding tonus as cause of axial elongation

I tried to search for any possibility to support the axial theories, although I had been against them. In order to explain emmetropization, it is necessary to prove that the ocular axis elongates due to tonus. This new theory is a compromise between Sato's theory and the axial theory. To analyse if this new theory is right or wrong, I examined phenomena in other parts of the body which are similar to the axial eye elongation. Since the length of a bone may correspond to the axial length of the eye, I measured the difference between the lengths of the dominant and recessive arms of several people but obtained no clear result. In sports medicine Saito (1935) found that, although functional muscular hypertrophy is certain and remarkable, functional bone elongation is uncertain or very small. Furthermore, we do not know if this functional bone elongation is caused by tetanus or tonus.

If the axial elongation of the eye was caused by tetanus, emmetropization could not be explained.

Thus it is certain that there is little or insignificant possibility for establishment of axial theories based on the normal phenomenon of tonus. After having made efforts in pursuit of possible establishment of accommodogeneous axial theories on school myopia, I have concluded that such pursuit has been fruitless.

CONCLUSION

To estimate accommodogeneous axial theories and Sato's theory on school myopia, 'emmetropization' (EM) was taken up. Sato's theory explained EM well, but axial theories could not at all. With the other six bases added (cf. Sato 1979) I have to conclude that no axial theory will be established neither at present nor in the future.

REFERENCES

Bayliss, W.M. Principles of general physiology. Tonus. p. 533. London (1927).

Cohn, H. Schulmyopie, Eine ätiologische Studie. Leibzig (1867).

Erggelet, H. Die Refraktion und die Akkommodation mit ihren Störungen. Sch.-Br. Hdb., 2: 562 (1932).

Saito, K. Sports and orthopaedy. Acta Soc. Orthopaed. Jpn. 9: 475–549 (1935).

Sato, T. Ein Beitrag zur Kenntnis der Refraktionskurve. Acta Soc. Ophthalmol. Jpn. 45: 2277–2291 (1941).

Sato, T. The 'tonus' of the ciliary muscle and its relation with the ocular refraction. Acta Soc. Ophthalmol. Jap. 46: 71–94 (1942).

Sato, T. The causes and prevention of acquired myopia. pp. 1–244. Yokohama, Japan (1957).

Sato, T. Probability of Sato's theory and the axial theory of the acquired myopia. Acta Soc. Ophthalmol. Jap. 81: 545–549 (1977).

Sato, T. A number of unreasonable ideas in traditional theories pertaining to myopia, derived from a common logical mistake. Acta Soc. Opthalmol. Jap. 82: 572–578 (1978).

Sato, T. 2nd Int. Conf. Myopia. International Congress Series No. 450, XXIII Concilium Ophthalmol., Kyoto, 1978, Excerpta Medica pp. 578–579 (1979).

Sato, T. Summary and criticism of Sato's theory on school myopia. Proc 2nd Int. Conf. on Myopia. Usuki Printings Ltd., Suita, Japan (1980).

Straub, M.Ü. die Ätiologie der Brechungsanomalien u. den Ursprung der Emmetropie. Graefes Arch., 70: 130–199. (1909).

Tscherning, M. Studien ü. die Ätiologie der Myopie. Graefes Arch., 29: 201. (1883).

Author's address:
T. Sato, M.D.
6–90, Onoecho
Naka-ku, Yokohama
231, Japan

ACCOMMODATION AND JUVENILE MYOPIA

Some findings in Danish material around the age of 18 years

H.C. FLEDELIUS

(Copenhagen, Denmark)

ABSTRACT

NPA-values were measured in 18-year-old persons (n = 137), and a nearwork-score was attempted (from interviews) concerning education, amount of nearwork and seeing habits during adolescence. Being part of a longitudinal study, the NPA-values could be weighted against (1) refraction at the age of 18, and (2) refractive *change* from ten to 18 years.

The 18-year NPA-scores were significantly higher in myopes than in emmetropes and hypermetropes (a paradox?, cf. discussion). Myopes also had higher nearwork-scores.

The myopes, being clearly superior accommodators, also showed the highest increase in refraction (from age of ten to 18). Anyhow, it is considered unjustified directly to conclude that the refractive change (towards myopia) is caused by accommodation.

INTRODUCTION

The association between educational level and prevalence of myopia has been known for at least a century (Tscherning 1882). Accordingly, near-work has been claimed as *the* factor in myopia pathogenesis.

Nevertheless such theories have been on the retreat until recently, because most evidence was meant to indicate that myopia predominantly (or solely) depends on hereditary factors.

Myopia research of the last decade has again brought near-work and accommodation (among other *extrinsic* factors) into focus. The present paper deals with accommodative power and near-work conditions in 137 18-year-old Danes, who had been the subject of ophthalmological follow-up from their age of ten.

MATERIAL AND METHODS

At 10-year assessment (n = 539, Fledelius 1976) the results of nearpoint of accommodation measurements (NPA, on the R.A.F. ruler) were given only roughly as normal or subnormal. This was a consequence of the fact that many 10-year olds accommodated until 4—5 cm from the eye. A finer grading of the results was therefore impossible, due to the way the data were actually collected. 'Everyday conditions' were aimed at, and concave lenses (to facilitate examiner's reading of the scale) were not inserted in a trial frame.

At 18-year follow-up (n = 137, 70 with a low birth weight (LBW), 67 full-term controls (FT)), monocular NPA readings could be more accurately recorded (because of the intervening loss of accommodative power), now using a more appropriate scale area of the R.A.F. ruler.

The dioptric value was read and converted to an 'emmetropic' reading, according to cycloplegic refractive value. An accommodation of 15 D *without* lenses was thus recorded as 13 D in case of myopia of two dioptres, or as 16 D when refractive value was + 1.0 D.

In most cases only right eye values were entered into calculations. In addition, however, a few left eyes were included, deriving from anisometropic eye pairs. This was considered as justified because the present *main* objective was an analysis of NPA as related to refractive value.

Information was gained (by interviews) about educational level, free-time activities and visual nearwork habits, and each had an attempted cumulated nearwork score.

RESULTS

Accommodative capacity ranged from 6.3 to 22.2 D. The distribution in the LBW-group (n = 70) does not differ from that of FT-controls (n = 67), and the mean values of the two birth weight groups are identical (12.2 D).

After pooling the results irrespectively of birth weight, a subdivision is made into the usual refractive groups of hypermetropia, emmetropia, and juvenile myopia. To avoid undue statistical noise, the pathologic group of 'myopia of prematurity' is kept entirely out of calculations.

Table 1 shows NPA mean values (± SD) and ranges in the three refractive groups. The tendency is obvious: With a 13.8 D mean value, the myopes are superior as compared with emmetropes ($p < 0.01$), and the hypermetropes have the lowest mean score.

The ranges of Table 1 further indicate, that myopia entails some *super* high scores, considerably above the scant 17 D upper limit of emmetropes and hypermetropes.

These super scores — applying to seven myopic eyes (13.5% of all) — might explain the quite superior mean value of the myopes. The difference between myopes and the rest is, however, retained, even after adjusting these super scores down to a more customary top score level of for instance 16 D. The superiority of myopes thus depends on the *full* distribution of NPA readings, and is not due merely to the skewing effects of a few extremely skilful myopic accommodators.

Next, myopes at age of 18 have shown refractive changes since age of ten which are clearly above the changes occurring in emmetropes and

Table 1. Accommodative power (NPA, in D) as related to refractive class. Number of eyes, mean values ± SD, and ranges are shown. The pathological group of 'myopia of prematurity' is let out of calculations.

	Number of eyes	Mean value and SD	Range of NPA, in D
Juvenile myopia	52	13.8 ± 3.18	(8.3–22.2)
Emmetropia	56	11.6 ± 2.43	(6.3–16.7)
Hypermetropia	29	10.7 ± 2.03	(6.6–14.8)

Table 2. Percentage distribution of three educational levels in juvenile myopia, in emmetropes and in hypermetropes.

	Juvenile myopia (n = 52)	Emmetropia (n = 56)	Hypermetropia (n = 29)
High school, university	38%	20%	3%
9–10 school years + basic school for trade and handycraft, *or*, apprentice with near work	46%	46%	62%
Basis only (8–9 years at unity school)	16%	34%	35%
Total	100%	100%	100%

hypermetropes (Fledelius 1980a, b). An association between accommodative power (at age of 18) and refractive change (from ten to 18) is thus probable, and a linear regression between the two parameters may be calculated.

With accommodative power on abscissa, and Δ Refr. on ordinate, the following equations are found:

$$\text{LBW: } y = 0.148x - 0.553; \quad r = 0.36$$

$$\text{FT: } y = 0.220x - 1.23; \quad r = 0.47$$

The slopes have a positive sign, and correlation coefficients differ significantly from zero, without, however, suggesting a *strong* correlation. With pooled values (LBW + FT), linear regression points to a scant one diopter teenage refractive change when NPA is 10 D (at age of 18), while a 20 D accommodative power coincides with a refractive change of about 2.8 D.

Table 2 shows the relation between refractive groups (as percentage, vertically read) and school background, the latter being divided into three classes. Minimum levels are exceptional in myopes (with only 16%) who conversely predominate in the upper end of the educational scale (38% of myopes). With only 3.5% in 'High school + University' the hypermetropes

Table 3. Cumulated near-work score in the sample. Percentage distribution of cumulated scores is given in juvenile myopia (left) and in emmetropia + hypermetropia (right). Distributions differ highly significant (χ^2, p ≪ 0.01).

			Juvenile myopia (n = 52)	Emmetropia + hypermetropia (n = 85)
Cumulated score	0−1	points	8%	33%
	2−3		15%	33%
	4−5		38%	22%
	6−7		25%	6%
	8−10		14%	6%
			100%	100%

are skewed away from the more sophisticated levels of education. The low number of hypermetropes in the sample is, however, to be kept in mind before unduly condemning the apparently fed-up-with-school hypermetropes.

Finally, a cumulated nearwork score (Table 3) was based on (a) school background (cf. Table 2), (b) school homework at the age level of 12−16, (c) free-time activities, and (d) nearwork (reading) distance when performing a + b + c. Cumulated scores ranked from one to ten in the sample. High scores (≥ 6) occurred in 39% of myopes (n = 52 eyes), 16% of emmetropes (n = 56 eyes), and only 3.5% of hypermetropes (n = 29 eyes).

DISCUSSION

Data collected by Duane were compiled in a classical graph to show the variation of accommodation with age (Duke-Elder 1949), according to which the 18-year-old has a mean amplitude of accommodation of 11.5 D. This is neatly reproduced in the present study. An 18-year mean value of 11.6 D is thus obtained, if the mean values of Table 1 are applied to a theor-etical population 'norm' consisting of 15% myopes, 45% emmetropes (0−0.9 D), and 40% with refractive values ≥ + 1.0 D.

The role of nearwork and accommodation in myopia pathogenesis is at present vigorously discussed. The present study adds some facts to this debate. Concerning accommodative power, the myopes of the sample are significantly superior as compared with emmetropes and hypermetropes.

The finding may seem paradoxical, because in young adult myopes there is no apparent need of the strong accommodation. From usual biological feed-back mechanisms one might even expect a 'lazy' accommodation, once myopia *has* developed.

In this connection, a comment is to be given on the parameters yet under study. *Refractive change* from the age of ten to 18 was based on truly longitudinal, quite accurate refractive value determinations (in cycloplegia), while accommodative power was measured reliably only at the *end* of the observation period. The crucial question: 'How was accommodative strain actually *during* adolescence? is not answered. Again, it is stated only that those who developed myopia during school years have a superior accom-modation *when* 18 years old.

106

The objective of the various nearwork scores is to fill this gap in information, but admittedly such data are indirect and often inaccurate. A rough estimate of nearwork during adolescence is obtained from the school levels referred to in Table 2, but the visual behaviour of the child (sustained accommodation?) cannot be ascertained. Keep in mind, for instance, that some teachers in their teaching prefer to use the black-board (distance vision conditions) while others do demand lots of reading and nearwork, both at school and when preparing lessons.

Further, myopic teenagers' spectacle habits vary much, at least in Denmark. Only a minor part wear their glasses *fulltime* (and usually they are not instructed to do so either). Many use glasses only when they optically need them, namely for distance, and not for close work. In particular this applies to low grade myopia, thus reducing the impulse for accommodation when performing the much incriminated nearwork.

Finally, a comment on the age at onset of juvenile myopia. In the present sample, the mean age was 11.5 years (± 3.0), and only one third started clinically (with glasses) *after* the age of 12. The majority thus had their recorded onset at an early age level, when the Danish unity school does not yet demand any important amount of reading. Correspondingly only nine out of 52 felt convinced, in retrospect, that they had had tough amounts of nearwork (school + free-time) when myopia actually occurred.

SUMMARY

A report is given on NPA findings in an 18-year-old Danish sample (n = 137) followed-up ophthalmologically since the age of ten. Focus is on NPA as related to refractive class (at age of 18) and refractive change (from ten to 18).

The present mean value (corrected, of 11.6 D) at age of 18 is in accord with classical standards of amplitude of accommodation. Juvenile myopes, however, score significantly better (13.8 D) than emmetropes (11.6 D) and hypermetropes (10.7 D).

An analysis of school background confirms the well-documented skewing of *myopes* towards higher educational levels, as compared with the other refractive classes.

A positive correlation is found between refractive *change* from age of ten to 18 and accommodative capacity at the latter age. This is discussed at some length. My observations prove only that myopes are indeed keen accommodators, although they might do well and unstrained at near distance with relaxed accommodation (*without* spectacles as many actually do).

No direct proof is rendered that developing juvenile myopia is actually *due* to this superior accommodative capacity.

REFERENCES

Duke-Elder, S., Textbook of Ophthalmology, vol. IV, H. Kimpton, London. p. 4424 (1949).

Fledelius, H.C. Prematurity and the Eye. Acta Ophthalmol. (Kbh.), Suppl. 128 (1976).

Fledelius, H.C. Ophthalmic changes from age of ten to 18 years. A longitudinal study of sequels to low birth weight. I., Refraction. Acta Ophthalmol. (Kbh.), 58: 889, (1980).

Fledelius, H.C. Changes in refraction and eye size during adolescence. Docum. Ophthalmol. Proc. Series 28: 63–69, 1981. Tscherning, M. Studier over myopiens aetiologi. Copenhagen (1882).

Author's address:
H.C. Fledelius, M.D.
University Eye Clinic
Rigshospitalet
Blegdamsvej 9
DK-2100 Copenhagen Ø
Denmark

MYOPIA OR EXPANSION GLAUCOMA

T. STUART-BLACK KELLY
(Bath, England)

ABSTRACT

The accepted reasons for myopia are compared with those supporting the concept of expansion glaucoma as the aetiology of myopia. Three types are apparent:
(1) Stress, or self inflicted vitreous glaucoma with temporary rises in IOP (simple myopia).
(2) Active anterior chamber glaucoma with continuous rise in IOP due to anterior chamber anomaly (malignant myopia).
(3) Inactive glaucoma rise in IOP (congenital myopia), having had previous rise in utero.
The change from being an untreatable, hereditary, domestic pet becoming worse annually, to being mostly a non-hereditary, self-inflicted Trojan Horse monster that can be arrested as soon as it is discovered, is discussed.

INTRODUCTION

The term myopia is very ancient. It signifies a common hereditary condition which we accept like the weather. We only treat it with distance glasses and damage our children even more. That damage is six times more than chronic glaucoma. With respect, I feel 'expansion glaucoma' would be a wiser and more helpful name than myopia. It would alert us and the parents to the monster that myopia really is. I exclude corneal and lenticular myopia.

I wish to show that chronic glaucoma and myopia are both due to a rise in IOP. By international convention any damage due to raised IOP is called glaucoma. In chronic glaucoma the eye is too mature to expand. In myopia it expands because it is young. Chronic glaucoma is therefore a non-expansion glaucoma and myopia is expansion glaucoma. In comparing the conditions:

The refraction in myopia shows axial change. In expansion glaucoma it indicates the extent of the disease.

THEORIES CONCERNING IOP AND MYOPIA PATHOGENESIS: SCHISIS BLOCK OR ZONULAR BLOCK

The accepted cause for *young* myopia is overgrowth of the dominant tissue, the retina. So the choroid and sclera must go on growing until the retina stops.

This does not explain young *adult* myopia, nor why the growth within the eye should damage itself, when no other part of the body does so, at so young an age, by normal growth.

Concerning intraocular pressure in myopes, the IOP has been found to be significantly raised, by 1.5 mm, when measured in the morning (expansion glaucoma, Perkins and Kelly, unpublished data 1974).

Barraquer (1974) showed the difference in applanation tonometry between hypermetropia and myopia. The most common pressure in hypermetropia was 10 mmHg and in myopia 19 mmHg. (These differ by 100 mgm/mm^2 in conventional compressive stress, but by 800 mgm/mm^2 in tangential scleral stress, to be discussed later).

Most important, two unexpected levels of aqueous block have now been found. The first may be described as at schisis level. It gives rise to malignant or pathological myopia or 5% of myopia. Evidence suggests that the second block is at the zonular level and accounts for 90% of myopia.

The schisis term is based on the following observations: In some parts of the angle the iris passes straight into the lower part of the trabecular area (Figure 1) instead of dipping into the recess. Processes pass from the surface of the iris to the trabecular area, difficult to see in fair people, as Curtin has said (1978). In some, these strands can be seen to bend forward, away from the angle (as in the left side of Figure 1). This suggests there is a transparent retinoschisis-like membrane on which the processes lie. Such a membrane was suggested by Gorin (1964). A schisis membrane cannot be seen unless a light strikes a break or a hole in it (Figure 1). A membrane like this must have reduced the outflow sufficiently to raise the IOP. This reduces the pulse amplitude and vascular flow, and over the years gradually expands the eye.

Contact lens wearing may influence this type of block (in the oral presentation, some clinical examples are given).

The second level of blockage is at the zonular level. On accommodation the ciliary body acts as a sphincter, pulling forward the thick anterior vitreous, concentrating the zonule, and closing the zonular gap. The aqueous outflow is blocked until the sphincter is released by voluntary demand, as in all parasympathetic sphincters. In this case the demand is for distant vision. Young (1975) has brilliantly shown this with his radiosonde, and accounted for the 90% self-inflicted myopes. Young (1977) has also shown that the depth and axial correlation in expansion myopia is consistent with IOP increase.

Curtin and Karlin, (1971) consider that progressive myopia should be considered a mechanical problem and Arcineagas (1980) consider it as well to be due to abnormal vitreous pressure.

In the rare congenital myopes the pressure must have acted in utero.

110

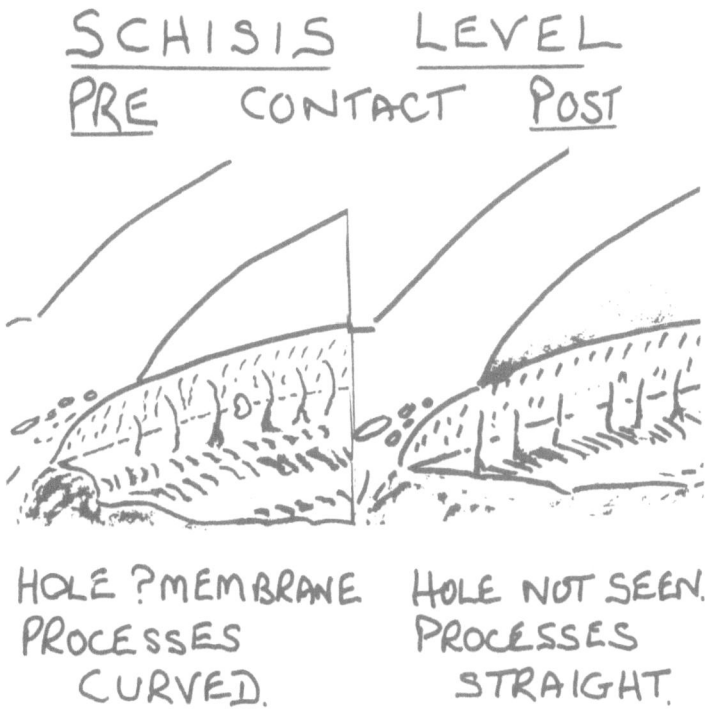

Fig. 1. Gonioscopy drawings of the 'schisis membrane', cf. text.

There is no active pressure after birth until either the accommodation is needed or a schisis block is present.

IOP INCREASE AND SCLERAL STRESS

The importance of the pressure increase was shown by Friedman (1966) because the tangential scleral stress, which is like the stress to tear apart the wall of a balloon, is 7.5 times higher at emmetropia than that of the compressive stress we associate with applanation. On accommodation the conventional stress of 204 mgm/mm^2 can be raised to 2244 mgm/mm^2. So it is easy to see why the soft sclera can expand like the wall of a balloon.

In Figure 2 the tangential scleral stress (TSS) lines and the compressive stress (CS) lines are compared for the same applanation. As you can see the CS is negligible. It is the TSS that really matters. The thick line is the incidence of retinal detachment of Perkins (1979) and probably most other complications, and marches with the TSS.

With a normal 50% rise in accommodation the normal stress changes from 204 mgm towards the 2244 mgm depending on how long it is in use. It is the long acting stress that starts the expansion. In a monkey it takes two months to start expanding.

111

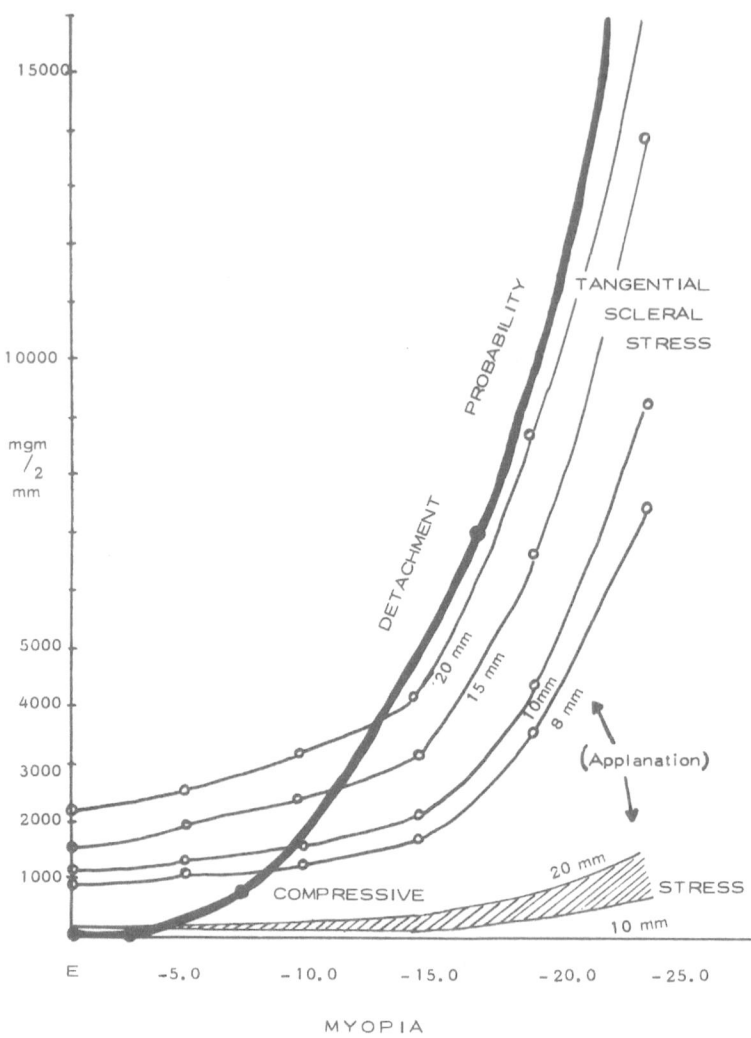

Fig. 2. Curves showing tangential and compressive scleral stress as a function of intra-ocular pressure.

OCULAR RIGIDITY, IOP AND CONTACT LENSES

During treatment ocular rigidity can become 'negative' and depend on the IOP as when near the moment of death. A case of rapidly increasing myopia in a girl was kept almost arrested for five years by bifocals and contact lenses (Figure 3). She was on continuous contact lens wearing combined with atropine to see if a reduction was possible, when she got something in her eye, took the contact lens out and saw me an hour later. The eye

112

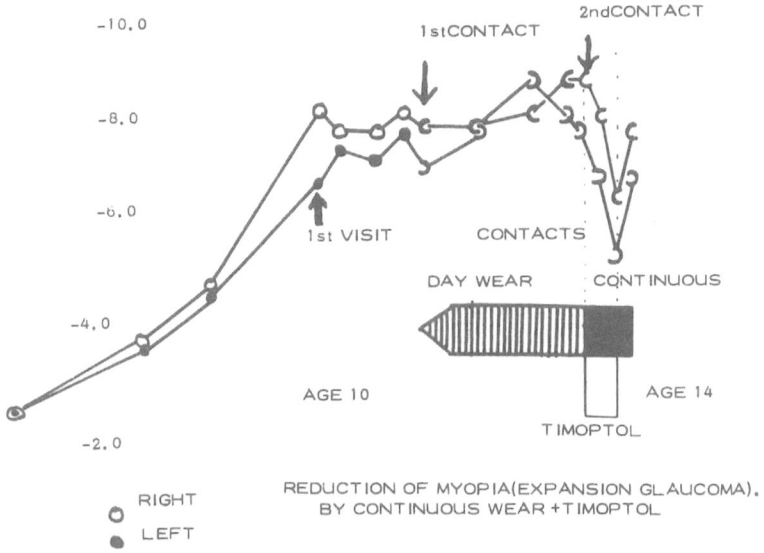

-10.0

1stCONTACT

2ndCONTACT

-8.0

-6.0

1st VISIT

CONTACTS

DAY WEAR

CONTINUOUS

-4.0

AGE 10

AGE 14

TIMOPTOL

-2.0

RIGHT

LEFT

REDUCTION OF MYOPIA(EXPANSION GLAUCOMA),
BY CONTINUOUS WEAR +TIMOPTOL

Fig. 3. Arrest of progressive myopia (expansion glaucoma) by contact lens and atropine, in a teenage girl. A reduction of myopia is seen when timoptol is added.

with no contact lens had the same refraction as in the previous month. But the eye with the contact lens had changed + 2.75 D. Her IOP's were 5 and 10 mmHg (Goldmann) respectively. So the contact lens had pressed into the eye at more than 5 mm lid pressure. On removal the refraction returned to that of the previous month. So the rigidity had become 'negative' – for want of a better term – while using the contact lens.

The damaged condition of the choroid and sclera can be assessed by comparing pulse amplitude with the emmetropic and hypermetropic amplitudes, as Langham has suggested (1980), seen in pneumotonograph pulsation.

In some cases of very low pressure, when the contact lens is removed the myopia is higher than it was. So the anemic choroid and sclera are stretching in spite of the contact lens and the low pressure. These may be beyond arrest, and emphasise that the earlier we recognise the schisis block the quicker we must arrest by contacts. One could say 'The lower the pulse amplitude, the lower the pressure needed to expand. Rigidity may be 'negative' below 10 mm Goldmann'.

ENVIRONMENTAL FACTORS

Let us next look at the effects of environment. Myopia has no evidence to offer for an environmental cause. But self-inflicted expansion glaucoma has.

Young (1977) has shown it can be induced in monkeys – and how.

113

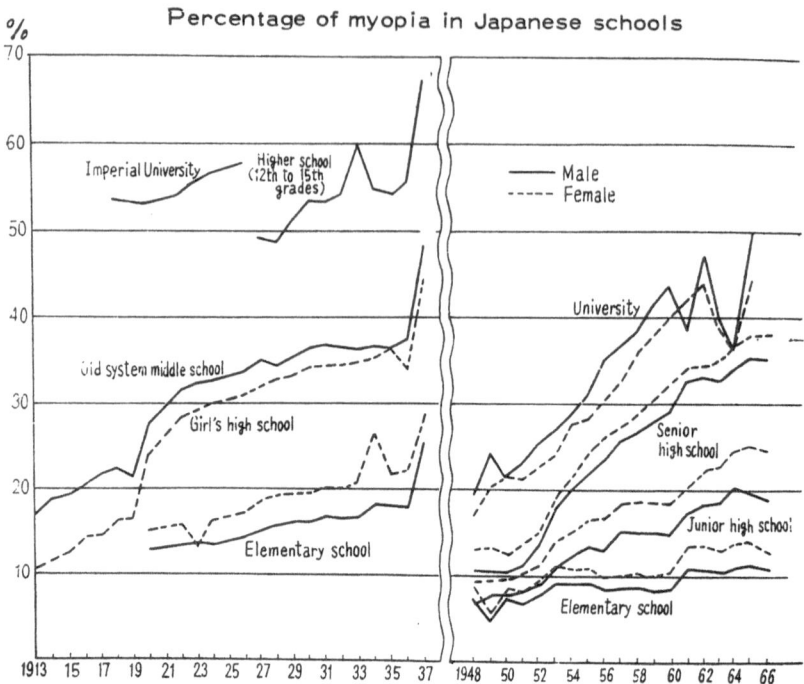

%
70

60

50

40

30

20

10

Percentage of myopia in Japanese schools

Imperial University   Higher school
(12th to 15th grades)

—— Male
----- Female

Old system middle school

Girl's high school

Elementary school

University

Senior high school

Junior high school

Elementary school

1913 15 17 19 21 23 25 27 29 31 33 35 37 1948 50 52 54 56 58 60 62 64 66

Fig. 4. Otsuka's classical graphs showing incidence of myopia in Japanese schools since 1913.

Young and Baldwin (1971) have shown how the illiterate Eskimos have no myopia but their grandchildren at school have 60%.

The effect of working for passing school examinations can be seen in graphs of my children.

In Japan and the USA TV has caused millions to become myopic.

The Japanese have been monitoring their myopia since 1913 in their schools (Figure 4). They have produced the most important myopia graph in history, Otsuka (1967). The higher the intellectual level of the school the higher the myopia. Then came the war and myopia dropped to the lowest that is usually found in country society. At the end of the war it all started again.

The fact that the Japanese Living Guidance and Daily Exercises have reduced defective vision in some schools, is evidence that the environment can cause myopia.

INDICATIONS FOR THERAPY, IN GENERAL. HEREDITY

Pathological myopia can start at less than −0.5 D, and is accepted as incurable. Myopia has only abiotrophy to offer as an explanation. In some it leads to blindness.

114

But expansion glaucoma shows that the cause is increased IOP. It shows that pathological or malignant myopia is simply the ruthless increase of axial length due to the constant small schisis block.

It appears up to now that over 95% can be arrested and so prevented from going on to blindness.

The complications are so serious, being more than chronic glaucoma, that they should be listed. The myopia outlook has nothing to offer for detachments, macular degeneration, glaucoma, and cataract, now shown to be 20%, and blindness, but expansion glaucoma treatment can avoid them all.

Next *heredity*. In expansion glaucoma the schisis block due to incomplete atrophy or splitting of the mesoderm, is difficult to prove as hereditary. In our school children I have only seen four families that have anything near a satisfactory proband.

For the zonular block the only hereditary factor seems to be the keenness to learn of the parents, that has naturally been passed on to the children. To prove any ocular heredity one would have to clear the environment of anything that might produce the zonular block.

Next *treatment*. The only treatment that myopia can offer is to give distance glasses and this makes 100% of the children worse over a four-year period.

But expansion glaucoma treatment can arrest nearly all young children and reduce the risk of complications as well, as seen in Bath bifocal and contact lens results (Kelly, *et al.* 1975), and Oakley and Young (1975). The executive bifocals of the latter acted much better than the wide angle bifocals used in Bath. As a result in Bath 84% have been arrested during the last four years, and the number is improving.

CONCLUDING REMARKS

Lastly if we compare chronic glaucoma with expansion glaucoma we find the non-expansion glaucoma in the over forties and the expansion glaucoma in the young. In general the high increase in IOP is in those above 40, there is no expansion, environment does not play a part, the pathology is due to pressure on the internal blood supply, other complications are few, heredity is common, and treatment is mainly to reduce the pressure.

On the contrary myopia or expansion glaucoma is the result of increased IOP in the *young* causing all cases to expand, environment plays a role, pathology is due to scleral expansion, the only heredity would appear to be in the 5% schisis block, and treatment arrests almost all cases.

We do not know what causes diabetes, but we always treat it, even though we are only arresting it. We do not yet know all the details of myopia, we may even be wrong in some, but we can arrest myopia safely, until the eye is so mature that it cannot expand any more.

In three of the developed areas for which we have some statistics – Japan, Europe and the USA – a total of 20 000 become myopic daily, mostly self-inflicted. We could arrest nearly all for an average cost of 150% more than they pay for damaging distance glasses. Treatment might eliminate all complications, and in our developed society possibly eliminate myopia within a generation. Surely treatment is a medical responsibility that should become legal.

Myopia conventionally describes a common hereditary pet found in most families for which it is supposed that nothing can be done. So myopia is a Trojan Horse Monster which Perkins (1979) has shown to be a major cause of blindness under 65.

But the name expansion glaucoma describes a damaging condition. It will alert the family to obtain treatment as soon as possible, as they would for diabetes.

May I plead to change the name of myopia to that of Expansion Glaucoma.

REFERENCES

Arcineagas, A. and Amaya, L.E., Biostructural Model of Human Eye. No. 954. Institut. Barraquer, Bogota (1980).

Barraquer, J. Coloquio Sobre Miopia. Bogota. Arch. Soc. Am. Opthalmol Optom. 10 (2) (1974).

Curtin, B. Personal Communication. Director Sprague Myopia Institute. Manhattan Eye & Ear Hosp. New York (1978).

Curtin, B.J., Karlin, D.B., Axial length measurements and fundus changes in the myopic eye. Am. J. Ophthalmol. 71: 42–53 (1971).

Friedman, B. Stress on Ocular Coats, Eye, Ear, Nose & Throat Mon. 45. 59. 1966.

Gorin, G., Developmental Glaucoma. Am. J. Ophthalmol. 58 (4): p. 572 (1964).

Kelly, T.S-B., Chatfield C., Tustin, G., Clinical assessment of arrest of myopia. Br. J. Ophthalmol. 59 (Oct. 1975).

Langham, J. Personal Communication.

Oakley, K.H. & Young, F.A. Bifocal Control of Myopia Am. J. Optom. & Physiol. Optics. 52 (11): 758 (1975).

Otsuka, J., Research in Myopia. Tomus 71. Acta Soc. Ophthalmol. Jap. (1967).

Perkins, E.S. Morbidity from Myopia. Sight Saving Review. University Iowa (Spring 1979).

Young, F.A., Visual Characterisation of Apes & Humans. Academic Press. New York. p. 207 (1977).

Young, F.A. & Baldwin W. Comparison of Cycloplegic and non cycloplegic refraction of Eskimos. Am. J. Optom. 48 (1971).

Young, F.A. Development and Control of Myopia in Human and Subhuman Primates. Contacto (Nov. 1975).

Author's address:
Dr. T. S-B. Kelly, M.D.
Linden, Weston Road
Bath
England

DISTENSABILITY OF THE YOUNG EYE

Considerations based on ultrasound examination of eyes with
previous trauma

H.C. FLEDELIUS
(Copenhagen, Denmark)

ABSTRACT

Prior to surgery, 24 consecutive patients with previous eye trauma were
referred for ultrasonic assessment of intra-ocular morphology. Besides,
bilateral axial *size* estimates were performed in most cases.

Out of 13 cases with significant eye size side difference, three were due
to involution (phthisis). In ten cases, however, the damaged eye was the
larger of the two. Ordinary anisometropia might explain one or two cases,
while a real post-traumatic distension was probable at least in eight. Elevated
IOP had been recorded in some of these (buphthalmic nature?).

The age at eye trauma had been 0, 0, 4, 6, 11, 12, 14, and 14 years.
The tendinous tunics of the eye can thus be stretched in relation to trauma
even at a rather high age.

INTRODUCTION

The present study was founded on the following premises:

*1. The distensability of the eye, as related to infantile, juvenile and adult
glaucoma.* The *infantile* eye gives way for an elevated intraocular pressure
(IOP). The scleral collagen is stretched, and the eye gets larger than it would
otherwise have been. In contrast, the *adult* eye resists such effects of an
elevated IOP.

The course of events — eye enlargement or not — depends on (among
other factors) the age level when the elevated IOP exerts its influence.

Accordingly, there must be a borderline age zone, which is probably in
childhood years, but may be somewhat later. To my knowledge, ophthalmic
literature has no exact notions concerning this 'critical' age level.

2. The growth curve of the normal eye. The eye follows the cerebral growth
pattern, with a marked increase in size during the first few years of life.
Growth then decelerates until the age of 10–13. In my 1976 thesis, a growth
curve of the eye was compiled from published data by various authors among

whom were Sorsby and coworkers (1961, 1970). They stated that eye size does not augment after the age of 13, except from that *minor* part of the refractive spectrum which has become, or becomes near-sighted.

In such persons, the tendinous tunic of the eye is – for scarcely known reasons – still able to stretch and bring about axial myopia. There is a juvenile distensability of the eye, related to the refractive state of (progressive) myopia.

3. Accidental observations during diagnostic ultrasonography revealed an axial elongation of some eyes that were examined because of opaque media due to earlier eye trauma. Thus, there is a post-traumatic distensability of the young eye, a course of events which shows some resemblance to the axial elongations described above cf. (1) and (2).

The present study was carried out to establish whether a post-traumatic eye distension might be a more common feature, and – if so – to what age classes such a feature is confined. Thus, information will be obtained concerning the mentioned borderline age zone of ocular distensability. The results may further apply to the more common enlargement of the eyeball related to developing juvenile myopia.

MATERIAL AND METHODS

During 1978, 24 eye trauma cases were referred to the ophthalmic ultrasound clinic of Rigshospitalet prior to some kind of reconstructive eye surgery. Evaluation by ophthalmoscopy was not possible due to opaque media, nor could refractive value be assessed.

A morphological evaluation by ultrasound (Kretztechnik 7000, Bronson-Turner B-scan) of the posterior eye segment was the primary objective, but an additional bilateral estimate of eye size was carried out in most cases.

Further, the ophthalmic history had to be checked. In some cases the history proved to be dubious concerning the nature of the initial eye lesion. This applied for instance to several immigrants (so-called foreign workers) with claimed eye lesions of early childhood.

RESULTS

The sample comprises a total of 24 consecutive trauma cases, referred for ophthalmic ultrasound examination during the year of 1978.

In 11, side differences were not stated, while 13 showed a significant difference concerning axial lengths of the two eyes.

In five of the former 11 with (presumed) equal eye size, ultrasound measurements had not even been considered because the traumas were fresh. Mostly, they were cases with intraocular foreign bodies, to be located by ultrasound prior to surgery *a chaud*.

Among the six cases with ultrasonographically documented *equal* eye size, the four had acquired their eye lesions after the age of 20. The two

118

Table 1. Tabulation of the 13 cases (out of the total 24) that showed a marked side difference in eye size related to eye trauma, as assessed by ultrasound measurement.

I.   3 cases: *Trauma eye smaller*
             Due to phthisical changes

II. 10 cases: *Trauma eye larger*
             (a) Two cases with dubious trauma history, true anisometropia?
             (b) *Eight remaining cases*

Sex	Age at trauma (years)	Eye disorder	Axial length side difference
m.	at birth	contusion	1.8 mm
m.	$\frac{1}{2}$	perf. injury	5.0 mm
m.	4	contusion	2.0 mm
m.	6	perf. injury	2.6 mm
f.	11	keratitis, uveitis	2.5 mm
f.	12	perf. injury	2.5 mm
m.	14	perf. injury	1.2 mm
m.	14	contusion	3.0 mm

remaining were boys aged 12 at the time of the trauma; they will be discussed later.

Table 1 shows the 13 cases with an *established side difference* in eye size. Three were due to phthisical changes and are of no interest in the present context.

In the remaining 10 cases, *the trauma eye was the larger of the two.* Trauma history was doubtful in two patients, which might represent cases of true anisometropia (independent of the history). One of the two, however, had weakening conditions during the first year of life (pleurisy and rachitis).

Perforating lesions or contusion of the eyeball were the underlying disease of the remaining seven cases. The last patient had unilateral dendritic keratitis, relapsing uveitis and secondary glaucoma, since the age of 11.

DISCUSSION

As a common feature, secondary glaucoma had been diagnosed in most of the cases with post-traumatic enlargement of the eye.

This applied also to one of the cases of documented equal size of the two eyes, a boy aged 12 who had his blind trauma-eye enucleated after one year. With a similar case (without recorded elevation of IOP, however) of the same age, the age of 12 might thus be *beyond* the limit of developing lesional distension of the eyeball.

This, however, could not be substantiated by the cases *with* post-traumatic eye enlargement, who showed – in four – an age at lesion of 11–14 years. A lesional eye distension thus seems possible even at an age so high and ocularly full-grown as 14.

An ocular distensability to occur so rather late may be due to eye wall plasticity associated with a *pubertal* ocular growth phase. This is contrary to the already quoted statements of Sorsby and co-workers cf. introduction,

119

(2), but it seems probable according to recent longitudinal data by myself (Fledelius 1980).

Finally, mention is given of several reports of a somewhat higher IOP-level of myopic eyes as compared with emmetropes and hypermetropes (most recently quoted by Gardiner 1979). A more general influence of IOP in myopia pathogenesis is thus suggested. The association seems, however, to be weak only. Based on own, yet unpublished data (from 137 18-year old Danes), no correlations could be ascertained between applanation tonometry readings on the one hand, and refractive value (and axial eye length) on the other.

CONCLUDING REMARKS

The present proportion of enlarged trauma eyes is far beyond expectancy, and eye changes triggered by the lesion are held responsible. At least in some eyes, the mechanism appears to be a glaucomatous ballooning of the ocular sheaths.

In the remaining eyes a glaucomatous phase cannot be ruled out, at some stage on the way to the present 'balanced' normotensive state, but ophthalmic recordings are lacking as direct support.

There may even be a more general association between the juvenile myopic axial eye length increment and the effects of a probably only slightly elevated intraocular pressure, and minor eye traumas *may* play a role this way.

The present ultrasound study signifies only that eyes may enlarge as a response to an elevated IOP – also at age levels (10–14) where juvenile myopia usually has its onset or shows progress.

If the mechanical resistance to IOP levels be of any importance in myopia pathogenesis *in general,* the study does not answer the relevant questions: Why *some* eyes seem to give way, while most eyes *resist* and keep their, from an optical view-point, dimensional harmony.

REFERENCES

Fledelius, H.C. The growth of the eye from the age of ten to 18 years. Paper read at SIDUO VIII Conference in Nijmegen, Sept. 1980 To appear in congress report (1981).
Gardiner, P.A., Epidemiology of myopia. In: Visual Handicap in children, Ed. V. Smith & J. Kern S.I.M.P. London-Philadelphia pp. 29–33 (1979).
Sorsby, A., Benjamin, B. & Sheridan, M., Refraction and its components during growth of the eye from the age of three. Medical Research Council SRS 301, London, H.M.S.O. (1961).
Sorsby, A. & Leary, G.A., A longitudinal study of refraction and its components during growth. Medical Research Council SRS 309. London, H.M.S.O. (1970).

Author's address:
H.C. Fledelius, M.D.
University Eye Clinic
Rigshospitalet
Blegdamsvej 9
DK-2100 Copenhagen Ø
Denmark

120

MYOPIA AND SCLERAL STRESS

E.S. PERKINS

(Iowa City, Iowa, U.S.A.)

INTRODUCTION

There are two main theories to account for the enlargement of the globe in myopia; the biological theory postulates that it is due to an overgrowth of the retina while the mechanical theory maintains that the eye enlarges as a result of an increased stress on the scleral envelope. Scleral stress can be calculated using Laplace's formula (Friedman 1966) if the axial length (or radius of the globe), the intra-ocular pressure and the scleral thickness are known and assuming that the eye is spherical in shape. If the mechanical theory is correct it would be expected that the degree of myopia and severity of pathological changes would show some correlation with the calculated scleral stress.

Axial length, intraocular pressure and scleral thickness was measured in 146 eyes with a range of refractive errors from 0 to -20.00 D and scleral stress calculated for each eye.

METHODS

Axial length was estimated by a modification of the optical method previously described (Perkins *et al.* 1976). The eye is observed through a measuring telescope while the subject changes fixation from one illuminated slit to another illuminated slit so arranged that the eye rotates through an angle of $40°$. The distance between the two corneal reflexes is measured by a scale in the telescope. The position of the image in relation to the apex of the cornea was considered to be at a distance of half the radius of curvature of the cornea as measured in the horizontal axis by the keratometer attachment for the Diag (Clement Clarke Ltd.) slit lamp. Knowing the distance between the two reflexes and their position relative to the apex of the cornea the radius of the axis of rotation of the eye can be calculated and the axial length estimated.

Intraocular pressure was measured with the Goldmann applanation tonometer.

Scleral thickness was estimated using a light scattering technique. A probe was designed containing a low intensity miniature incandescent bulb surrounded by a perspex cone 5 mm in external diameter. When the probe is applied to the sclera, light is scattered from the central area beneath the bulb and collected by the perspex cone which acts as a light guide. The intensity of the scattered light is measured by a photo-diode after passing through a blue filter to exclude red light. Calibration on 28 different areas of four enucleated eyes showed a linear relationship between the amplified output of the photo-diode and measurements made with a measuring telescope after incising the sclera along the meridian measured. The correlation coefficient between the directly measured values and the output of the photo-diode was + 0.94 and the slope of the regression line was used for calibration of the output of the probe. Measurements on living eyes were made approximately 12 mm from the limbus in the lower temporal quadrant of the globe.

Calculation of scleral stress.
Scleral stress was calculated from the formula $\rho = PA/4t$ ρ = scleral stress, P = intraocular pressure. A = axial length and t = scleral thickness.

PATIENT POPULATION

Subjects were drawn largely from patients attending the General Clinic for routine eye examination and refraction but some patients attending the Retina Clinic were also seen. The patients selected did not represent a truly random sample of the clinic population as selection was biased towards higher refractive errors. For statistical purposes the refraction was considered as the spherical equivalent of the distance prescription.

All patients had an ophthalmoscopic examination and eyes were classified on the fundus appearances into three groups: normal, with no evidence of myopic changes; grade I in which typical myopic crescents were present at the disc and grade II in which there was evidence of retinal thinning, pigmentary or lattice degeneration, macular lesions, retinal holes or retinal detachment. Fourteen out of 30 eyes in grade II also showed myopic crescents.

Table 1. Mean refractive errors and standard deviations (dioptres).

Age	Normal		Grade I		Grade II	
9–15	(18)	− 2.69 ± 1.61	(2)	− 5.00 ± 0.35	(2)	− 14.75 ± 0.35
16–40	(33)	− 3.19 ± 4.37	(39)	− 5.99 ± 2.63	(13)	− 7.56 ± 5.87
Over 40	(18)	− 2.71 ± 2.54	(6)	− 5.5 ± 1.5	(15)	− 7.68 ± 3.79

Table 2. Proportion of eyes with refractions greater than − 4.0 D.

Age	Normal	Grade I	Grade II
0–15	4/18	2/2	2/2
16–40	6/33	30/39	11/13
40 +	2/18	5/6	13/15
Totals	12/69	37/47	26/30
% > 4.0 D	17%	79%	87%

Incomplete data. In 12 eyes the axial length was not measured but for the purposes of calculation was derived from the refraction and the slope of the correlation curve between refraction and axial length. In 18 eyes scleral thickness was not measured and the mean thickness of all eyes measured (0.5 mm) was used in the calculations.

RESULTS

1. Refraction

Table 1 shows the mean refraction of the eyes according to age and grading of fundus appearances. The mean refractive error increases with the severity of the fundus changes and the difference between the normals and grade I and grade II is statistically significant for the two older age groups.

Table 2 shows the proportion of eyes in each group with a refractive error greater than -4.0 D. Only 17% of eyes with a normal fundus had a refraction greater than -4.0 D compared with 79% and 87% for grades I and II respectively.

2. Axial length

Table 3 shows the mean axial length for eyes in each group. As with refractive error there is an increase in mean axial length with severity of fundus changes, and the difference between normals and grade I and grade II is statistically significant for the age group 15–40 and between normal and grade II for the age group over 40 years.

There was a highly significant correlation between the degree of myopia and the axial length. The correlation coefficient for male eyes was $+0.56$ ($p < 0.001$) and for female eyes $+0.667$ ($p < 0.001$) but the slope of the linear regression line was less than expected (0.24 for female and 0.16 for male eyes) suggesting that the method used underestimates the axial length in myopic eyes.

Table 3. Mean axial lengths and standard deviations (mm).

Age	Normal	Grade I	Grade II
9–15	22.88 ± 1.09	23.95 ± 0.07	24.15 ± 0.2
16–40	23.33 ± 3.55	24.73 ± 1.27	25.13 ± 1.36
40 +	24.0 ± 0.9	24.4 ± 0.82	24.64 ± 1.35

Table 4. Proportion of eyes of axial length equivalent to -4.0 D or more.

Age	Normal	Grade I	Grade II
9–15	3/18	0/2	0/2
16–40	12/33	24/29	11/13
40 +	6/18	4/6	14/15
Total	21/69	33/47	25/30
%	30%	70%	83%

Table 5. Mean intraocular pressures and standard deviation (mm Hg).

Age	Normal	Grade I	Grade II
9–15	15.94 ± 2.68	17.5 ± 0.7	14 S.D. 0.0
16–40	16.16 ± 4.2	16.2 ± 2.55	15.36 ± 2.1
40 +	14.78 ± 3.75	16.3 ± 3.38	18.73 ± 2.94

Table 4 shows the proportion of eyes in each group with an axial length equivalent to over -4.0 D as calculated from the slope of the linear regression line for male and female eyes separately. The proportion of eyes with an axial length greater than this equivalent value is similar to that found for refractive errors greater than -4.0 D, except that the percentage of eyes with normal fundi is higher than the percentage of such eyes with refractive errors greater than -4.0 D.

3. Intraocular pressure

The mean and standard deviations of the applanation readings of eyes in each group are shown in Table 5. The only significantly different mean is that of the 40 + grade II group.

4. Scleral stress

There was no statistically significant correlation between the degree of myopia and the calculated figure for scleral stress. Table 6 shows the mean scleral stress for the different groups. The only statistically significant difference is between the normal and grade II eyes in the oldest age group ($p < 0.05$).

There was no significant correlation between refractive error and scleral thickness as measured by this method. It is possible therefore that this method is unreliable in the living eye and in case this was responsible for the failure of the scleral stress measurements to show a correlation with

Table 6. Scleral stress. Means and standard deviations (mm Hg).

Age	Normal	Grade I	Grade II
9–15	199.4 ± 14.1	197	211
16–40	212 ± 60.8	206 ± 45	211 ± 51.6
40 +	178 ± 44.8	214 ± 43	219 ± 63.2

Table 7. Scleral stress using mean value for scleral thickness. Means and standard deviations (mm Hg).

Age	Normal	Grade I	Grade II
9–15	173.4 ± 51.8	208.5 ± 7.8	170
16–40	197 ± 34.5	204.5 ± 28.8	191.5 ± 41.6
40 +	179.8 ± 39.9	185.2 ± 32.8	236.7 ± 36.9

the degree of myopia the scleral stress was recalculated using the mean figure of 0.5 mm for each eye, which agrees well with measurements made in enucleated eyes (Table 7).

When scleral stress was calculated in this way (P x AL/2) there was a small but statistically significant correlation between refraction and scleral stress (r = 0.196, p < 0.02). Again there was a significant difference between normal and grade II eyes in the oldest age group but at a higher level of significance (p < 0.001) and also a significant difference between grade I and grade II in this age group (p < 0.002).

Unfortunately, even in these groups in which there were statistically significant differences in the mean values, the standard deviations were large so that it was not possible to choose any figure for scleral stress which gave a satisfactory dividing line between normal and pathological fundus appearances.

DISCUSSION

These results support clinical observations that myopic refractive errors in excess of − 4.0 D are associated with an increased incidence of pathological changes in the fundus. A cut-off point of − 4.0 D gives a fairly good separation between patients without any fundus changes and those with fundus changes, if a myopic crescent is accepted as a pathological condition. The incidence of more severe degenerative changes increases with the refractive error but it is not possible to choose a cut-off point which effects a satisfactory separation between eyes with a myopic crescent only and those with other retinal changes.

Axial length measurements also showed a correlation with the degree of myopia and the severity of the fundus changes as has been previously demonstrated by Karlin and Curtin (1976).

It was disappointing to find that scleral stress calculated from axial length, intraocular pressure and scleral thickness showed no correlation with the degree of myopia. There was a just statistically significant difference between the mean values for the normal and grade II eyes in the 40 + age group, probably because the mean intraocular pressure of the eyes in this group was higher (Table 5) than the other eyes.

When the scleral stress was calculated using a mean value of 0.5 mm for scleral thickness there was a small but statistically significant correlation between refraction and scleral stress, and although the mean values for scleral stress were higher in the eyes with myopic crescents and retinal changes from patients in the oldest age group, it was not possible to effect a satisfactory division between normal and pathological eyes using the figures for scleral stress.

The parameters in the calculation of scleral stress are axial length, intraocular pressure and scleral thickness. Axial length showed a good correlation with the refractive error but in percentage terms the variation in axial length is small (approximately 25%) over the range of errors encountered. Intraocular pressures had a large range (over 100%) so that unless there was some correlation between refraction and intraocular pressure a combination of axial length and intraocular pressure could not achieve a greater correlation with refraction than axial length alone.

The other parameter in the calculation of scleral stress is the thickness of the sclera. Using the method of scleral scatter and measuring at a point 12 mm from the limbus there was no correlation between refraction and scleral thickness. It is not surprising therefore that the inclusion of this parameter did not increase the correlation between refraction and scleral stress. Perhaps if it had been possible to measure the sclera at the posterior pole the results would have been different as this is the region of the globe which shows the most marked thinning in myopic eyes. By using a mean value of 0.5 mm for scleral thickness instead of the measured values, there was a statistically significantly higher scleral stress in the eyes showing the most marked degenerative changes in the older age group, but this difference is at least in part due to the higher levels of intraocular pressure found in these eyes (see Table 5). If the enlargement of the globe in myopic eyes was due to abnormal stretching forces on the sclera the highest scleral stress would be expected to be present in the younger age groups when the most rapid enlargement takes place.

It is possible that the failure to show a correlation between the degree of myopia and scleral stress was due to the methods used for the calculation of axial length and scleral thickness. This study was intended to be a pilot study using quick and easy methods and if the results had been encouraging more sophisticated methods would have been used in a further series of eyes. Certainly the estimation of scleral thickness is predisposed to errors in the *living* eye the extent of which is difficult to determine in the absence of any other method of measurement. The optical method of measuring axial length correlates quite well with ultrasonic measurements but undoubtedly has a higher scatter and probably underestimates the axial length in myopic eyes. On the basis of the present results it seems that the calculation of scleral stress is unlikely to have any greater clinical value than the degree of refractive error or the axial length in assessing the risk of degenerative fundus changes occurring in myopic eyes.

It is possible that the sclera of myopic eyes is more easily distensible than that of emmetropic eyes even though the force of the intraocular pressure is no higher than normal. The ocular rigidity of myopic eyes is lower than that of emmetropic eyes but experiments on enucleated eyes (Perkins 1980) suggest that the difference can be accounted for by the increased volume of the eye and that it is not due to a greater distensibility of the sclera itself. Ocular rigidity as measured clinically can only measure rapid changes, and it is possible that the sclera of myopic eyes may behave normally to rapid changes of intraocular pressure and yet exhibit *creep* in the face of a normal pressure.

SUMMARY

Measurements of refraction, axial length, intraocular pressure and scleral thickness were done on 146 eyes with a range of refractions from + 1.0 D to -20.0 D spherical equivalent. Axial length measurements showed a good correlation with the degree of myopia but there was no significant correlation between refraction and intraocular pressure or scleral thickness.

The eyes were classified into those with no evidence of pathological changes (normal), those with a myopic crescent only (grade I) and those with more severe degenerative myopic changes (grade II). Eighty-seven percent of eyes in grade II, 79% of eyes in grade I and only 17% of normal eyes had a refractive error greater than -4.0 D. Eighty-three percent of eyes in grade II, 70% in grade I and 30% of normal eyes had an axial length greater than that equivalent to -4.0 D.

Scleral stress calculated from PA/4t, where P = intraocular pressure, A = axial length and t = scleral thickness did not show any correlation with refractive error or severity of degenerative changes except that the mean scleral stress of grade II eyes from patients over 40 years of age was significantly higher in this group.

CONCLUSIONS

The measurement of scleral stress by the methods used did not seem to be related to the development of myopia and only showed some correlation with the severity of myopic degenerative changes in the oldest age group. Scleral stress values did not produce any clear cut guide as to the development of degenerative changes.

Refractive errors greater than -4.0 D gave a fairly good separation between eyes with and without fundus changes. Axial length also separated the normal eyes from eyes with fundus changes but with a greater overlap than refractive error.

The results give little support to the theory that the myopic eye enlarges as a result of mechanical stress on the sclera.

REFERENCES

Friedman, B., Stress upon the ocular coats: effects of scleral curvature, scleral thickness and intraocular pressure. Eye, Ear, Nose & Throat Monthly. 45: 59–66 (1966).
Karlin, D.B., Curtin, B.J., Peripheral chorioretinal lesions and axial length of the myopic eye. Am. J. Ophthalmol. 81: 625–634 (1976).
Perkins, E.S., Hammond, B., and Milliken, A.B., Simple method of determining the axial length of the eye. Br. J. Ophthamol. 60: 266–270 (1976).
Perkins, E.S., Ocular volume and ocular rigidity. Submitted for publication. (1980).

Author's address:
Professor E.S. Perkins, M.D., Ph.D.
University of Iowa Hospitals & Clinics
Iowa City,
Iowa 52262
U.S.A.

A STUDY ON THE EFFECT OF SOME STEROID HORMONES IN DEGENERATIVE MYOPIA

C. BALACCO-GABRIELI and R. TUNDO

(Bari, Italy)

ABSTRACT

Continuing their study of the ethiopathogenesis of high myopia, the authors have determined serum cortisol, testosterone, 17 β-estradiol, progesterone and urinary 17-KS and 17-OHCS, in a group of 55 males and 32 fecund females with high myopia (above − 10 D); the patients were strictly selected, excluding from the study all cases with signs of systemic disease.

The results showed in both sexes an increase in serum cortisol level, as compared with a control group. Further there was a reduced serum testosterone in males, and an increased 17 β-estradiol in females, however only in the first half of the menstrual cycle. Progesteron showed no change.

The present results indicate a pathogenetic correlation between changes concerning glucocorticoid and sexual steroids and reduced resistance of the sclera in high myopia.

INTRODUCTION

Apart from a notable elongation of the anterior-posterior axis of the eye-ball, degenerative myopia is characterized by a progressive deterioration of the posterior segment of the eye.

For some years now, degenerative myopia has been considered not only as a pathological process, but as a genuine disease in its own right, the causes of which can be traced back to a complex morbid condition.

In previous studies, Balacco-Gabrieli *et al.* (1972−1978) have underlined the importance of certain hormonal factors in the pathogenesis of this disorder. In a mixed group of young subjects, they recorded a reduced daily urinary excretion of 17 ketosteroides (17-KS) and an increased daily urinary excretion of mucopolysaccharides. These results were subsequently confirmed by Avetisov *et al.* (1976).

The present paper constitutes a further contribution to the etiopathogenetic study of degenerative myopia with reference to steroid hormones.

MATERIALS AND METHOD

The study was based on 87 subjects, all with myopia higher than 10 D, not known to suffer from any other endocrine, vascular, neoplastic or ocular disease. Of the subjects studied, 55 were males between the ages of 20 and 50, and 32 were females between the ages of 20 and 45. None of them had taken hormone-based medicine for at least six months before the tests.

The comparison, a 'control group' consisting of 573 non-myopic subjects (433 women and 140 men) was also studied.

In the male sample the following were measured:
(a) the basic level of serum testosterone and cortisol;
(b) the functional reserve of the suprarenal cortex (as the response to a quickly injected ACTH stimulus);
(c) the daily urinary secretion of 17-ketosteroid (Drekter *et al.* 1952) and 17-hydroxicorticoid (Liu 1964).

Concerning the females, all of whom were fertile, the investigations were conducted on the 12th and 22nd day of their menstrual cycles:
(a) the basic level of serum cortisol;
(b) the functional reserve of the suprarenal cortex;
(c) the daily urinary excretion of 17-KS and 17-OHCS.

The levels of progestorone and 17-β-estradiol were the only to be measured in both phases of the menstrual cycle.

The blood samples were taken between eight and nine o'clock in the morning.

The evaluation of the results (using the average of two readings) was carried out with the 't' of Student and with variance-analysis.

The amounts of cortisol, testosterone, progesterone and 17-β-estradiol were measured with the radioimmunological method (R.I.A. Kit, Sorin, Italy).

RESULTS

The average basic level of cortisol in those suffering from degenerative myopia was significantly higher than that of the 'control group' (Table 1, 2), but there was no difference between the groups regarding the percentual increase of cortisol after the injection of ACTH.

In the group of myopic males, however (Table 1), the serum testosterone level and the daily urinary excretion of 17-KS and 17-OHCS were significantly reduced in comparison with the males of the 'control group'.

· No statistically significant difference was recorded between highly myopic females and female controls regarding the urinary excretion of 17-KS and 17-OHCS, the level of progesterone (in both phases of the menstrual cycle) and the level of 17-β-estradiol (in the second phase of the cycle only).

In the follicular phase, however, the content of 17-β-estradiol was significantly higher in the myopic women.

130

Table 1. Hormone analysis in females with high myopia as compared with controls, with indication of significant differences.

♀	Serum Basal	Cortisol After ACTH	Urinary 17-OH	Steroids 17-Ks	Progesterone 1° Half	Progesterone 2° Half	17-β Estradiol 1° Half	17-β Estradiol 2° Half
	mcg/100 ml		mg/24^h		ng/ml		pg/ml	
Controls n = 433	12.4 ± 2.9	28.0 ± 6.0	3.15 ± 1.94	5.33 ± 2.76	0.27 ± 0.10	2.72 ± 1.7	104 ± 42	228 ± 69
High Myopia n = 32	16.43 ± 5.61	27.5 ± 6.97	2.53 ± 1.67	5.39 ± 2.84	0.25 ± 0.17	3.61 ± 1.29	176 ± 99	209 ± 91
	x	N.S.	N.S.	N.S.	N.S.	N.S.	x	N.S.

P < 0,001

131

Table 2. Hormone analysis in males with high myopia as compared with controls, with indication of significant differences.

♂	Serum Basal	Cortisol After ACTH	Urinary 17-OH	Steroids 17-Ks	Testosterone
	mcg/100 ml		mg/24^h		ng/ml.
Controls n. = 140	13.9 ± 3.8	27.7 ± 5.4	4.16 ± 1.79	7.76 ± 3.15	4.19 ± 1.21
High Myopia n. = 55	16.30 ± 5.38	28.08 ± 7.74	3.38 ± 1.65	5.69 ± 2.04	3.07 ± 0.95
	x	N.S.	xx	x	x

x $P < 0.001$
xx $P < 0.01$

DISCUSSION

The results leave us the following facts to interpret:
(1) the increased quantity of cortisol circulation in high myopia of both sexes;
(2) the reduced quantity of serum testosterone and of 17-KS in the urine of males suffering from myopia;
(3) the increase of 17 β-estradiol in myopic females, however, only in the first half of the menstrual cycle.

Experimental physiology has brought to light the fact that cortisol produces its effects on the connective tissue only when it is present in excess, *inhibiting* the production and the metabolism of mucopolysaccharides, the activity of fibroblasts and thereby the formation of precollagenous tissue, collagenous tissue and, in particular, elastic fibres.

A confirmation of this inhibition is provided by observations in human pathology, in states with increase in glucocorticoid level, whether this is due to pathology of the suprarenal-hypothalamus-hypophysis axis, or for iatrogenous reasons (by medication).

In males, testosterone undoubtedly has an effect on collagenous tissue which appears to be opposite to the effect of cortisol, in *facilitating* the formation and metabolism of mucopolysaccharides, the activity of fibroblasts and thus the formation of collagenous tissue and elastic fibres.

In females, the effect of estrogen on the metabolism of collagenous tissue is identical to that of testosterone in men.

Analysing the results in males we can see that two conditions occur (an increase in cortisol and a decrease in testosterone) which both tend to produce an inhibition of the metabolism of collagenous tissue.

The changes in the myopic females on the other hand, are not comparable to that of the males, and much harder to interpret. The high cortisol content contrasts with the high level of 17 β-estradiol, even if this is limited to just one phase of the menstrual cycle.

In this context it is stressed that when estrogen is present in excess, or when it is not counterbalanced by an adequate production of progesterone, it can induce an increase in the volume of extracellular liquid due to retention of sodium, chloride and water. This is supported by studies carried out to investigate the effects of estrogen on connective tissue. They have shown that an excess of the hormone can induce hydration and a tendency to fibril-dissociation with a consequent blockage of fibrillogenesis. (Digman *et al.* 1956, Preedy and Aitken 1956).

Concerning myopic females, it seems realistic to hypothesize that interference with the metabolism of collagenous tissue, should be attributed mainly to an excess of cortisol. In addition, estrogen may periodically exert an influence of probably minor importance.

In apparent contrast with our findings are the results of recent studies carried out by Carnevalini *et al.* (1977) who describe an increased response of growth hormone (HGH) to injection of arginine in young patients suffering from serious degenerative myopia.

It is well-known that the action of sexual hormones on collagenous tissue manifests itself only in case of a certain level of HGH. The increase of HGH can therefore be interpreted as a mechanism compensating for a deficit of the other sexual hormones. The markedly deviating secretion of these hormones, which are among the most active regarding metabolism of collagenous tissue, seems to justify the hypothesis of a certain pathogenetic association with a reduced resistance of the sclera, producing the pathologic myopic deterioration of the posterior pole of the eye-ball.

REFERENCES

Avetisov, E.S., Winezkaja, M.I., Sawizkaja, N.F. Einige Stoffwechselwerte für saure Mukopolisaccharide bei der Myopie. Klin. Mbl. Augenheilk. 168: 750–754 (1976).

Balacco-Gabrieli, C. Indagine preliminare sui 17-chetosteroidi nella miopia degenerativa. Boll. Soc. It. Biol. Sper. 48: 241 (1972).

Balacco-Gabrieli, C. I 17-KS nelle miopia degenerativa. Boll. di Oculistica. 53: 195–203 (1974).

Balacco-Gabrieli, C., Scorcia, G., Asciano, F. Les mucopolysaccharides urinaires dans la myopie degencrative. Ann. d'Oculist. (Paris), 210: 147 (1977).

Balacco-Gabrieli, G., Santoro, G., Santoro, M., Abaticchio, G., Vavalle, G., Giorgino, R. Plasmatic and urinary steroids in the high myopia. Note I. Testosterone, 17-OH, 17-KS. Boll. Soc. Ital. Biol. Sper. 54: 975 (1978).

Balacco-Gabrieli, C., Santoro, G., Santoro, M., Scardapane, R., Tundo, R., Giorgino, R. Plasmatic and urinary steroids in the high myopia. Note 2. Cortisol, 17-OH, 17-KS (males). Boll. Soc. Ital. Biol. Sper. 54: 978 (1978).

Balacco-Gabrieli, C., Santoro, G., Santoro, M., Lattanzi, V., Di Gioia, C., Giorgino, R. Plasmatic and urinary steroids in the high myopia. Note 3. Cortisol, 17-OH, 17-KS (prolific females). Boll. Soc. Ital. Biol. Sper. 54: 981 (1978).

Balacco-Gabrieli, C., Santoro, G., Santoro, M., Bellizzi, M., Giorgino, R. Plasmatic and urinary steroids in the high myopia. Note 4. Progesterone, 17 β-estradiol, 17-OH, 17-KS. Boll. Soc. Ital. Biol. Sper. 54: 984 (1978).

Carnevalini, A., Givannini, E., Micheli, W., Mucci, M.P. Determinazione dell'ormone somatotropo (HGH) in soggetti giovani con miopia degenerativa. Relazione al 58° Congresso S.O.I. Roma (1977).

Digman, W.S., Voskhian, J., Assali, N.S. Effect of estrogens on renal hemodynamics and excretion of electrolytes in human subjects. J. Clin. Endocrinol. Metab. 16: 1032–42 (1956).

Drekter, I.J., Heisler, A., Scism, G.R., Stern, S., Pearson, S., Mc Gavack, T.H.J. Clin. Endocr. Met. 12: 55 (1952).

Liu, H.C. A modified procedure for the estimation of total 17-Hydroxy-corticosteroids (Porter Silberchromogens) in urine. Clin. Chem. 10: 103–115 (1964).

Preedy, J.R.K., Aitken, E.H. The effect of estrogen on water and electrolyte metabolism. J. Clin. Invest. 35: 423–29 (1956).

Key words: Myopia, Serum cortisol, testosterone, progesterone, 17 β-estradiol, Urinary 17 KS, 17 OHCS.

Senior author's address:
Prof. C. Balacco-Gabrieli, M.D.
Universita di Bari,
Via Putignani 128
Bari 70122
Italy

THE HEMODYNAMICS OF THE MYOPIC EYE: RHEO-OCULOGRAPHIC FINDINGS

A. GIOVANNINI, S. COLOMBATI and C. CILIBERTI

(Bologna, Italy)

ABSTRACT

With the technique developed at our clinic, rheo-oculography has proven to be a sensitive means for the sphygmodynamic investigation of the eye (rheo-oculography with a definite time constant) and is the only means available in clinical practice for blood flow measurements, even if semi-quantitative (rheo-oculography with an infinite time constant).

Forty-five patients with pathological axial myopia, 32 patients with simple myopia and 26 controls were examined with our technique. From the results there emerged a clear, statistically significant, rheo-oculographic picture of pathological axial myopia characterized by flow indexes that were consistently lower than both the controls and the patients with simple myopia. The ocular pulse showed a marked reduction in amplitude, a clear decrease in speed, and a convex descending branch on the rheo-oculogram. These characteristics appear to correspond well in functional terms to the anatomicopathological alterations of the retinochoroidal vessels.

INTRODUCTION

With the technique developed at our Clinic (Cristini *et al.* 1975), rheo-oculography proved to be a sensitive means for the sphygmodynamic investigation of the eye (rheo-oculography with a definite time constant), and, although only semiquantitative, is the only means available in clinical practice for blood flow measurements (rheo-oculography with an infinite time constant, Giovannini and Puglioli 1977). Our rheo-oculographic method is described in previous papers (Cristini *et al.* 1975a, b).

MATERIAL AND METHODS

Forty-five patients with pathological axial myopia having between 18 and 26 diopters of myopia and an age between 18 and 51 years, 32 patients with simple myopia and 26 controls were examined with our technique.

Table 1. Rheo-oculographic findings. Average values and independent statistical variables of sphygmous amplitude, sphygmous speed and blood flow.

	Sphygmous amplitude (in mm)	Sphygmous speed (ascending phase, in % of cycle)	Blood flow (cc/min/100 cc tissue)
Normals (n = 26)	11,9 ± 3,1	26,4 ± 1,8	1,4 ± 0,2
Simple myopia (n = 32)	10,9 ± 2,9	27,5 ± 1,8	1,3 ± 0,2
High myopia (n = 45)	4,7 ± 1,8	39,3 ± 4,7	1,0 ± 0,2

Table 2. Rheo-oculographic findings. Minimal and maximal values recorded.

	Sphygmous amplitude (mm) Min Max	Sphygmous speed (per cent) Min Max	Blood flow (cc/min/100 cc tissue) Min Max
Normals	8–18	23–30	1,1–2,1
Simple myopia (n = 32)	6–18	23–30	1,0–1,8
High myopia (n = 45)	2–8	33–50	0,8–1,4

The patients were exempt from general and other ocular diseases and showed normal systemic and opthalmodynamographic pressure values, so that the observed sphygmous alterations were due exclusively to the chorio-retinal vessels. In addition to the recordings under basal conditions, we used the Amyl nitrite test (Cristini and Giovannini 1979) to verify the entity of the so-called functional reserve by stimulating the 'mechanogenous' vasal reactions (Rodenhauser 1963) in the presence of a normal rheo-oculographic behaviour, or the possible presence of a reversible functional quota in case of a rheo-oculographic deficit. We did not include the responses of those patients who presented marked variations in cardiac frequency, or in arterial blood pressure.

RESULTS AND DISCUSSION

Results are summarized in Table 1 which shows average values and independent statistical variables of sphygmous amplitude, sphygmous speed and blood flow for normal controls, patients with simple myopia, and patients with high myopia. Sphygmous amplitude is expressed in millimeters, related to the same calibration; sphygmous speed expresses in percent the relationship between duration of the ascending branch and the overall wave cycle; blood flow is expressed in cc/min/100 cc of tissue.

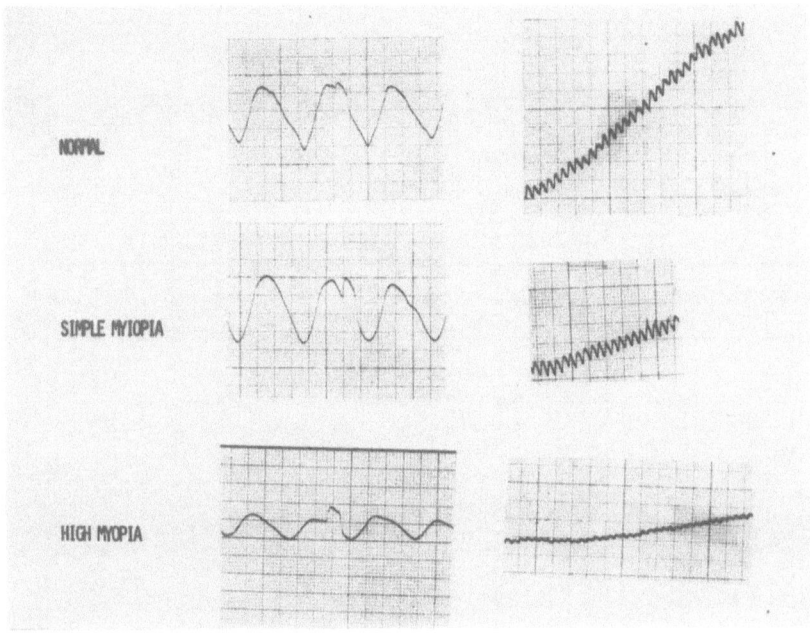

Fig. 1. Left row: ocular pulse (rheo-oculogram with determined time constant) Right row: rheo-oculogram with infinite time constant.

Table 2 shows minimal and maximal values recorded. The analysis of these tables shows that high myopia has the following sphygmographic features:

(a) reduction of sphygmous amplitude
(b) increase in the duration of the ascending branch and decrease of sphygmous speed.
(c) flattening of the curve summit
(d) reduction of blood flow.

Figure 1 illustrates the paradigmatic behaviour of the ocular pulse and of the blood flow in simple myopia, in high myopia and in controls: while simple myopia shows ocular pulse and blood flow comparable to those of the controls, high myopia shows a clear flow reduction and hyposphygmia.

Also, we have observed a clear-cut difference between patients with high myopia and the other two groups regarding the amyl nitrite test. In fact, as can be seen in Figure 2, while the controls and the patients with simple myopia show an increase in sphygmous amplitude after amyl-test, those with high myopia displayed a clear reduction of the sphygmous amplitude.

It is worth remembering that the amyl rheographic test can be useful in the early diagnosis of glaucoma (Cristini and Giovannini 1979): the glaucomatous eye displays in fact a decrease in the sphygmous amplitude after the test, contrary to the normal subject.

137

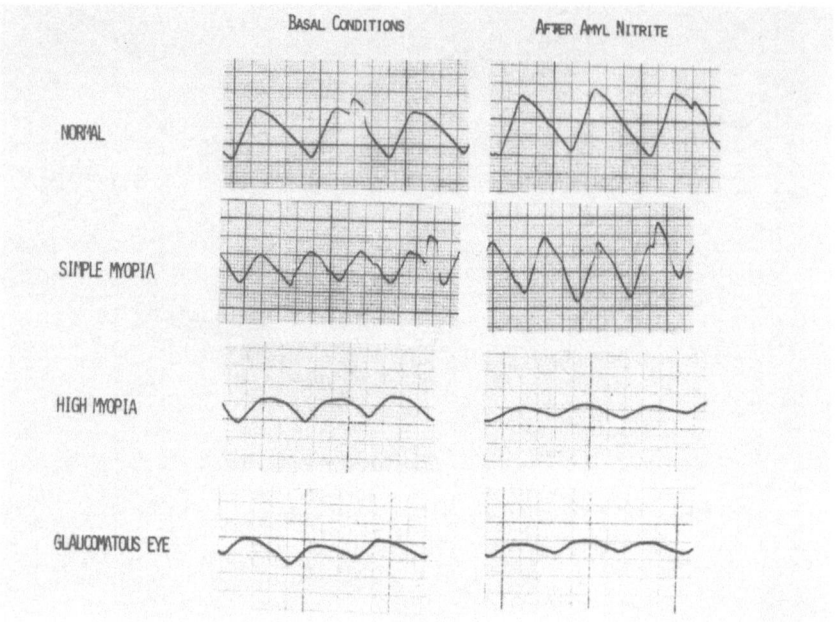

Fig. 2. Amyl-nitrite test in normal, in simple myopia, in high myopia and in glaucoma. Left row: basal conditions. Right row: after amyl test. Note that in the normal and in simple myopia the inhalation of amylnitrite produces a clear increase in the sphygmous amplitude, while the behaviour in high myopia and in glaucoma is just the opposite.

Such a test is therefore not reliable in the early diagnosis of glaucoma in cases associated with high myopia.

To conclude, the rheo-oculographic behaviour observed in high myopia appears to correspond well in functional terms to the pathological alterations of the retino-choroidal vessels.

It is interesting to note the analogy between the rheo-oculographic behaviour of the highly myopic eye and of the glaucomatous eye.

REFERENCES

Cristini G., Meduri R., Garbini G.C., Giovannini A.: A new method for determining the blood quantity in the eye. Albrecht v. Graefes Arch. Klin. Exp. Ophthalmol. 197: 1–11 (1975).

Cristini G., Meduri R., Giovannini A., Semeiologia reografica bulbare. Ann. Ottalmol. Clin. Ocul. CI, 319–334 (1975).

Cristini G., Giovannini A., Rheography in early stages of glaucoma. In 'Glaucoma Update' Ed. G.P. Halberg New York Inter Optic Publications Inc., 31–34 (1979).

Giovannini A., Puglioli R., Rheo-oculography in clinical practice. Agg. Ter. Oftalmol. 29: 45–63 (1977).

Rodenhauser J.: Uveadurchblutung und Augeninnendruck. Buch. Augen. Beih. Klin. Augen. 17: 42 (1963).

Senior author's address:
Senior Dott. Alfonso Giovannini,
Clinica Oculistica I
University of Bologna
Via Massarenti 9,
40100 Bologna
Italy

CALCIUM, CHROMIUM, PROTEIN, SUGAR AND ACCOMMODATION IN MYOPIA

B.C. LANE

(New York, N.Y., U.S.A.)

ABSTRACT

Persons with increasing myopia statistically invest more diopter-hours in closework accommodation, have abnormal hair concentrations of chromium and calcium, and consume excessive protein and sugar. Myopes, as a class, whether or not their myopia is increasing, statistically are deficient in chromium as measured in nape hair of 120 subjects. Young myopes, ages 7–17, at their greatest period of bone growth and vulnerability to myopic increase, tend to mishandle body calcium significantly more than emmetropes.

INTRODUCTION

For the first time, we can now link (a) deficiency of the trace metal chromium (Cr) and (b) overconsumption of denatured protein to the development of myopia. In addition to these radical discoveries, this new study has produced new, strong, statistically significant support for old theories that earlier had received only sketchy corroboration. For example, this study was able to reconfirm that increase in myopia is associated statistically with:
  (a) not the hours per se of sustained reading and closework, but the diopter hours or diopter-log hours of sustained stimulus to accommodation (Lane 1973, 1980);
  (b) consumption of refined carbohydrates in high ratio to total carbohydrate consumption (Bardiger and Stock 1972; Young 1975; Young *et al.* 1973); and
  (c) derangement in calcium metabolism or intake (Knapp 1939; Laval 1938; Law 1934).
More than a century ago, the German ophthalmologist, Hermann Cohn (1883, 1892), promulgated myopia-prevention hygienes based on reducing the stimulus to sustained closework accommodation, principally by use of head restraints, sloped desks and improved lighting to prevent a too-close working distance.

Doc. Ophthal. Proc. Series, Vol. 28,
ed. by H.C. Fledelius, P.H. Alsbirk and E. Goldschmidt
© *1981 Dr W. Junk Publishers, The Hague*

Cohn presumed that sustained accommodation resulted in elevation of the baselines of pressure within the eye, and hence in elongation of the eyeball, thus, as a servomechanism, reducing the need, eventually, for so much accommodation.

When later studies (Hess and Heine 1898; Hess 1909; Yamamoto 1954; Armaly and Rubin 1961) proved that the immediate effect of accommodation was a lowering of this intraocular pressure (IOP) as measured at the anterior chamber of the eye, Cohn's hypothesis was considered 'disproven.'

In 1973, at the Glaucoma Section of the annual meeting of the Association for Research in Vision and Ophthalmology, Lane (1973, 1980) reported that the effect of daily-repeated, sustained closework accommodation, repeated for more than two weeks, was opposite to the short-term effect as measured at the cornea, and did, in fact, result in elevation of IOP. In 1973, in agreement with other investigators, Lane (1980) found that besides being sensitive to accommodative stresses, IOP changes are influenced by nutritional deficits and physical activity.

But until the present study the only nutritional elements clearly defined as related to myopic development were blood calcium and vitamin D deficiency (Knapp 1939; Laval 1938; Law 1934) and disordered mucopolysaccharide metabolism (Vinetskaya and Savitskaya 1976).

METHOD

I selected 120 consecutive nutrition workups from my patient files for use in this study. Four United States laboratories had computed each patient's food ingestion from dietary questionnaire data provided by each patient and had used optical-emission spectroscopy for 19 elements and atomic-absorption spectroscopy for a 20th to determine the mineral absorption in nape-of-neck hair samples provided by each patient. Refractive findings for at least two dates approximately framing the hair-tissue test date were recorded for non-presbyopes where this data was complete.

This was a retrospective study with essentially double-blind data collection assuring freedom from investigator bias and from placebo effect.

In order to look at the correlates to 'change in refractive power relative to the retina,' the study compared the data for three groups on the basis of change within two years: Group One data was for eyes increasing in refractive power relative to the retina. I shall call this 'increasing in myopia, etc.,' since it could refer either to increasing in myopia or decreasing in hyperopia. The second data group represented eyes 'decreasing in myopia, etc.' The third group, a control group, was the comparison group for eyes not changing more than a quarter-diopter in two years.

It is clear that other factors besides nutrition are associated with the increasing myopia, etc., in the study sample. For example, there is a significant *interaction* effect between Habitual Relative Add (HRA) and whether the myopia is increasing (etc.) or decreasing (etc.).

The Habitual Relative Add is the habitual near-vision refractive 'correction' or Rx glasses or contact lenses, if any, minus the distance

142

Table 1. Habitual relative add (HRA) § scores for eyes changing in refractive power ⩾ 0.5 D/2 yrs.

Group	Median HRA (diopters)	Mean HRA (diopters)	Std Dev (diopters)
↑ MYO or ↓ HYP	+ 0.25	+ 0.6875*	± .596
↓ MYO or ↑ HYP	+ 1.25	+ 1.257	± .419
No change	+ 0.875	+ 0.870*	± .616
No change EMM	+ 0.875	+ 0.9286*	± .220

§ ages 7–42, HRA relative to controlling eye, where the HRA = (the habitual near Rx in spherical-equivalent diopters) minus (the distance ametropia in spherical-equivalent diopters).
Note. – Significantly different means vs ↓ Myopia group: *$p < 0.05$.

vision ametropia. For example, a person habitually wearing no lenses to read, but who is a 1-diopter myope at distance, would be considered as having a + 1.00 diopter HRA.

RESULTS AND DISCUSSION

It turns out that the non-strabismic binocular persons increasing in myopia (etc.) have a median Habitual Relative Add (HRA) of only + 0.25 D, while the non-strabismic persons decreasing in myopia (etc.) have a median and a mean of + 1.25 D, as in Table 1, and despite the interaction of nutrition, this difference is significantly different for increasing hyperopia vs increasing myopia.

The effect of stimulus to accommodation is apparent. [We can better appreciate its correlation with behavioral studies if we look at the product of the logarithm of the accommodative stimulus multiplied by the logarithm of hours spent daily at sustained closework – as I showed in a study in 1977 on functional photophobia (Lane 1978). The value of the accommodative stimulus is given by the average working-distance accommodative stimulus minus the HRA.]

When we look at refractive *change* and mineral absorption in hair tissue we found in the study that the highest levels of calcium absorption in hair are associated with – to our initial surprise – increasing myopia. Next highest calcium levels in hair are associated with the other extreme of *decreasing* myopia, and the lowest, more normal concentrations of calcium in hair are found in the no-change group. At first this may seem contrary to the literature hypothesizing the importance of calcium in the prevention of myopic increase. But high hair calcium characteristically occurs when calcium is being spilt into hair tissue at the expense of other body tissues – a condition often corrected with supplemental vitamin B_6, vitamin D and calcium complex. It should be noted that elevated hair calcium may reflect a vitamin B_6 deficiency [often associated with heavy consumption of animal protein that has been denatured by cooking to internal temperature exceeding 60° C (140° F)]. Vitamin B_6 lowers hair calcium and hair magnesium.

143

Table 2. Refractive strata & mineral absorption in hair tissue.

Mineral	Age range	Initial median (ppm) Myopia	Emmetropia	Hyperopia
Calcium	7−17	585	173**	210*
	18−35	450	350	350
Chromium[§]	7−17	0.14	0.24*	0.40***
	18−38	0.10	0.30	0.24**

Note. − Significantly different distribution vs Myopic group:
[§] Excl. strabismics.
*p < 0.05 by Mann-Whitney.
**p < .01, Mann-Whitney
***p = .001, Mann-Whitney test

Table 3. Refractive strata & calcium absorption in hair tissue.

Initial mean & standard deviation (ppm) Ages 7−17			
Myopia	Emmetropia	Hyperopia	Non-myopia
573.8	208.6**	276.0	240.5*
± 348.8	± 100.9	± 182.1	± 145.0

Note. − Significantly different means vs Myopic group:
*p < 0.05
**p < 0.02

Chromium absorption in hair tissue of persons increasing in myopia (etc.) is virtually a third of the level absorbed in persons decreasing in myopia (etc.) when median values are compared.

Instead of looking at the direction of refractive *change,* if we now look at the refractive *strata* (Table 2), we find that calcium absorption in hair in school-age children, ages 7−17, is lowest for *emmetropes* and highest for myopes, but that it tends to average out after age 18. The evidence is that the syndrome of excessive spilling of calcium into the hair during the high-bone-growth years is associated with both distensibility and contractibility of the sclera, while normal levels of calcium in the hair are associated with structural stability of the sclera. In Table 3 we see that the standard deviation for the distribution of calcium concentration relative to a mean value for emmetropia is distinctly tighter than for myopia and hyperopia, suggesting that emmetropia is characterized by a relatively narrow distribution of calcium concentration about a mean of 208.6 calcium parts per million (ppm) [1 ppm = 0.1 mg%], that myopia and hyperopia are not so tightly defined about mean values of calcium. It appears that normal well-controlled calcium metabolism may be essential to the maintenance of emmetropia.

Also in Table 2, we see that chromium level in myopes is extremely low regardless of age. It is as if myopes per se are constitutionally more subject to myopia than non-myopes. This robust systematic effect of

Table 4. Refractive strata & chromium absorption in hair tissue.

Initial mean & standard deviation (ppm)			
Myopia	Emmetropia	Hyperopia	Non-myopia
0.142	0.666*	0.450**	0.534***
± 0.065	± 0.926	± 0.641	± 0.761
(22)	(17)	(27)	(44)

Note. – Significantly different means vs Myopic group:
*$p < 0.05$
**$p < 0.02$
***$p < 0.001$

chromium shines through with great strength despite the 'noise' due to interactions with accommodative-stress effects and the error factors that we can expect in a study of this nature. In Table 4 we see that the standard deviation for the distribution of chromium concentration relative to a mean value is distinctly narrow in range for myopia around a mean of 0.142 ppm – suggesting that most myopes have lowered chromium level virtually as a hallmark of their myopia. But low chromium levels can be found non-definitively in other refractive strata, since the chromium standard deviation for non-myopia is quite wide.

In order for an emmetrope to become a myope of significance it appears that at least two of three conditions need to be in process during the period of myopic increase:

(a) calcium mishandling, especially during a period of high growth rate or bone repair – probably resulting in scleral distensibility;

(b) tissue-chromium depletion – apparently resulting in IOP elevation, as reported in this investigator's companion study (Lane 1981);

(c) daily repeated, sustained stimulus to accommodation and accommodative fatigue syndrome – apparently involving elevated IOP as a surrogate mechanism to lenticular accommodation, as reported in this investigator's companion study (Lane 1981).

The importance of trace amounts of chromium as a cofactor potentiating insulin at ciliary muscle sites, enabling sustained energy exchange for sustained accommodation, and similarly, its importance in sugar metabolism – these functions of chromium may be the key here in the development of myopia, rather than any structural effect of chromium in eye tissues. Chromium depletion has long been recognized as a consequence of ingestion of sucrose. Chromium deficiency in myopes may be principally an index of sugar consumption and associated demineralization and devitaminization. In my companion study (Lane 1981) we find that chromium depletion is associated with elevation of IOP.

We see in Table 5 that in metropolitan New Jersey, U.S.A., the ratio of protein intake to the RDA (Recommended Daily Allowance) for protein intake is highest in persons increasing in myopia – protein-ratio levels almost fantastically high in terms of human need for protein – whereas myopes not changing refractively have a far lower ratio of protein intake than hyperopes who are not changing refractively. Myopes intrinsically do not

Table 5. Refractive change & ratio of protein intake to RDA.

↑ Myopia or ↓ Hyperopia	No change		↓ Myopia or ↑ Hyperopia
	Myopia	Hyperopia	
	Protein ratio medians		
3.22*	0.93**	2.32	2.03

Note. – Significantly different distributions by Mann-Whitney test.
*$p = 0.025$, compared to ↓ Myopia, etc. sample.
**$p = 0.001$, compared to Hyperopic No-Change group.

consume more protein than hyperopes, except statistically when the myopia is increasing.

When Gardiner (1958) reported on the experimental effect of adding animal protein to the diet of British children to reduce the rate of myopic progression, both Dr. Gardiner and his readers may have missed the point that the protein supplement he was using for the experimental group – calcium caseinate – [a calcium-protein complex] – delivers calcium in an easily utilized form and counters an otherwise expected calciuretic effect.

A calciuretic effect [documented in a series of studies since 1968 (Linkswiler 1976; Margen *et al.* 1974)] results in the spilling of calcium into the urine and presumably into the hair when large amounts of cooked protein are ingested.

Although these new findings appear to be in conflict with the older literature on the role of protein in myopia reversal, the new data does make sense. Why? – because exaggerated, denatured protein intake increases the body's requirements for vitamins (especially B_6 and pantothenic acid – both utilized in regulation of IOP) and for minerals – and this elevated demand for vitamins is aggravated by excessive consumption of simple sugars and other refined carbohydrates which do not carry with them enough vitamins and minerals required for their own digestion and assimilation.

As to refined carbohydrate ingestion, by far, the principal nutritional factor associated with myopia is the *ratio* of simple *refined* carbohydrates to *total* carbohydrates, as we see in Table 6. For hyperopes, the mean percentage of refined carbohydrates (CHOs) to total CHOs ingested is 9.6%. For myopes, the mean percentage of refined CHOs to total CHOs is 35.3%, with $t = 5.78$ and $p < 0.001$.

Table 6. Mean % refined carbohydrates to total CHOs ingested as associated with refractive strata.

Group	Initial mean (%)	Std Dev (%)	t	df	p
Myopes	35.27	± 14.82	5.78	31	< .001
Hyperopes	9.61	± 8.27			
Emmetropes	27.31	± 23.44	2.51	29	< .05

146

CONCLUDING REMARKS

In my opening paragraphs I hinted at a rationale to explain these effects of nutrition and accommodation as factors in myopia development. The key seems to be 'nutritionally instigated rise in IOP.'

The author's new findings concerning these IOP relationships are discussed in more detail in a companion paper (Lane 1981), extending on the discoveries documented in his 1973 study (Lane 1980).

It is not important in this brief synopsis to show how these findings on myopia development fit in with what is known of the effect of nutrition on IOP – except to note that this data fits splendidly.

In summary, persons with increasing myopia do *not* spend more hours at closework, but do statistically invest more *diopter*-hours in closework accommodation. Statistically, they have abnormal hair concentrations of chromium and calcium, and they consume excessive amounts of cooked, overprocessed protein and sugar. Hence, we find the most common form of myopia is triggered by sustained accommodation and deficit-inducing diets.

REFERENCES

Armaly, M.F. & Rubin, M.L.: Accommodation and applanation tonometry. Arch. Ophthalmol. 65: 415 (1961).

Bardiger, M. & Stock, A.L.: The effects of sucrose-containing diets low in protein on ocular refraction in the rat. Nutr. Soc. Proc. 31: 4A (1972).

Cohn, H.: The hygiene of the eye in schools. (Translated, edited by W.P. Turnbull) London, Simpkin, Marshall & Co. (1886) (Originally published in German 1883).

Cohn, H.: Lehrbuch der Hygiene des Auges. Vienna, Urban & Schwarzenberg (1892).

Gardiner, P.A.: Dietary treatment of myopia in children. Lancet, No. 1: 1152 (1958).

Hess, C.: Vergleichende Untersuchungen über den Einfluss der Accommodation auf den Augendruck in der Wirbelthierreihe. Archiv für Augenheilkunde, 63: 88 (1909). Cited by T. Sato: The causes and prevention of acquired myopia. Tokyo, Kanehara Shuppan pp. 2 & 218 (1957).

Hess, C. & Heine, L.: Arbeiten aus dem Gebiet der Accommodationslehre: IV. Experimentelle Untersuchungen über den Einfluss der Accommodation auf den intraocularen Druck nebst Beiträgen zur Kenntnis der Accommodation verschiedener Säugethiere. Graefes Arch., 46: 243 (1898) Cited by T. Sato: The causes and prevention of acquired myopia. Tokyo, Kanehara Shuppan, pp. 2 & 217 (1957).

Knapp, A.A.: Vitamin D complex in progressive myopia: Etiology, pathology and treatment: Preliminary study. Am. J. Ophthalmol., 22: 1329. (1939).

Lane, B.C.: Elevation of intraocular pressure with daily sustained reading and closework. Glaucoma Section Session II. Ann. Meeting Program of the Assoc. for Res Vision and Ophthalmol Abstract (2) p. 44. (May 5, 1973).

Lane, B.C.: Lowering of functional photophobia threshold with daily, sustained closework accommodation. Eastern Seaboard Invitational Skeffington Symposium on Visual Training 23: 64 (1978).

Lane, B.C.: Elevation of intraocular pressure with daily, sustained reading and closework stimulus to accommodation. (Master's Thesis State University of New York, State College of Optometry, 1973) University Microfilms International Ann Arbor, Michigan & London, Publication No. 13–14: 525 (1980).

Lane, B.C.: Elevation of intraocular pressure with daily, sustained closework stimulus to accommodation, lowered tissue chromium and dietary deficiency of ascorbic acid (vitamin C). Docum. Ophthalmol. Proc. Series 18: 149–155 (1981).

Laval, J.: Vitamin D and myopia. Arch. Ophthalmol., 19: 47 (1938).

Law, F.W.: Calcium and parathyroid therapy in progressive myopia. Trans. Ophthalmol. Soc. United Kingdom, 54: 281 (1934).

Linkswiler, H.M. Calcium. In: Nutrition reviews' present knowledge in nutrition (4th ed) Ed. D.M. Hegsted New York, The Nutrition Foundation p. 232 (1976).

Margen, S., Chu, J.-Y., Kaufmann, N.A. & Calloway, D.H.: Studies in calcium metabolism: I, The calciuretic effect of dietary protein. Am. J. Clin. Nutrition, 27: 584 (1974).

Vinetskaya, & Savitskaya,: (1976). Cited by E.S. Avetisov in personal communication #3 to Francis A. Young (April, 1980).

Yamamoto, Y.: Change in the ocular pressure caused by the stimulus of induced current to the ciliary body. Acta Ophthalmol Jap, 58: 1458 (1954).

Young, F.A.: The development and control of myopia in human and subhuman primates. Contacto, 19(6): 16 (1975).

Young, F.A., Leary, G.A., Zimmerman, Z.R. & Strobel, D.A.: Diet and refractive characteristics. Am. J. Optom & Arch. Am. Acad Optom 50: 226 (1973).

Author's address:
B.C. Lane, O.D., M.S.
16 North Beverwyck Road
Lake Hiawatha, New Jersey 07034
U.S.A.

ELEVATION OF INTRAOCULAR PRESSURE WITH DAILY SUSTAINED CLOSEWORK STIMULUS TO ACCOMMODATION LOWERED TISSUE CHROMIUM AND DIETARY DEFICIENCY OF ASCORBIC ACID (VITAMIN C)

B.C. LANE

(New York, N.Y. U.S.A.)

ABSTRACT

Sustained closework accommodative stimulus results in elevated intraocular pressure (IOP), especially aggravated when tissue chromium is low and vitamin C ingestion does not exceed the US Recommended Daily Allowance. The requirement for tissue chromium in control of IOP is age-related and appears to be essential for sustained accommodation and strong ciliary-muscle function, probably as a co-factor potentiating insulin. IOP elevates as if in an effort to reduce sustained, daily-repeated accommodative stimulus by axial elongation of the eye in the presence of deficient levels of (a) chromium, (b) vitamin C, and (c) binocular-accommodative-amplitude skill-level as measured in terms of Positive Relative Accommodation — measured binocularly with negative lenses at 40 cm from the eyes.

INTRODUCTION

Hermann Cohn (1883, 1892) hypothesized that sustained, detailed closework accommodation caused intraocular-pressure (IOP) elevation and subsequent axial elongation and myopia. But by 1898, Hess and Heine (1898) showed that the short-term effect of accommodation was not elevation of IOP, and other studies confirmed actual lowering of IOP (all measured at the anterior chamber) with *short-term* accommodation.

In 1973, at the Glaucoma Section of the annual meeting of the Association for Research in Vision and Ophthalmology, Lane (1973, 1980) reported that the effect of daily-repeated, sustained closework accommodation, repeated for more than two weeks, was opposite to the short-term effect as measured at the cornea, and did, in fact, result in elevation of IOP. In 1973, in agreement with other investigators, Lane found that besides being sensitive to accommodative stresses, IOP changes are influenced by nutritional deficits and physical activity.

In 1979, further supporting this accommodation-induced-hypertension concept, Francis Young (1979) reported a pressure-flow gradient within the primate eye in direct response to accommodation, causing increased

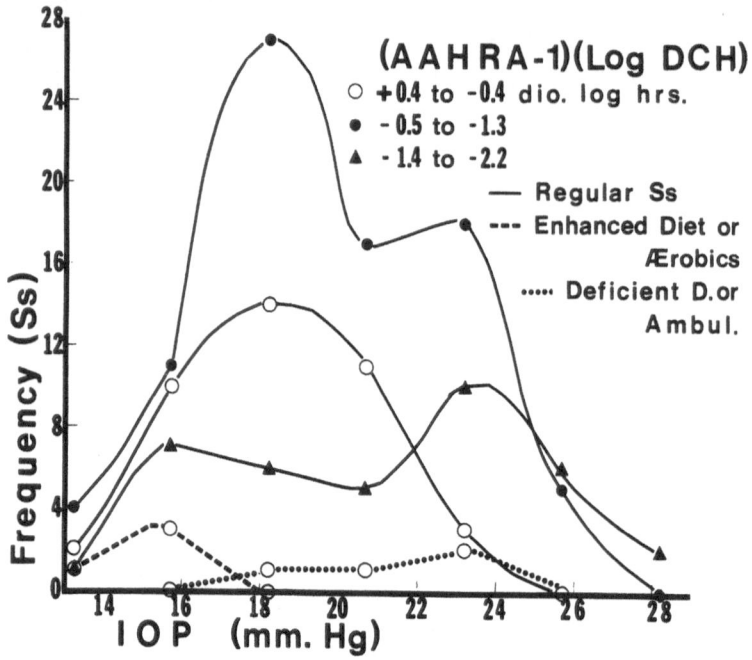

Fig. 1. Frequency distribution of subjects with high, medium, and low ranges of accommodative-stimulus-hours [(AAHRA-1) (Log Detailed Closework Hours)] with regard to the higher-pressure-eye IOP. The *low*-accommodative-stress group presents a normal-valued, bell-shaped distribution curve. Higher accommodative-stress groups have bimodal IOP response. The effect of extremes of nutrition and physical conditioning on IOP are indicated by broken curves for the low-accommodative-stress group. (Schiøtz tonometry, subjects ⩾ 40 years old.)

pressure in the vitreous, gradually transferred forward to the anterior chamber aqueous, with increased IOP eventually measured at the cornea.

MATERIAL AND METHODS

Out of 107 consecutive nutrition-workup patients (ages 7–76) selected for the study only 32 had eligible tonometric recordings after excluding all those persons with histories of medication or eye surgery known to influence IOP.

The study is retrospective, with double-masked data collection assuring freedom from investigator bias in scoring findings.

Nape-of-neck hair samples were examined for mineral absorption by spectroscopy (atomic absorption and optical emission techniques).

Computerized trace-mineral analysis and computerized dietary inventories (to produce quantifiable data for statistical evaluation) were tabulated for each patient. Tonometry was performed a.m. Goldmann; refractive values were given in spherical-equivalent form.

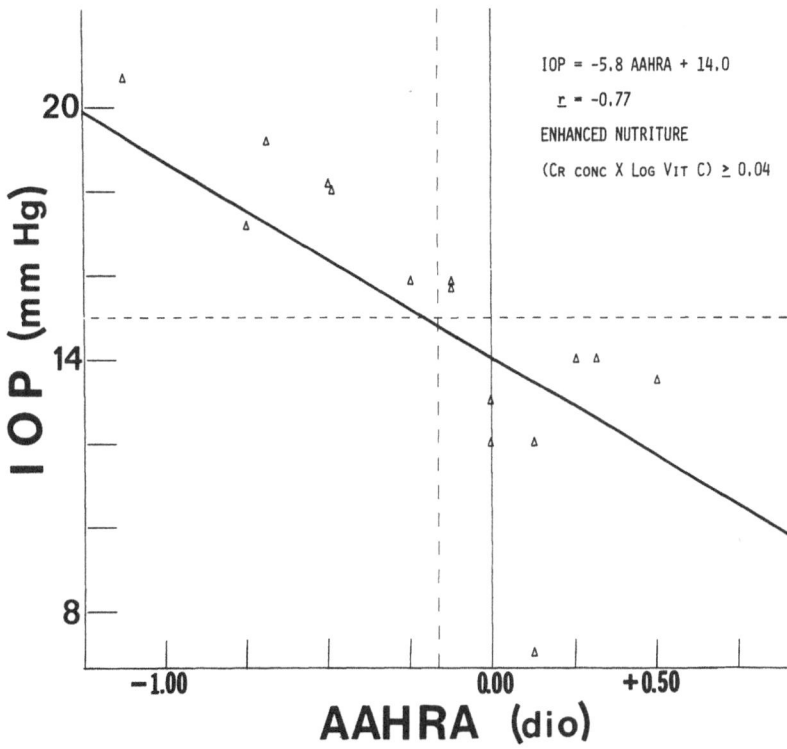

IOP = -5.8 AAHRA + 14.0

$\underline{r} = -0.77$

ENHANCED NUTRITURE

(Cr conc X Log Vit C) $\geq$ 0.04

Fig. 2. Correlation of controlling-eye IOP with Age-Adjusted Habitual Relative Add (AAHRA) for subjects with enhanced nutriture such that (Cr concn mg% in hair X log vit C intake mg) $\geqslant$ 0.04 mg% log mg. Broken lines indicate mean scores for IOP and AAHRA. All subjects with closework Rx's deemed adequate or more than adequate in plus dioptrics had IOPs below the mean. All subjects with inadequate closework Rx's had IOPs above the mean. Pearson $r = -0.77$. (Goldmann tonometry, subjects 26–59 years old.)

The IOP data of the near-point 'controlling eye' (cf. Lane 1980) was chosen for the study, because the nearpoint 'controlling eye' IOP data correlates best with nutriture factors in this study. Importantly, the controlling eye is the eye for which the accommodative level is actively and optimally set when the eyes are not co-equal partners.

Daily-repeated, sustained accommodative-stimulus stress was assessed with reference to the 'Age-Adjusted Habitual Relative Addition' (AAHRA), measured in diopters. The AAHRA is defined in short form as =

[(habitual near Rx prosthesis) − (distance vision ametropia)] minus (the median dioptric addition expected for the subject's age).

RESULTS

On the background of more extensive publication elsewhere (e.g. Lane, in press), the presentation of results is condensed to Tables 1–3 and Figures 1–3:

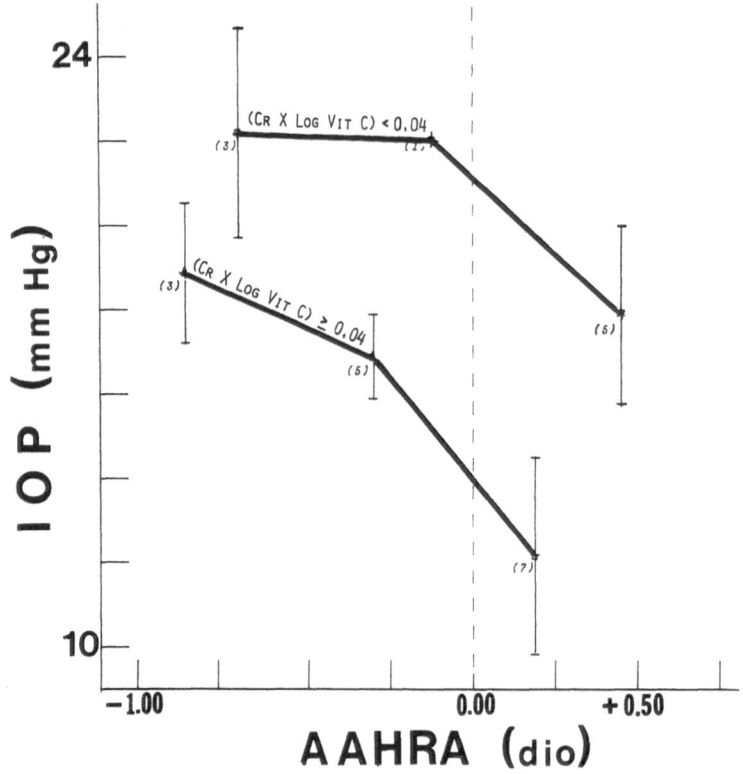

Fig. 3. Variation in controlling-eye IOP in relation to Age-Adjusted Habitual Relative Add (AAHRA) compared for deficient-nutriture group [(Cr concn X log vit C intake) < 0.04] vs enhanced-nutriture group [(Cr concn X log vit C intake) ≥ 0.04]. Vertical bars indicate range for ± 1 std dev IOP. IOP is elevated both by accommodative stimulus and by poor nutriture. Here we see graphically both the separation in IOP scores provided by nutriture and the effect created by accommodative-stimulus stress and AAHRA. The lower 39% of nutriture scores fall into the deficient-nutriture category in this sample. (Goldmann tonometry, ages 26–59.)

SUMMARY AND IMPLICATIONS

This study confirmed the author's (Lane 1973, 1980) 1973-study finding that the long-term effect of daily *sustained* accommodative stimulus is elevation of intraocular pressure (IOP).

New discoveries revealed by the present study include the following:

(1) IOP elevation is more closely correlated with increased stimulus to accommodation to the controlling eye – as if, according to the author's hypothesis, to elongate the eyeball to adjust as a servo-mechanism for the relative failure or difficulty of the controlling eye in fully responding to accommodative stimuli.

(2) IOP elevation in the controlling eye is closely associated with:

152

Table 1. IOP means for habitual vit C intake.§

Vit C intake (mg)			IOP (mm Hg)	
Group	Mean	Std Dev	Mean	Std Dev
< 85	74.6	± 6.8	22.33*	± 2.02
> 150	1205.0	± 1061.0	15.15*	± 3.40

*$p < 0.001$, $t = 4.58$ for difference between means; $df = 31$.
§ Ages 26–74, IOP for controlling eye.

Table 2. Difference in mean IOP with nutriture level ages 26–59.

Nutriture level	Controlling-eye IOP		N	t
Cr X log Vit C (mg% log mg)	Mean (mm Hg)	Std Dev'n (mm Hg)		
Enhanced (⩾ 0.045)	14.77	± 3.33	14	3.69*
Deficient (< 0.045)	19.65	± 2.84	10	

*$p < 0.01$

Table 3. Difference in mean IOP with accommodative stimulus ages 26–59.

Age-adj'd hab'l rel add (Diopter)	Controlling-eye IOP		N	t
	Mean (mm Hg)	Std Dev (mm Hg)		
Full-plus add: + 1 ⩾ AAHRA ⩾ 0	14.54	± 3.66	12	3.36*
Inad.-plus add: 0 > AAHRA ⩾ − 1	19.07	± 2.79	12	

*$p < 0.01$

    (a) decreasing tissue Cr concentration – possibly because of the importance of Cr in potentiating insulin in the process of mediating glucose metabolism required for long-sustained closework accommodation;

    (b) decreasing habitual ingestion (or body pool) of vitamin C (ascorbic acid or ascorbate), with physiological effectiveness proportional to the *logarithm* of the weight of ascorbic acid habitually ingested. [Habitual intake of less than 85 mg vitamin C per day is cause for concern!]

(3) Axial myopic increase requires both:

    (a) increased IOP, as may be triggered by decreased tissue Cr concentration and as related inversely to logarithm of vitamin C habitual ingestion, and as triggered by long-sustained, daily-repeated closework accommodative stimulus, but also as may become manifest secondary to many mechanical and biochemical factors; and

    (b) increased scleral distensibility—as occurs with calcium mishandling, often as related to excessive consumption of cooked protein or oxalates.

(4) Myopia progression is prevented by:

    (a) reducing stimulus to closework accommodation with:

        (i) plus-dioptric spherical addition lenses approximating the age-expected median add;

        (ii) redesign of the visual task and/or furnishings to allow for increased working distance;

    (b) increasing the amplitude of binocularly-fused Positive Relative Accommodation (PRA), especially with biofeedback training, but also with nutritional enhancement and other measures.

The confirmation of the long-term effect of accommodative stimulus on IOP renders more understandable the theories attempting to explain axial-elongation myopia, and even the transition from crystalline-lens myopia to axial myopia as debated by Sato (1957, 1964) and by Otsuka (1964).

In the light of this confirmation, the therapies advocated almost three decades ago to reduce IOP by underprescribing plus dioptrics (Lebensohn 1952) are no longer tenable. Additionally, this study has provided new insights into the importance of chromium as related to normal functioning of the visual system, as earlier independently suggested in this investigator's companion study (Lane 1981) in nutrition and myopia. Most importantly, new adjunctive hygienes can be identified and prescribed for the conservation and enhancement of vision and the prevention of myopia.

REFERENCES

Cohn, H. The hygiene of the eye in schools. (Transl. and ed W.P. Turnbull) Simpkin, Marshall & Co. London, (1886), (Originally published in German, 1883).

Cohn, H. Lehrbuch der Hygiene des Auges. Urban & Schwarzenberg, Vienna, (1892).

Hess, C. & Heine, L. Arbeiten aus dem Gebiet der Accommodationslehre: IV. Experimentelle Untersuchungen über den Einfluss der Accommodation auf den intraocularen Druck nebst Beiträgen zur Kenntnis der Accommodation verschiedener Säugethiere. Graefes Arch. 46: 243 (1898). Cited by T. Sato: The causes and prevention of acquired myopia. Kanehara Shuppan Tokyo, pp. 2 & 217 (1957).

Lane, B.C. Elevation of intraocular pressure with daily sustained reading and closework. Glaucoma Section Session II. Annual Meeting Program of the Assoc. for Res. Vision and Ophthalmology (Abstract) (2) p. 44 (May 5, 1973).

Lane, B.C. Nutrition and myopia. Lecture to the Myopia Symposium, American Academy of Optometry, Boston, Massachusetts, December 10, 1978. Reported in, Nutritional factors linked to development of myopia. Optometric Observer 4 (1): 1 & 5 (1979).

Lane, B.C. Elevation of intraocular pressure with daily, sustained reading and closework stimulus to accommodation. (Master's Thesis, State University of New York, State College of Optometry. 1973) University Microfilms International Ann Arbor, Michigan & London, Publication No. 13–14: 525 (1980).

Lane, B.C. Calcium, chromium, protein, sugar and accommodation in myopia. Docum. Ophthalmol. Proc. Series 28: 141–148 (1981).

Lane, B.C. Deficit nutritive, accomodative stimulus and ocular hypertension. Am J. Optom & Physiol Optics. In press.

Lebensohn, J.E.: Minus lenses as an effective adjuvant in the control of juvenile glaucoma. Am. J. Ophthalmol. 35: 1029 (1952).

Otsuka, J. My opinion on the cause and treatment of myopia. Paper presented at First Int Conf Myopia, New York (September 1964).

Sato, T. The causes and prevention of acquired myopia. Kanehara Shuppan Tokyo, (1957).

Sato, T. Acquired myopia. Paper presented at First Int Conf Myopia, New York (September 1964).

Young, F.A., Tanner, K.N., Leary, G.A. & Chatburn, C.C. Accommodation and fluorescein movement in monkey eyes. Invest. Ophthalmol. & Visual Sci. 18 (ARVO Suppl.) 13 (1979).

Author's address:
B.C. Lane, O.D., M.S.
16 North Beverwyck Road
Lake Hiawatha, New Jersey 07034
U.S.A.

THE RELATIONSHIP BETWEEN REFRACTIVE ERROR AND SCORES ON THE MINNESOTA MULTIPHASIC PERSONALITY INVENTORY

T. GROSVENOR

(Houston, Texas)

ABSTRACT

The Minnesota Multiphasic Personality Inventory (MMPI) was administered to 70 third year University of Houston optometry students, and the results were compared to the subjects' refractive errors. The MMPI consists of 566 test items, each item being a statement which the subject is asked to mark as true or false as applied to himself or herself. The test is scored in terms of ten scales: Hs (hypochondriasis), D (depression), Hy (hysteria, Pd (psychopathic deviate), Mf (masculinity-femininity, Pa (paranoia), Pt (psychasthenia), Sc (schizophrenia), Ma (hypomania) and Si (social introversion). Linear correlation coefficients between refractive error and each of the MMPI scales were determined, considering males and females separately, and the significance of each correlation coefficient was determined. It was found that the coefficients for the females for the Pd (psychopathic deviate) and Sc (schizophrenia) scales were significant at the 0.05 confidence level, whereas none of the correlation coefficients for males was found to be significant at this level. The results of the study are discussed in terms of the nature of the MMPI test and are compared to those of previous studies comparing refractive error and personality.

INTRODUCTION

A growing body of literature supports the assertion that personality characteristics of myopes differ from those of emmetropes and hyperopes. Many of the early reports were made strictly on the basis of observations: perhaps the earliest of these was that of Thorington who, as reported by Baldwin (1964) remarked in the year 1900 that myopes were introverted and shy, had few friends, and preferred indoor activities. A more recent observation was that of Gesell, *et al.* (1949) who reported that 'The pronounced myope ... gathers all experience unto himself and is in consequence better oriented within himself, but not so facilely oriented to his physical or social milieu.'

The first investigation designed for the purpose of relating refractive error to specific personality traits was that of Schapero and Hirsch (1952) who administered the Guilford-Martin Temperment Test to 119 optometry students and compared the results to spherical equivalent refractive error. These researchers concluded that myopes tended to have inhibited dispositions and overcontrol of emotions, tended to be inert and disinclined to motor activity, but scored high in social leadership; while hyperopes tended to have happy-go-lucky, carefree dispositions and to engage in vigorous activity but scored high in social passiveness. Schapero and Hirsch, however, warned that the degree of association was so slight as to be of no predictive value.

Additional studies showing relationships between myopia and personality traits have been reported by Van Alphen (1946) using the Rorschach test; by Young and his co-workers (1967, 1975, 1976) using the Edwards Personal Preference Test, the Strong Vocational Interest Inventory, the Omnibus Personality Inventory and the Gough Adjective Check List; and by Shultz (1966) using the Minnesota Multiphasic Personality Inventory (MMPI). In the Shultz study, the MMPI was administered to 131 clinical patients and hospital employees, with the result that a statistically significant finding occurred for only one of the 10 MMPI scales: hyperopes scored significantly higher on the Pd (psychopathic deviate) scale than emmetropes, while comparisons of myopes and hyperopes and of myopes and emmetropes resulted in no significant difference on this scale or on the other nine scales.

THE MINNESOTA MULTIPHASIC PERSONALITY INVENTORY

Hathaway and McKinley (1967) have described the MMPI as having been designed to provide 'an objective assessment of some of the major personality characteristics that effect personal and social adjustment', with the point of view of assaying 'those traits that are commonly characteristic of disabling psychological abnormalities.' The test consists of ten scales, each identifying a specific abnormality, which were developed by contrasting more than 800 patients from the neuropsychiatric division of the Minnesota University Hospitals with 700 'normal' individuals who visited University Hospital patients and were thus considered to be representative of the Minnesota population.

The ten scales are Hypochondriasis (Hs), Depression (D), Hysteria (Hy), Psychopathic deviate (Pd), Masculinity-femininity (Mf), Paranoia (Pa), Psychasthenia (Pt), Schizophrenia (Sc), Hypomania (Ma) and Social introversion (Si).

The test itself consists of a booklet containing 556 test items, each item consisting of a statement which the subject is instructed to mark as true or false as applied to himself or herself. The subject may leave a test item blank if he or she feels that the item does not apply, but is encouraged to leave as few spaces blank as possible.

SUBJECTS AND PROCEDURES

The MMPI was administered, during a regular class period, to 70 third year University of Houston optometry students. Due to the threatening nature

158

of many of the test items, students were instructed not to identify themselves by name but only by refractive error (sphere power, cylinder power and cylinder axis for right and left eyes) and by age and sex. The answer sheets were scored manually, using the templates supplied by the publisher.

Data for only 64 of the 70 subjects were usable, since six subjects failed to specify sex. Of the 64 subjects, 46 were males and 18 were females. Data were analyzed separately for the two sexes. Refractive error was specified in terms of spherical equivalent refraction for the right eye of each subject. For each of the 10 MMPI scales, linear correlation coefficients were determined between spherical equivalent refraction and raw MMPI scores.

RESULTS

Refractive Error Distribution

The refractive error distribution for the 64 subjects is shown in Table 1. It is of interest that 46 of the 64 subjects (or 72%) were myopes, and that only three subjects (5%) were in the + 1.00 D to + 1.87 D category. Although not indicated in Table 1, the highest hyperope, a female, had a spherical equivalent refraction of only + 1.37 D.

Table 1. Refractive Error Distribution.

Spherical Equivalent Refraction (R.E.)	Males	Females	Total
+ 1.00 D to + 1.87 D	0	3	3
Plano to + 0.87 D	10	5	15
− 0.12 D to − 1.00 D	8	3	11
− 1.12 D to − 2.00 D	7	1	8
− 2.12 D to − 3.00 D	6	3	9
− 3.12 D to − 4.00 D	7	1	8
− 4.12 D to − 5.00 D	3	0	3
− 5.12 D to − 6.00 D	3	2	5
− 6.12 D to − 7.00 D	1	0	1
− 7.12 D to − 8.00 D	1	0	1

Correlation Coefficients

Coefficients of correlation between refractive error and raw scores for each of the MMPI scales are shown in Table 2. The significance of each of the correlation coefficients was determined, and it was found that the correlations for females for the Pd (psychopathic deviate) and Sc (schizophrenic) scales were significant at the 0.05 confidence level, whereas none of the correlation coefficients for males was significant at this level. The + signs for the above correlations (+ 0.44 for Pd and + 0.45 for Sc) indicate that these traits tend to be associated with increasing hyperopia or decreasing myopia.

It should be emphasized that the relationships found here are not particularly strong relationships, and as with those reported by Schapero and

Table 2. Correlation Coefficients Between Refractive Error and each of the 10 MMPI Scales.

Scale	Males (N = 46)	Females (N = 18)
Hs hypochondriasis	0.13	0.29
D depression	0.11	0.26
Hy hysteria	0.01	0.10
Pd psychopathic deviate	0.00	0.44*
Mf masculinity-femininity	0.14	−0.12
Pa paranoia	0.00	0.18
Pt psychasthenia	−0.14	0.36
Sc schizophrenia	0.01	0.45*
Ma hypomania	−0.07	0.30
Si social introversion	0.03	0.16

*significant at the 0.05 confidence level

Hirsch are not strong enough to be of predictive value. It is of interest that in the Shultz study which also used the MMPI, the only significant relationship found was a significantly higher score on the Pd (psychopathic deviate) scale for hyperopes as compared to emmetropes (both sexes being considered together).

DISCUSSION

It is of interest that even though the 'conventional wisdom' of myopia (as indicated by the observations of Thorington and of Gesell et al) tells us that myopes are shy, introverted and introspective people, neither the present study nor the Shultz study resulted in significant relationships between refractive error and the Si (social introversion) scale of the MMPI. The lack of such a relationship may be explained partially on the basis of the method used to derive the Si scale. As described by Welsh and Dahlstrom (1960) this scale was validated on a group of University of Wisconsin female students during the years 1944–1945 (when few male students were available) and was based on the extent to which the subjects were involved in extra-curricular activities in high school or college: girls who scored *high* on the Si scale were found to be those who engaged in from four to six extra-curricular activities, whereas those who engaged in only one or two extra-curricular activities were found to score *low* on the Si scale. This being the case, a much more direct method of determining social introversion might be to simply ask the subject how many extra-curricular activities he or she engaged in, in high school or college!

The conventional wisdom of myopia *was* supported by the studies of Schapero and Hirsch (1952) and of Bedell and Young (1976), Schapero and Hirsch finding that myopes tended to have inhibited dispositions while hyperopes tended to be happy-go-lucky and carefree, and Bedell and Young finding that myopes exhibited introverted personality patterns while hyperopes tended to be extroverted. However the finding of Schapero and Hirsch that myopes scored high in *social leadership* while hyperopes showed a tendency for *social passiveness* is difficult to rationalize with the picture of the myope as an introvert and the hyperope as an extrovert.

Perhaps the conventional wisdom of myopia itself should be called into question. Observations that myopes are shy and introverted may well apply less to 'corrected' myopes than to uncorrected myopes: inability to succeed at baseball and other games or inability to recognize one's classmates on the playground may well be causes of shy and introverted behavior.

For the first few children in the classroom who appear in school wearing glasses (these are the children who will become the *highest* myopes), the 'correction' of myopia with glasses is sure to be greeted with shouts of 'four-eyes', further reinforcing previously acquired introvertive patterns. In contrast, the children who will become myopic later in their school years or even in college (the moderate and low myopes) are spared this embarrassment since glasses are commonplace in the upper grades of school and in college.

Even the higher myopes, once they have survived the ravages of elementary school, have reason to face the world more confidently than their myopic parents did. Whereas previous generations of myopic high school and college students were forced to wear 'ugly' glasses or to view the world dimly – a choice still preferable to some myopes – the present-day availability of fashion frames and contact lenses may well remove the major cause of shyness and introversion.

The preceding discussion is consistent with the contention that myopia is the cause, rather than the result, of personality traits. To the extent that personality traits may cause myopia or to the extent that myopia and personality traits may spring from a common underlying factor, the conventional wisdom of myopia may retain a degree of validity.

REFERENCES

Baldwin, W.R. Some Relationships Between Ocular, Anthropometric and Refractive Variables in Myopia, unpublished doctoral dissertation, Indiana University, Bloomington, Indiana (1964).

Bedell, S.L. & Young, F.A. Personality, physical characteristics and refractive error. Am J Optom. 53: 735–739 (1976).

Gesell, A., F.L. Ilg & G.E. Bullis Vision, its Development in Infant and Child, Hoeber, New York (1949).

Hathaway, S.R. & McKinley, J.C. Manual, Minnesota Multiphasic Personality Inventory, Psychological Corp., New York (1967).

Schapero, M. & M.J. Hirsch The relationship of refractive error and Guilford-Martin temperment test scores, Am. J Optom. 29: 32–36 (1952).

Shultz, L.B. Personality and physical variables as related to refractive errors, Am. J Optom. 37: 551–571 (1960).

Van Alphen, G.W.H.M. On Emmetropia and Ametropia (supplementum ad Ophthalmogica, Vol. 142), S. Karger, Basel & New York (1961).

Welsch, G.S. & W.G. Dahlstrom Basic Readings on The MMPI in Psychology and Medicine, Univ. of Minn. Press, Minneapolis, 184–185 (1960).

Young, F.A. Personality and myopia, Am. J Optom. 44: 192–198 (1967).

Young, F.A., Singer, R.M. & Foster, D. The psychological differentiation of male myopes and nonmyopes, Am. J Optom. 52: 679–686 (1975).

Author's address:
Professor T. Grosvenor,
College of Optometry
University of Houston
Houston, Texas 77004

MYOPIA AND THE EXTRAOCULAR MUSCLES

P.R. GREENE

(Cambridge, Mass. U.S.A.)

ABSTRACT

Axial myopia is a common ocular problem characterized by the fact that the posterior sclera has apparently stretched out of shape over a period of several years. The debate persists as to whether myopia is an inherited or acquired disorder. During the last few years, several new laboratory techniques have surfaced which can create large amounts of myopia in normal experimental animals. In an attempt to find a mechanical explanation common to both human and laboratory myopia, this paper examines the stresses experienced by the posterior sclera as a result of accommodation, convergence, vitreous pressure, and the extraocular muscles. The conclusion is that convergence, and more generally, the tension in the extraocular muscles, are mechanically much more important than accommodation because of the sizeable increase in vitreous pressure. The oblique muscles, because of their attachment sites at the back of the globe near the optic nerve entrance port, have the capability of producing local stress concentrations which may be very important in understanding pathological myopia.

INTRODUCTION

From literature, a great deal of information has been collected (cf. Greene 1980) around the general subject of myopia (axial, pathological, and experimental) and there is no *a priori* reason to assume that there is but one causative factor at work in these various cases. Moreover, there is no reason to preferentially look for a mechanical explanation, as opposed to say, a biochemical or genetic explanation. Nevertheless, because the net result in all cases is a distorted sclera, and because myopia can be imposed on otherwise normal experimental animals, it seems reasonable to explore the possibility of a common mechanical cause.

This is the purpose of the present paper. Analyses are made of the mechanical stress on the spherical eye ball exerted by the external eye muscles (including the obliques) with special regard to the tensile stress

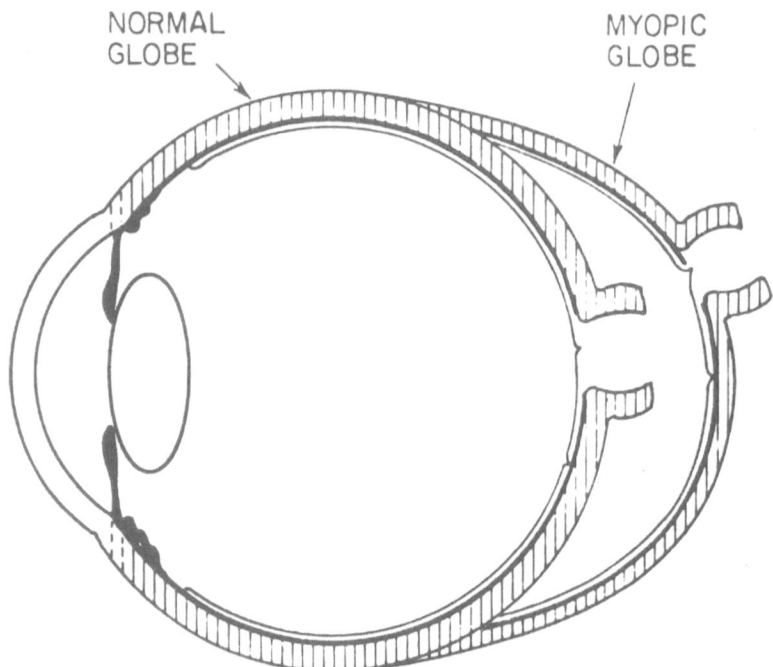

NORMAL
GLOBE

MYOPIC
GLOBE

Fig. 1. Geometry of the axially myopic globe superimposed on the normal emmetropic globe. Sketch shows the prolate geometry and scleral thinning characteristic of the posterior half of the axially myopic eye. Also note that the degree of implied stretching is greater on the temporal side. This sketch represents a horizontal section through the left globe, viewed from above. (Modified after Southall 1961).

in the posterior sclera and the 'stress concentration factor' related to the optic nerve entrance port.

RESULTS

Being published in detail elsewhere (Greene 1980), the main results will here be strongly condensed, as given by Table 1 and Figures 1–6.

DISCUSSION

This paper presents a review of the mechanical phenomenon which are most likely to cause axial, pathological, and experimental myopia. The calculations argue that the oblique muscles can exert significant amounts of localized tensile stress on the posterior sclera, and, with the increase in vitreous pressure attendant with convergence, this concentrated stress may be sufficiently large to permanently stretch the sclera out of shape. It has been shown in vitro that when elevated stress is applied for moderate durations of time, the sclera will creep permanently out of shape (Greene and McMahon, 1979).

164

Table 1. Mechanical Stress in Sclera Near Oblique Muscle Attachments in g/mm² as a Function of Muscle Force and Attachment Width.

Muscle Attachment	Muscle Force in grams			
Width in Millimeters	10g	20g	30g	40g
5 mm	1.0	2.0	3.0	4.0
7 mm	0.71	1.43	2.13	2.84
9 mm	0.56	1.12	1.68	2.24
11 mm	0.45	0.90	1.35	1.80
14 mm	0.36	0.71	1.08	1.44

Note: this table assumes a scleral thickness of 1.0 mm. A useful number to compare these tabulated values with is the stress imposed by normal intraocular pressure. For a globe of radius 12 mm, IOP of 15 mmHg, and scleral thickness of 1.0 mm, the stress is 1.2 g/mm².

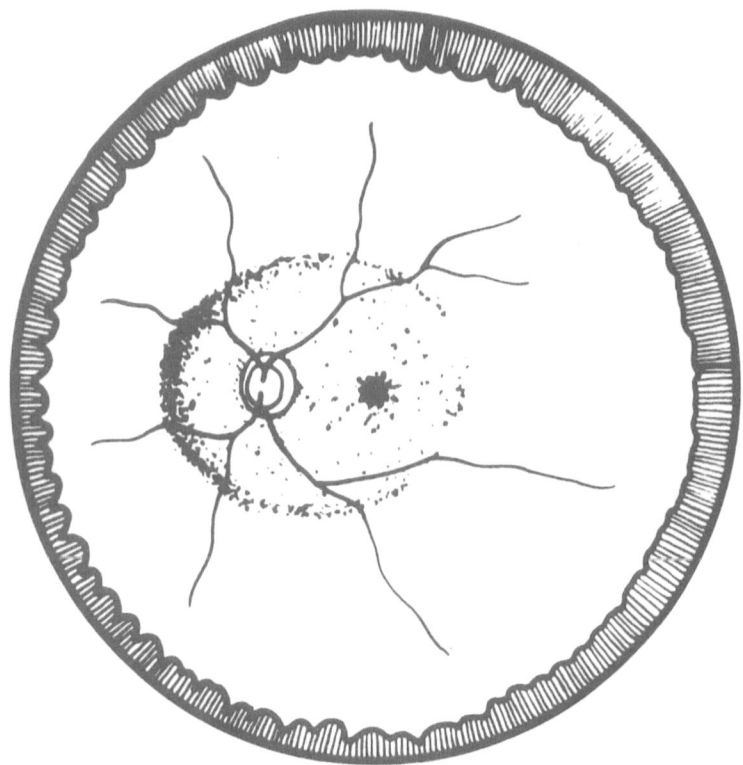

Fig. 2. Fundus sketch of the posterior staphyloma from an eye with pathological myopia. Fundus of the left eye, viewed from the front, is shown. Shaded area represents the localized herniation or out-pouching characteristic of this problem. The staphyloma varies from one individual to the next in size, shape, depth, abruptness of the margin, and associated changes in the optic nerve and retinal vessels. (Modified after Curtin 1977).

165

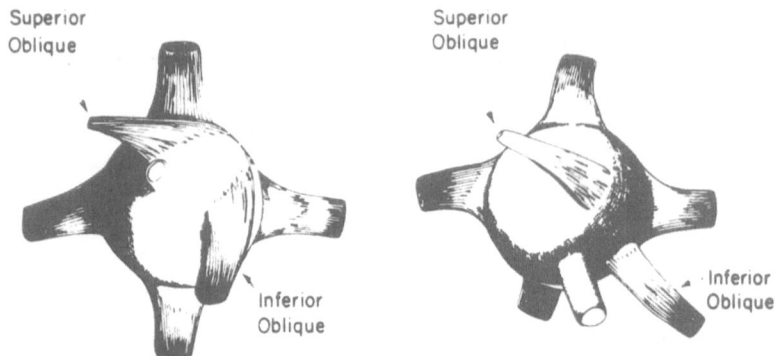

Fig. 3. Two slightly different views of the posterior aspect of the normal human globe showing the attachment locations of the superior and inferior oblique muscles. Note that the attachment widths and locations with respect to the optic nerve can vary. (Modified after Sobotta 1957).

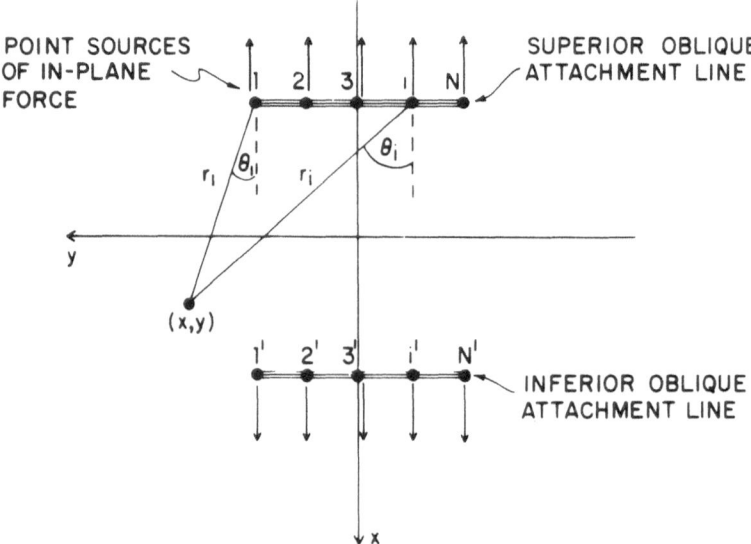

Fig. 4. Co-ordinate system for the computer program which models plate stretching due to the antagonistic pull of the superior and inferior oblique muscles. A line of N point sources, each of equal strength, is used to model the pull of each oblique muscle on the sclera. A separate (r, θ) co-ordinate system is attached to each point source of force, in order to calculate its contribution at the point (x, y) in the plane.

The important mechanical and geometric parameters are: the width of the oblique muscle attachment lines, the separation distance of these attachment lines, the tension in the obliques, both statically and during convergence, the location of the oblique attachment lines with respect

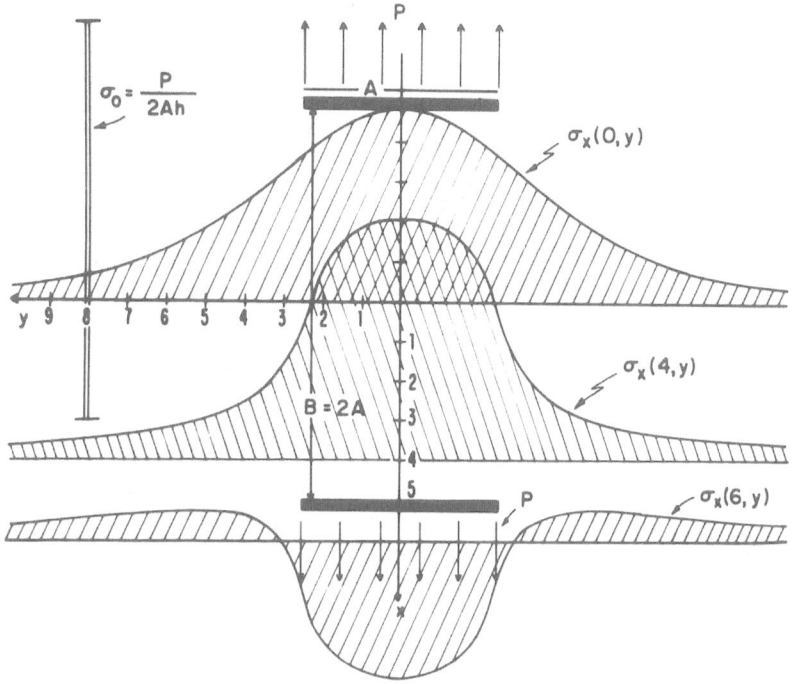

Fig. 5. Results of the plate-stretching computer program showing the distribution of stress at 3 different traverse locations with respect to the oblique muscles. For this particular case, the muscles are separated by a distance equal to twice their width. Note that in all cases, the stress field diffuses considerably off the centerline. Also note that in some regions, the stress field changes sign from tensile to compressive stress.

to the optic nerve entrance port, the thickness of the posterior sclera, the intrinsic mechanical properties of the posterior sclera, and finally, the vitreous pressure, both statically and during convergence. A knowledge of all of these parameters allows one to calculate the local mechanical stress (in g/mm^2) experienced by the posterior sclera at both the leading and trailing edges of the oblique attachment lines, before and during convergence, and to estimate the likelihood of permanent scleral distortion. The very worst case is realized by narrow attachment lines, high tension in the obliques, oblique attachments close to the optic nerve, a thin posterior sclera, a sclera with a high propensity to creep, and finally, high vitreous pressure.

These calculations make a prediction which may be useful for the *management of pathological myopia.* Since the posterior staphyloma in pathological myopia seems to occur because of a stress concentration near and around the optic nerve entrance port, and since the sclera is also locally weak, the recommendation is to relieve this stress concentration by relocating or flaring the oblique attachment sites. In particular, the inferior oblique

167

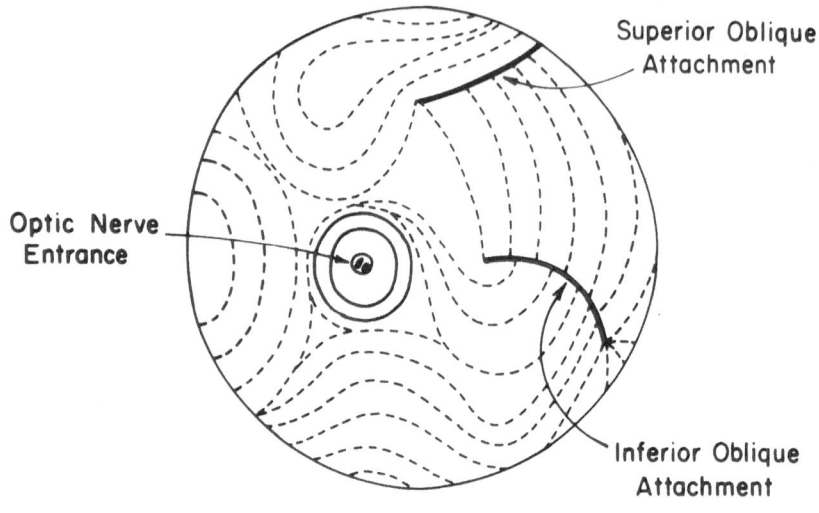

Superior Oblique
Attachment

Optic Nerve
Entrance

Inferior Oblique
Attachment

POSTERIOR VIEW OF RIGHT EYE

Fig. 6a. Schematic diagram showing primary fibril bundle orientation in the posterior sclera. Note that the sclera seems to have responded to the structural demands placed on it by the antagonistic pull of the superior and inferior oblique muscles.

attachment should be moved anteriorly, since it is often depicted in anatomy texts as being very close to the optic nerve. Moving one, or preferably both oblique attachments anteriorly accomplishes two things: first, it moves the most intense part of the oblique stress field away from the optic nerve, so that the stress concentration effect is minimized, and second, it reduces the static tension on the obliques. However, this procedure may prove difficult in that it may lead to alignment problems with the eyes.

Another surgical possibility for reducing the stress imposed on the sclera by the obliques is to flare the end of the muscle or ligament, so as to increase the attachment width, and thereby decrease the local mechanical stress. A third surgical possibility is to slacken the tension on both the medial and lateral rectus muscles, so that convergence can occur without a dramatic rise in vitreous pressure. This surgical alternative is particularly attractive, because it can be done without altering the alignment of the eyes.

Lastly, there is the subject of *practical diagnostic techniques* which can be used in a clinical setting for the purpose of predicting the course of events for an individual with progressive myopia. Quantitative information about the oblique muscles and the medial recti would seem to be important, specifically, the location of the attachment sites, their widths, and in addition, their resting tension and tension during convergence. Measurements of changes in vitreous pressure statically and during convergence would be very useful.

168

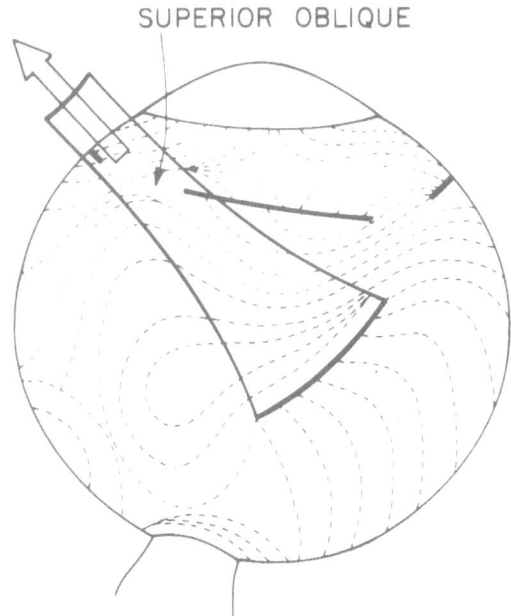

SUPERIOR OBLIQUE

Fig. 6b. Fibril bundle directions as viewed from the top of the right eye. To a certain limited extent, the same effect of altered fiber directions can be detected near and around the superior rectus, but the effect is less pronounced than with the superior oblique. (Modified after Hogan *et al.* 1971).

REFERENCES

Curtin, R.J. The posterior Staphyloma of Pathologic Myopia, Trans. Am. Ophthalmol. Soc. 75, 67 (1977).

Greene, P.R., and McMahon, T.A., Scleral Creep vs. Temperature and Pressure in vitro, Exp. Eye Res., V29, 1979 pp. 527–537.

Greene, P.R.: Mechanical considerations in myopia: Relative effects of accommodation, convergence, intraocular pressure and the extraocular muscles. Am. J. of Optom. Physiol. Optics 57: 902–914 (1980).

Hogan, M.J., et al. Histology of the Human Eye, an Atlas and Textbook, W.B. Saunders Co., Philadelphia (1971).

Sobotta, M.J. Atlas of Descriptive Human Anatomy, Hafner Publishing Co., New York (1957).

Southall, J.P.C. Introduction to Physiological Optics, Dover, New York (1961).

Author's address:
Assist. Professor Peter R. Greene, Ph.D.
Dept. of Biomedical Engineering
Johns Hopkins University
317 Maryland Hall
Baltimore, Maryland 21218
U.S.A.

INTRAOCULAR PRESSURE DYNAMICS ASSOCIATED WITH ACCOMMODATION

F.A. YOUNG

(Pullman, Washington and Houston, Texas, USA)

ABSTRACT

Anterior chamber pressure drops when a human or monkey accommodates while vitreous chamber pressure rises when a monkey accommodates. Since the monkey eye is very similar to the human eye, the rise in vitreous chamber pressure may also occur in the human eye. Measurement of fluorescein transport time from vitreal injection to appearance at the edge of the pupil is related to accommodation. With cycloplegia the movement takes 12 min; with normal eye conditions 30 min; under eserine 80 min; under eye contact induced accommodation fluorescein does not appear as long as accommodation is maintained. The implications of this effect are considered.

INTRODUCTION

Armaly and Rubin (1961) have reported that the intraocular pressure, as measured by applanation tonometry, drops when a person accommodates and remains down if accommodation is maintained. The stimulus used for accommodation was a Landolt ring at 25 cm Accommodation was relaxed by placing a 4.0 D plus lens in front of the eye viewing the target. Tonometry was done on the nonviewing eye. The drop in pressure begins almost as soon as the 4.0 D lens is removed but required an average of 2.7 min for younger subjects (20–25 years) to reach the maximum average drop of 4.5 mm Hg. Older subjects (45–55 years) required an average of 4.0 min to reach an average drop of 2.3 mm Hg. While we have not measured the response to accommodation in monkeys over time, there is a similar drop in anterior chamber pressure when the monkey accommodates.

Coleman and Young (1972) measured the differential pressure in the anterior and in the vitreous chambers when the ciliary muscle of chimpanzee, baboon, monkey and cat eyes was stimulated electrically. The experimental design used simultaneous manometry of the two chambers and recorded the differential output of the double transducers. Unfortunately, it was very difficult to maintain the patency of the manometer in the vitreous chamber since the vitreous would plug the manometer in a minute or two

The records that were obtained, particularly with cats, clearly indicate a gradient with an increase in vitreous chamber pressure and a decrease in anterior chamber pressure when the ciliary muscle is stimulated.

Young (1975) later used a surgically implanted radiosonde transducer which was designed by Collins (1967) to measure pressure changes in the monkey eye. This unit, which is slightly smaller than an aspirin tablet, was inserted into the vitreous chamber and floats to the top of the eye. The unit requires no connections since it is activated by radio frequency impulses beamed into the eye by an intermittent source. The source acts as a receiver and the output from the transducer is amplified and displayed on an oscilloscope. Through the use of this unit, pressure was measured in one eye of each of two Macaca nemestrina (pigtail) monkeys. The pigtail monkey has a very strong eye-contact response and will continue to look at the eyes of a human as long as the human will look at the monkey. Using a man's eye contact as a stimulus for a chaired monkey, we found that the pressure increased linearly as the man moved from 20 ft to 1 ft from the monkeys face. When the man stared at the monkey continuously for 45 min, the elevated pressure remained constant. When the man backed away from the monkey but maintained eye contact, the pressure linearly returned to its initial value of approximately 12 mm Hg. The increase in pressure appeared to be 6–7 mm Hg at the 1 ft distance.

If the similar pressure-drops in the anterior chambers of the man and monkey eyes under accommodation and the general similarity of the two eyes are acknowledged, the likelihood is high that there is a similar increase in pressure in human vitreous when the human accommodates even though this has not been measured. In order to have two separate pressures in the two chambers of the eye simultaneously and, apparently reciprocally, there must be some type of mechanism to support this effect.

Suzuki (1973) has reported the X-ray observed movement of water-soluble radiopaque materials injected directly into the vitreous chamber of the cat eye. The water-soluble material dispersed slightly and moved forward toward the lens, around the edge of the lens, between the lens and the iris into the anterior chamber, and out of the eye. Oily radiopaque material moved forward toward the anterior vitreous and stopped; it remained in the vitreous for the hour observation time.

Jacobsen (1977) reported that in the eye of the owl monkey the vitreous structure is more clearly demarcated than in man or pigtail monkeys. The owl monkey vitreous has a thick peripheral structured layer, like the shell of an egg, with an aqueous-like liquid in the center of the vitreous. The outer ring allows water soluble material to pass through but will not pass high molecular weight substances.

It appears that the hyaloid membrane and its associated elements may act like a differentially permeable membrane under certain conditions. If it should stop the normal movement of fluid (aqueous?) from the vitreous chamber into the anterior chamber when the eye accommodates strongly, it could result in a build up of pressure in the vitreous chamber and a simultaneous drop in anterior chamber pressure. The change in pressure in the vitreous chamber may also play a role in the process of accommodation.

The purpose of the present study is to evaluate the effect of accommodation on the movement of fluorescein from the vitreous chamber of the pigtail monkey eye into the anterior chamber.

METHODS

Pigtail monkeys were anesthetized with Ketamine at a dosage level of one mg/lb. After the anesthesia took effect, 0.5 ml of injectable fluorescein was injected into the vitreous chamber as near to the center as possible. After injection the monkey was placed in a restraining chair to permit observation of the eye under ultraviolet light. The time required for the dye to enter the anterior chamber over the edge of the pupil was measured for a variety of conditions.

(1) General anesthesia only – two animals.
(2) General anesthesia plus one drop of 2% and three drops of 1% Cyclogyl.
(3) General anesthesia plus two drops of 0.5% eserine in two monkeys, one with an iris and one with a Tornquist type iridectomy.
(4) General anesthesia for instillation and chairing, but animal was alert for observation. Two animals – one normal and one with vitrectomy. Condition (2) involved only one animal and a total of seven animals were used, and only one eye was used. Two observers carried out the observations.

RESULTS

The results are presented in Table 1. In general there was close agreement in the time required for the dye to appear at the edge of the pupil under similar conditions but there were differences between the normal and vitrectomized eyes. The fluorescein generally appeared to spread throughout the vitreous as far as could be seen by looking through the dilated pupil on the animal under Cyclogyl. In the case of the vitrectomized eye the spread was very rapid taking only two or three minutes, compared with the usual 10 to 12 min of spreading. The animals in Condition (4) were examined under the eye contact condition so that they were accommodating normally without the effects of any drugs.

DISCUSSION

The fluorescein appeared at the edge of the pupil in 25 to 30 min for the two monkeys under general anesthesia. This time is consistent with that reported by Gloor (1970) for the movement of fluid from the vitreous into the anterior chamber of 30 min. Since there is the possibility that the eye is in a state of partial accommodation while under anesthesia, this finding may be contrasted with that found under Cyclogyl.

Table 1. Time expiring between injection of fluorescein in the vitreous chamber of pigtail monkey eyes under different treatments and its appearance at the edge of pupil of the eye.

Treatment	Monkey 1 – time	Monkey 2 – time	Comments
General anesthesia only	25 min	30 min	
General anesthesia & Cyclogyl	12 min		
General anesthesia & eserine	81 min	75 min	Monkey 2 iridectomy
Alert Animal	70 min	66 min	Staring 60 min Monkey 2 vitrectomy

When the animal was under both general anesthesia and Cyclogyl, the dye appeared at the edge of the pupil in only 12 min, instead of the 25 and 30 min required for the monkeys under general anesthesia without Cyclogyl. Since the animal could not accommodate under the dosage level of Cyclogyl used, the more rapid movement when accommodation is prevented suggests that accommodation must be active in the animals under general anesthesia only. This finding also suggests that the most effective way to measure intraocular pressure may be under a cycloplegic.

As may be expected, the eserine causes a very strong miotic effect as well as an accommodative response. To control for the possibility that the fluorescein did not appear because of the joint effect of miosis and accommodation in blocking the movement of fluid between the iris and lens, we used an animal with an iridectomy which prevented the iris from responding to the eserine. Under these conditions the movement of the dye around the edge of the lens could be observed. The time of appearance of the fluorescein was similar in the two eyes. In the normal eye the pupil had dilated to about 4 mm before the dye appeared at the edge of the pupil. Since the time intervals are close whether the iris is present or not, the iris would appear to have little or no effect on the movement of the fluid in the eye.

Condition (4) provides the best evidence of the role of accommodation in affecting the movement of fluid in the eye. As long as eye contact was maintained no fluorescein appeared at the pupil. Since normal accommodative responses were more effective in raising the pressure in the vitreous chamber (as measured with the radiosonde device) than eserine or pilocarpine, it is likely that it is also more effective in blocking fluid movement in the eye. Although we stopped staring at the monkey after an hour and a quarter, it is probable that if this staring had been continued longer the blockage would also have continued.

The vitrectomized animal had a similar response to the eye contact as that of the normal monkey – no fluorescein appeared until after the eye contact had been broken. After breaking eye contact the fluorescein appeared slightly quicker in the vitrectomized eye than in the normal eye, but the vitrectomy did not basically effect the blockage of fluid movement demonstrated in all of the eyes examined.

It is possible that the drop in anterior chamber pressure results from the decrease in the amount of fluid entering the anterior chamber from the vitreous chamber. It is also possible that the fluid which moves from the vitreous chamber into the anterior chamber is aqueous humor. The movement appears to occur in one direction only, from the vitreous chamber into the anterior chamber. If this is so, the aqueous humor must be deposited in the vitreous chamber rather than in the posterior chamber. The fact that in severe myopia the volume of the eye may almost double without a serious loss of eye pressure suggests that aqueous humor is entering the vitreous chamber to fill the increased volume since no new vitreous can develop.

Further, the increase in pressure in the vitreous chamber may be involved in the increase in size of the vitreous chamber which appears to play the major role in the development of both 'Emmetropization' and myopia. Unpublished longitudinal studies of children and monkeys using ultrasound and phakometry indicate, that the increase in the size of the vitreous chamber is the major change occurring when the refractive characteristics of the eyes start to move toward myopia.

The pressure changes in the vitreous chamber may also play a role in the process of accommodation since the back lens surface could be molded by the increase in pressure more effectively than the front lens surface. Unpublished phakometric studies now indicate that the back lens surface contributes almost twice as much to the total vergence of light and is second only to the cornea in its refractive power. The attachment of the hyaloid membrane to the back lens surface may play a major role in the development of the greater lens power of the back lens surface. There is some evidence from children phakometry that the back lens may have several curvatures rather than the simple, monotonic curve of the front lens surface.

Finally, there is a possibility that the blockage of fluid movement plays a role in low tension glaucoma, in the development of high myopia as well as low myopia, and in the general deterioration of the choroid and retina, since the pressure levels are high enough to have some effect on the blood flow through the choroid.

REFERENCES

Armaly, M.F. & Rubin, M.L. Accommodation and applanation tonometry. Arch. Ophthalmol. 65 (3): 415–423 (1961).

Coleman, D.J. & Young, F.A. Measurement of vitreous-aqueous pressure gradient during ciliary muscle stimulation. Paper presented at Assoc. Res. Vision and Ophthalmol. Meeting, Sarasota, Fla. (April, 1972).

Collins, C.C. Minature passive pressure transensor for implanting in the eye. IEEE Trans. Bio-Medical Engineering, 14 (2): 74–83 (1967).

Gloor, B.P. Physiology of the vitreous. In: Adler's Physiology of the Eye Ed. Moses, R.A. St. Louis, C.V. Mosby Co. 311–332 (1970).

Jacobsen, B. Personal communication (1977).

Suzuki, H. Observations on the intraocular changes associated with accommodation; an experimental study using radiographic technique. Exp. Eye Res. 17 (2): 119–128 (1973).

Young, F.A. The development and control of myopia in human and subhuman primates. Contacto, 19 (6): 16–31 (1975).

Author's address:
Professor F.A. Young, Ph.D.
Primate Research Center, Washington State University
Pullman, Washington 99164
U.S.A.

A STUDY OF EXPERIMENTAL MYOPIA AFTER ENCIRCLING OPERATION

Y. BABA and A. SAWADA

(Miyazaki, Japan)

ABSTRACT

Myopia or increase in myopia after encircling operation for retinal detachment is not completely elucidated. To clarify the features of the induced myopia, the axial length was measured with Digital Biometric Ruler 300, and changes in refractive power were studied with Rodenstock refractometer for six months after encircling operation in rabbit eyes. In all cases myopia could be produced. The amount of myopia was directly proportional to the tightness of encircling. The axial length was likewise elongated almost proportional to the tightness of encircling. The relationship between these changes and the passage of time is discussed. Furthermore, increase of vitreous length and decrease of corneal curvature radius were important features.

INTRODUCTION

Myopia or increase in myopia after an encircling operation for retinal detachment has not been completely elucidated (Rubin 1975; Burton *et al.* 1977; Larsen and Syrdalen 1979). It is the purpose of this paper to clarify the true character of induced or increased myopia and to investigate the role of both refractive and axial factors in producing refractive changes.

MATERIAL AND METHODS

Changes in refraction were measured with Rodenstock's refractometer. Axial length and the length of ocular dimensions were measured with Digital Biometric Ruler 300. Changes in the radius of corneal curvature were measured with Bausch and Lomb's keratometer. These measurements were done for six months after encircling operations with silicone rods. The right eyes of pigmented rabbits were operated on and the left eyes were used as controls.

To determine the reliability of measurements, the refractive power, axial length and the length of ocular dimensions, and the radius of corneal

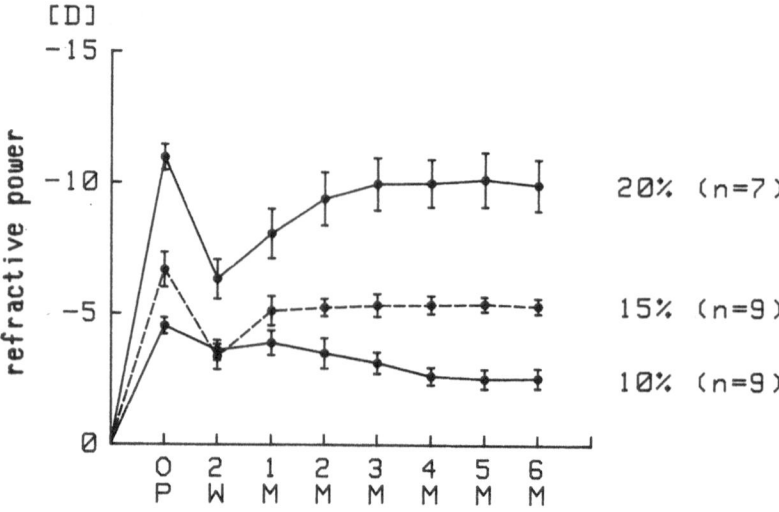

Fig. 1. Changes in refraction after encircling operations with different tightness.

curvature were measured ten times before the encircling operation on all 25 rabbits used in experiments. Values in each animal were stable and standard deviation was very small. No significant difference was found in the two eyes of each subject. These results show that the measurement procedures were precise and that contralateral eyes are valid as controls.

Dimensional changes occurring after an encircling operation depend greatly on the tightness of encirclement. Tightness was regulated by the length of the silicone rod sutured on the sclera. Rabbits were divided into three groups, based on the tightness of encirclement, namely 10%, 15% and 20%. Tightness of 10% means that encircling was done with the silicone rod of the length of 90% of the total circumference at the equator. In encircling operations with 15% tightness, encircling was done with the length of 85% of the total circumference. In 20% tightness encircling was done with the length of 80% of the total circumference. Nine rabbits with a tightness of 10%, nine with 15%, and seven with 20% were successively measured for six months.

RESULTS

Refraction

Figure 1 shows changes in refractive power from the controls after the encircling operation with various degrees of tightness. Immediately after the operation myopia developed markedly in all eyes in proportion to the tightness of encircling. During the first two weeks the degree of myopia reduced with a relative rapidity. Thereafter, the degree of myopia started to increase again in eyes in which the encircling was more tightly done

178

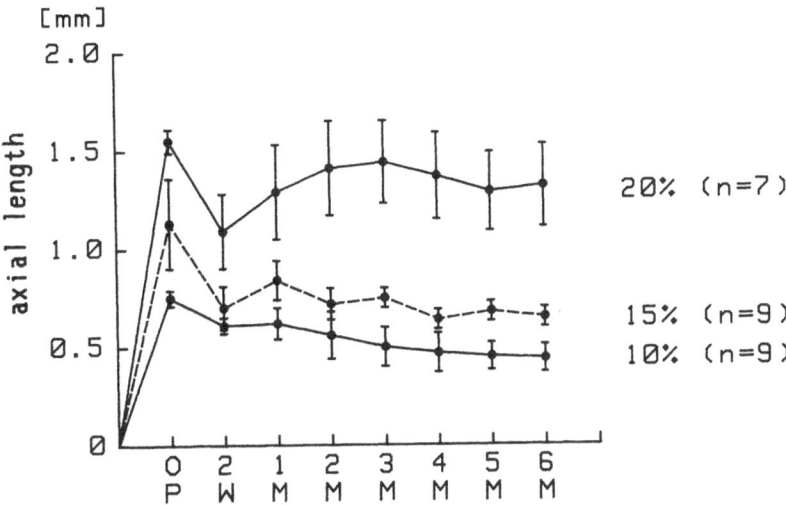

Fig. 2. Changes in axial length after encircling operations with different tightness.

(15% and 20%). At two months the variation in the degree of myopia was small, and thereafter the degree ceased to vary. At six months myopia was present in proportion to the tightness of encirclement.

What factors produced these changes in the degree of myopia in course of time after the encircling operation? Were these factors changes in axial length or in radius of corneal curvature?

Axial length

First, changes in axial length and the length of its components will be discussed as the main factor producing myopia or increase of myopia.

Figure 2 shows changes in axial length (as compared with the control eye of the animal) after encircling operation with various degrees of tightness. Immediately after the operation, axial length was markedly elongated in all eyes in proportion to the tightness of encircling. The degree of elongation then tended to decrease during the first two weeks in all groups. Thereafter, in the groups with the tightness of 15% and 20%, elongation started to increase again. However, elongation stopped to increase in the groups with 10% and 15% tightness at two months. The difference between the three groups remained statistically significant during the rest of the observation period.

Axial length is composed of corneal thickness, anterior chamber depth, lens thickness and vitreous length. Changes in any of these dimensions have a greater or lesser effect on axial length.

Central corneal thickness

The cornea thickened in all groups with different tightness of encirclement immediately after encircling. However, after four days the thickness returned

179

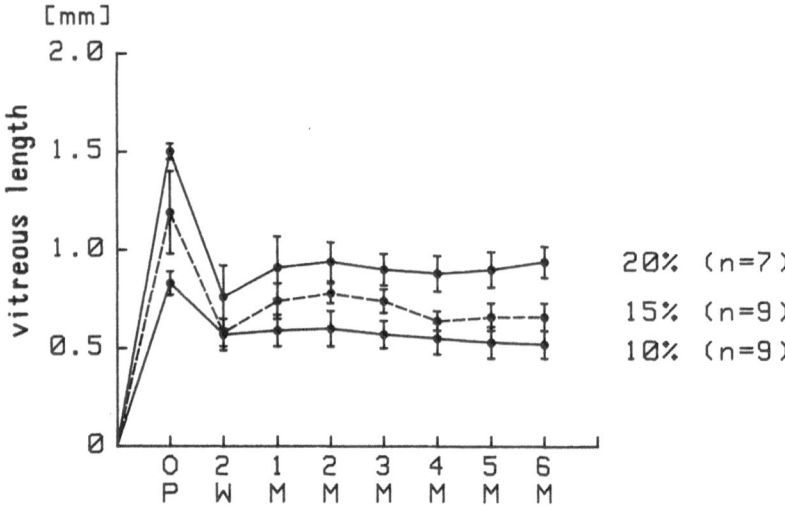

Fig. 3. Changes in vitreous length after encircling operations with different tightness.

to the preoperative value. Thereafter there was no significant difference between the three groups with different tightness. In comparison with controls there was no significant difference either.

Anterior chamber depth

Changes in the anterior chamber depth were also controversial (Fiore and Newton 1970; Hartley and Marsh 1973; Burton *et al.* 1977; Larsen and Syrdalen 1979). Immediately after encircling, anterior chamber depth was reduced in the three groups with different tightness. In groups with weak and mild tightness (10% and 15%), reduction of anterior chamber depth was present at six months, though it was slight. However, in some eyes in the group of strong tightness (20%), anterior chamber depth increased at two weeks. After two months marked increase of the depth was seen in three of seven rabbits. It is worth noting that strong myopia was produced in these 3 rabbits.

Lens thickness

Lens thickness in all groups did not change immediately after encircling. At four days after encircling, lens thickness started to increase in all groups. At two weeks the increase of lens thickness was in proportion to the tightness of encirclement. After that the increase of lens thickness tended to reduce. At six months in the group of weak tightness (10%), no difference was found in comparison with controls. In groups of mild and strong tightness (15% and 20%), a slight increase of lens thickness was still present.

180

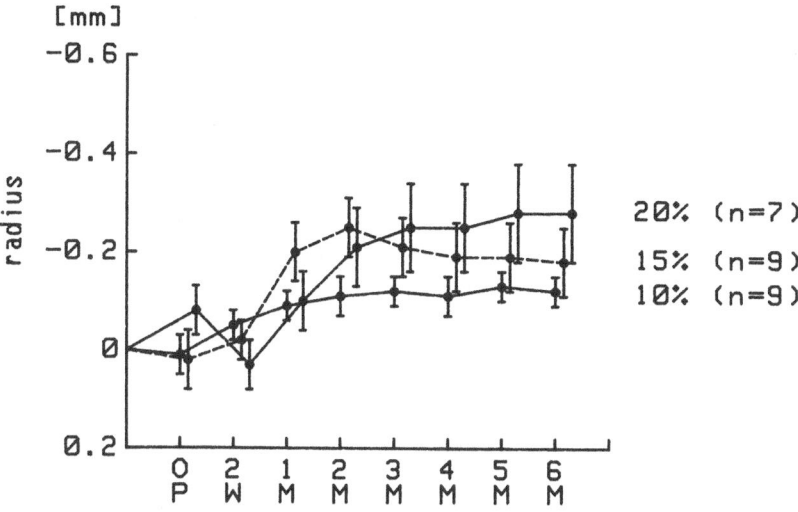

Fig. 4. Changes in the radius of corneal curvature after encircling operations with different tightness.

Vitreous length

The most important component of axial length is vitreous length (Larsen and Syrdalen 1979). Figure 3 shows changes in vitreous length after encircling operation with various degree of tightness. Immediately after the operation, vitreous length was markedly elongated in all eyes in proportion to the tightness of encirclement. The degree of elongation in vitreous length tended to decrease during the first two weeks in all groups. Thereafter, the degree of elongation tended to increase again up to two months after encirclement. Following this, vitreous length values were stabilized. At six months the elongation of vitreous length was present in proportion to the tightness of encirclement in all groups.

Other refractive components

Second, other refractive factors will be discussed, of which radius of corneal curvature is one of the most important. In the groups with tightness of 10 and 15%, the radius did not change immediately after encirclement, as shown by Figure 4, but from the second day to one week the radius tended to decrease. In the group with the tightness of 20%, the radius got smaller immediately after encircling. Two weeks later, the radius had returned to the value before surgery. Thereafter, the corneal radius value decreased relatively fast and reached a minimum value. At three or four months the range of variation became small and the values were stable. At six months reduction of the radius was present in proportion to the tightness of encirclement in all groups. There was remarkable similarity between the

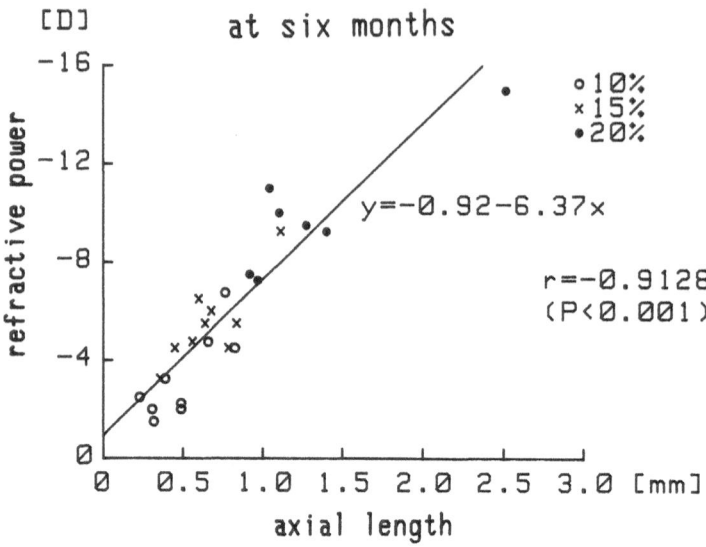

Fig. 5. Correlation between changes in refraction and those in axial length at six months after encircling operations with different tightness.

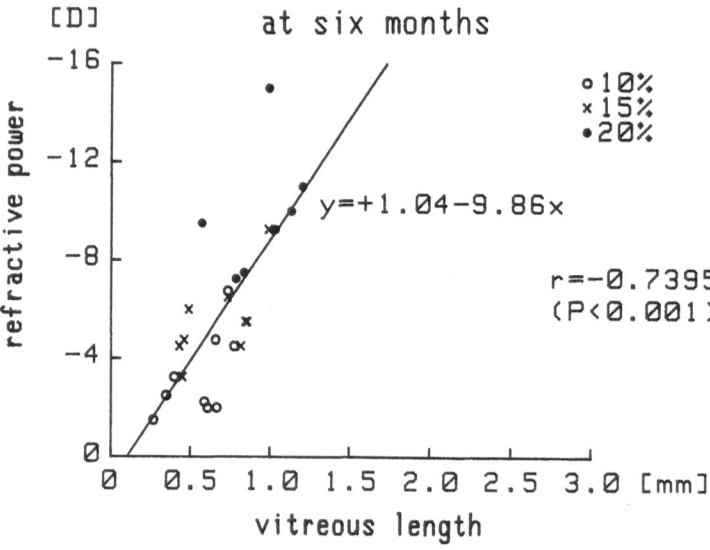

Fig. 6. Correlation between changes in refractive power and those in vitreous length at six months after encircling with different tightness.

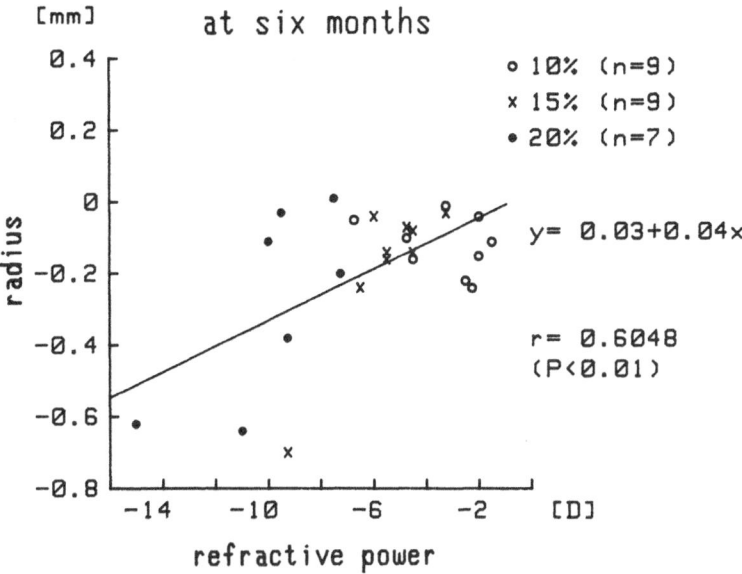

Fig. 7. Correlation between changes in the radius of corneal curvature and those in axial length at six months.

vatiation curve in the refractive state and that in the radius of corneal curvature, except immediately after encircling.

Correlations between the changes observed

At six months after encircling, the amount of changes in the various refractive components were found to be correlated as follows:

Between degree of myopia and axial elongation a strong correlation was proved, as shown by Figure 5. The correlation coefficient r was −0.91.

Among the other components the vitreous length also had a strong correlation with changes in refraction, as shown in Figure 6. The coefficient was −0.74.

Figure 7 shows a strong correlation between changes in radius of corneal curvature and refractive change. The coefficient was 0.60.

Figure 8 shows a strong correlation between changes in corneal curvature radius and changes in axial length, the coefficient being −0.58. Axial length increased, as the radius of corneal curvature decreased.

Another factor determining the refractive state after encircling is thickness of the lens and/or its position. Figure 9 shows measurements of components of axial length at six months after encircling with different degrees of tightness. As anterior chamber depth decreased, vitreous length increased. Taking it into consideration that changes in lens thickness were very small, as described before, it is suggested that the lens shifted forward after the encircling operation. Forward shift of the lens might have some influence on the change in refraction.

183

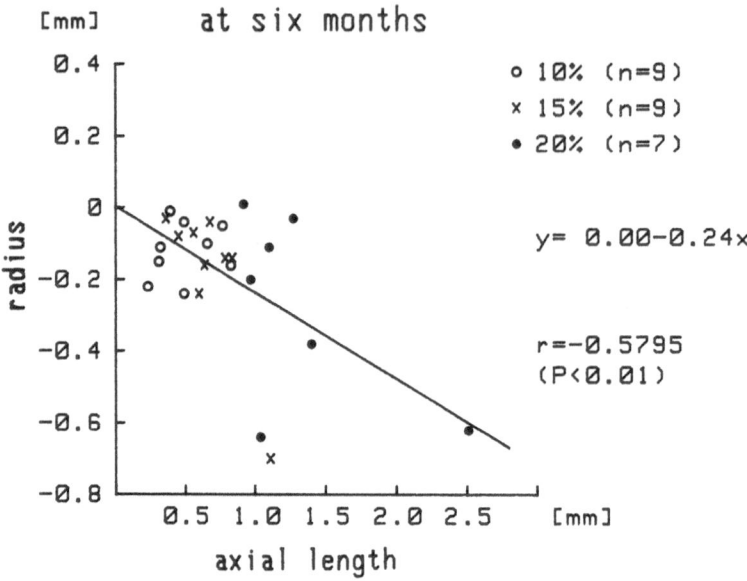

Fig. 8. Correlation between changes in the radius of corneal curvature and those in axial length at six months after encircling operations with different tightness.

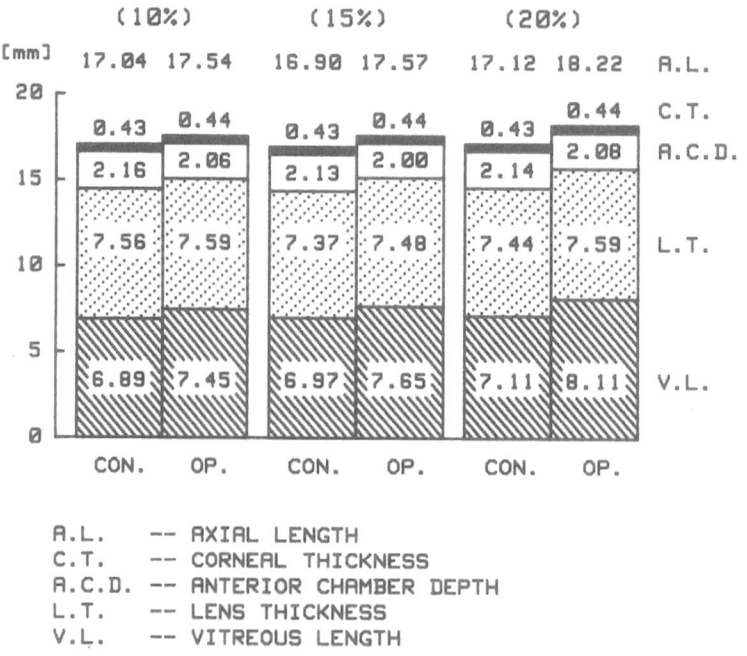

A.L. — AXIAL LENGTH
C.T. — CORNEAL THICKNESS
A.C.D. — ANTERIOR CHAMBER DEPTH
L.T. — LENS THICKNESS
V.L. — VITREOUS LENGTH

Fig. 9. Measurements of the various axial dimensions at six months after encircling operations, as related to degree of tightness (10, 15, and 20%).

The amount of reduction in the radius of corneal curvature at six months after encircling was 0.12 mm at 10% tightness, 0.18 mm at 15% tightness and 0.28 mm at 20% tightness. The stronger the tightness at encircling, the more the radius of corneal curvature decreased. It is definitely shown that the reduction of the radius of corneal curvature is concerned in producing myopia.

CONCLUDING REMARKS

From the above-mentioned results in experimental myopia in pigmented rabbits after encircling band surgery with different tightness, the following conclusions can be drawn:

(1) The degree of myopia which developed immediately after the encircling operation (at the equator) was proportinal to the degree of tightness of encircling.

(2) At six months after encircling, myopia in proportion to the degree of tightness was still present.

(3) Variation in the degree of myopia was influenced by elongation of vitreous length as an axial factor, and by decrease in the radius of corneal curvature as a refractive factor.

REFERENCES

Burton, T.C., Herron, B.E. & Ossoinig, K.C.: Axial length changes after retinal detachment surgery. Am. J. Ophthalmol. 83: 59 (1977).
Fiore, J.V. & Newton, J.C.: Anterior segment changes following the scleral buckling procedure. AMA Arch. Ophthalmol. 84: 284 (1970).
Hartley, R.E. & Marsh, R.J.: Anterior chamber depth changes after retinal detachment. Br. J. Ophthalmol. 57: 564 (1973).
Larsen, J.S. & Syrdalen, P.: Ultrasonographic study on changes in axial eye dimensions after encircling procedure in retinal detachment surgery. Acta Ophthalmol. 57: 337 (1979).
Rubin, M.L.: The induction of refractive errors by retinal detachment surgery. Trans. Am. Ophthalmol. Soc. 73: 452 (1975).

Authors' address:
Department of Ophthalmology
Miyazaki Medical College
5200 Kihara, Kiyotake, Miyazaki 889–16
Japan

ATROPINE AFFECTS LID-SUTURE MYOPIA DEVELOPMENT

Experimental studies of chronic atropinization in tree shrews

J.A. McKANNA and V.A. CASAGRANDE

(Nashville, Tennessee, USA)

ABSTRACT

The abnormal development of the eye and its optics caused by neonatal lid-suture in the tree shrew *Tupaia glis* parallels human myopia from several aspects.

To test the intersecting feedback loop hypothesis, we have attempted to block accommodation in lid-sutured eyes in the animal mentioned, by daily treatment with 1% atropine sulfate in sterile 0.9% NaCl, inserted under the fused lids through PE 10 tubing.

In general, atropine-treated lid-sutured eyes have not developed the anomalies (axial elongation and high myopia) characteristic of untreated eyes. Variability of results, however, limits the statistical significance of data on refraction and axial length.

On the other hand, the effects of atropine on the ciliary zonule of both lid-sutured and open atropinized eyes seems to be consistent. In both types, the zonule fibers are 20–30% more numerous than normal. The zonule in the atropine-treated eyes comprises a greatly increased number of elastic-fiber microfibrils. Taken together, these data indicate that atropine, by blocking accommodation, decreases tendencies for axial elongation and increases zonule development. Such results complement the lid-suture data in suggesting that accommodation influences ocular development, and thereby support the intersecting feed-back loop hypothesis.

INTERSECTING FEEDBACK LOOP HYPOTHESIS

The abnormal development of the eye and its optics caused by neonatal lid-suture in the tree shrew *Tupaia glis* parallels human myopia from several aspects. Correlation of data revealing axial elongation, lenticular hypoplasia, and zonular dysplasia in the myopic lid-sutured eye (McKanna and Casagrande 1978) led to an hypothesis of ocular maturation that describes an intersecting feedback loop mechanism whereby visual activity can influence coordinated development of both axial and refractive elements. By describing a role for physiologic activity influencing the development of both axial and refractive elements, the hypothesis offers a synthesis of several major theories of acquired myopia development and emmetropization (Sato 1957; Sorsby, *et al.* 1961; van Alphen 1961).

METHODS

According to the intersecting feedback loop hypothesis, excessive accommodation would be predicted to cause increased axial elongation and decreased lens and zonule development – the anomalies observed in lid-sutured myopic eyes (McKanna and Casagrande 1980). To test the intersecting feedback loop hypothesis, we attempted to *block accommodation in lid-sutured eyes* by daily treatment with 1% atropine sulfate in sterile 0.9% NaCl solution. The atropine was administered to lid-sutured eyes through PE10 tubing inserted under the fused lids through a drainage aperture situated at the nasal angle. Control non-deprived animals received monocular treatment on identical schedules.

The parameters under study are: refraction, axial elongation as well as number and size distribution of zonule fibers.

RESULTS AND DISCUSSION

In general, atropine-treated eyes develop optics similar to their non-treated controls, and the lid-sutured *atropinized eyes* do not become myopic. The developmental response to atropine cycloplegia is not completely straightforward, however, because in two cases out of 12, non-deprived atropinized eyes have required 0 to + 2D correction while the non-treated eye of the same animal fell in the normal range of + 5 to + 8D (relative values; not corrected to compensate for small globe size). These unexpected results could be explained by reduced sensitivity to atropine, allowing the treated eye to accommodate during refraction under atropine cycloplegia. To test this possibility, we intend to repeat these experiments using other cycloplegics at the time of refraction.

Regardless of the optics of the treated eye, the effects of atropine on development of the ciliary zonule have been consistent with the intersecting feedback loop hypothesis. Using scanning electron microscopy, quantitative comparison of 25 µm thick meridional sections from both lid-sutured and non-sutured atropinized eyes with sections from their normal control eyes reveals an increased number of zonule fibers in the treated eyes.

The delicate meridional sections, prepared from epoxy-embedded specimens using the 'de-poxy' technique and the phase separation protocol for critical point drying (McKanna and Lempka 1980), allow inspection of the zonule fibers along their entire course from ciliary body to lens as shown in Figures 1 and 2. The great resolution of the scanning electron microscopy allows preparation of high magnification micrographs of the fibers (Figures 3 and 4).

We have made series of micrographs to create a continuous montage from anterior to posterior of the zonule, and have used the BIOQUANT II

188

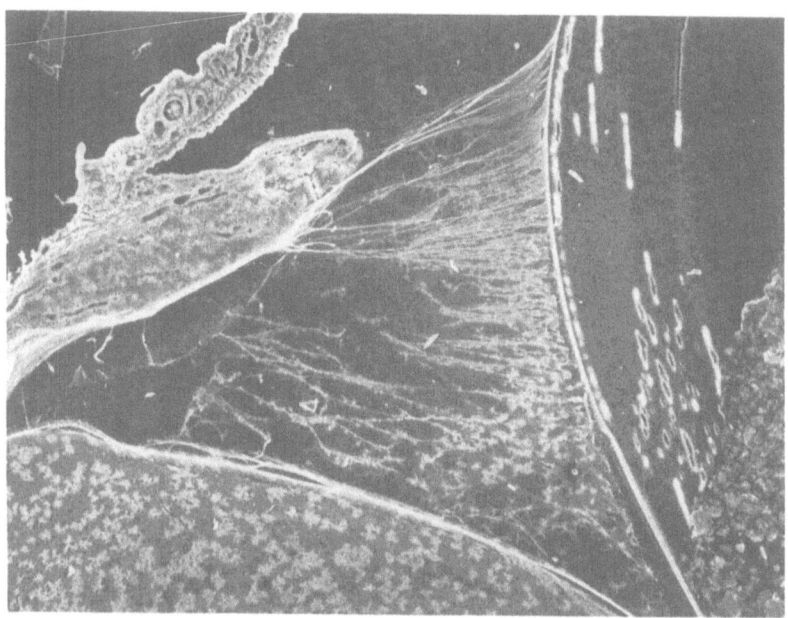

Fig. 1. Left eye, non-treated control.

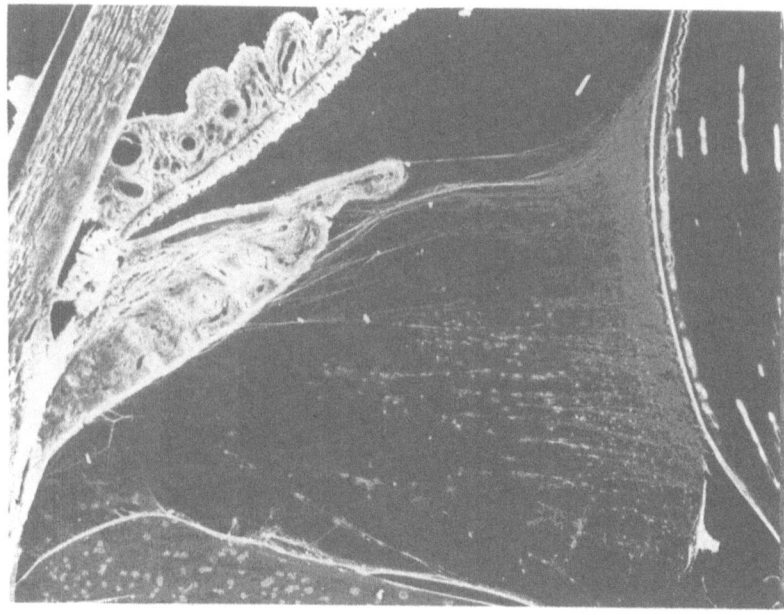

Fig. 2. Right eye, lid-sutured at day 7 and atropinized from day 28 to age 13 months.
Figs. 1 and 2. Meridional sections, 25 μm thick, from tree shrew eyes. × 100.

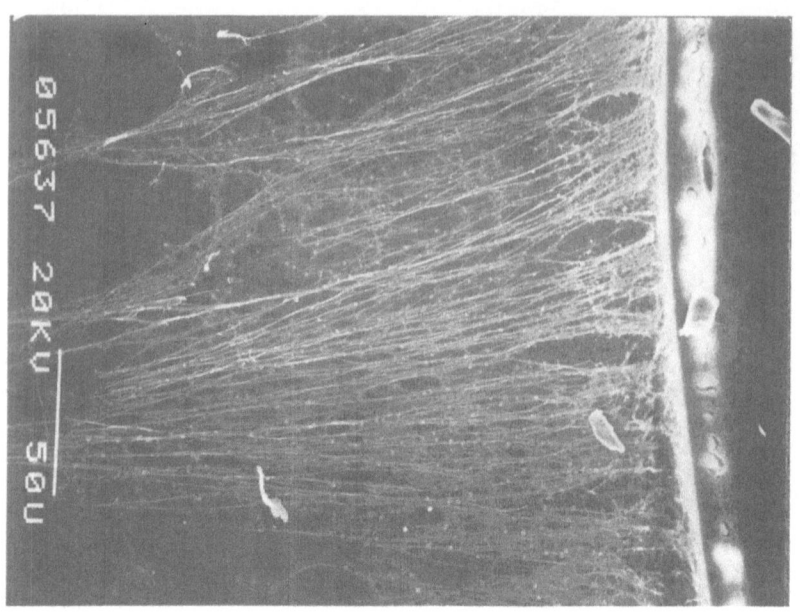

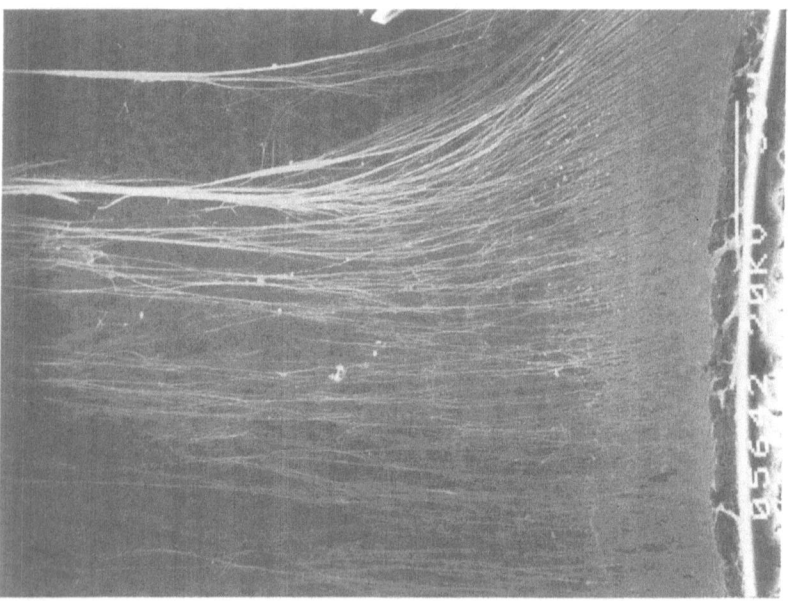

Figs. 3 and 4. Higher magnification SEM of zonules from specimens in Figs. 1 and 2, respectively. Quantitative measurements, made along a line 10 μm from the zonular lamella from micrographs at five thousand magnification, reveal a greater number of fibers in the atropinized zonule (Fig. 4). × 430.

190

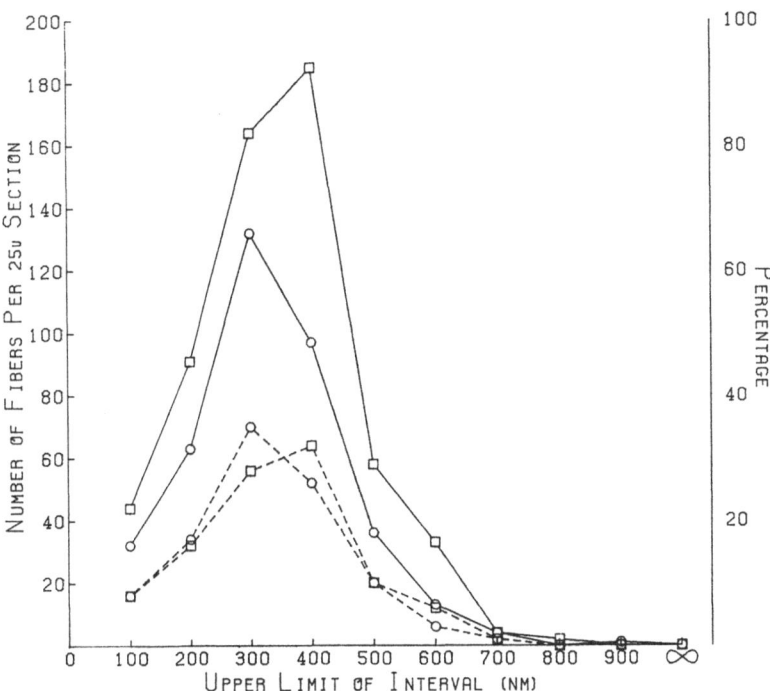

Fig. 5. Quantitative size distribution for fibers in sections from normal control (circles) and non-sutured atropine-treated (squares) eyes. Solid lines connect points representing actual numbers of fibers in each class; the treated eye has many more fibers. Dashed lines connect points representing percentages of fibers in each class; percentages are similar, indicating normal size distribution for zonule fibers in the treated eye.

computerized image analysis system to measure the diameter of all fibers in each of many serial sections. Comparison of the quantitative results from typical sections from a 13-month-old non-deprived tree shrew that received monocular atropine treatments from day 28 are presented graphically in Figure 5. The zonule section from the normal eye contained 378 fibers while that from the non-sutured atropinized eye had 581. This difference of 56% is obvious in the size frequency distribution graph (solid lines); however, the dashed lines connecting points representing the percentages of fibers in each size interval reveal that the percentages are virtually identical in the two eyes. Because these patterns hold for serial sections, we conclude that the atropine treatment has resulted in hyperplasia of the zonule.

A possible explanation of these results could be that the increased zonule tension caused by chronic cycloplegia has resulted in increased synthesis or increased stability of the fiber subunits. Since the fiber subunits resemble elastic fiber microfibrils on ultrastructural, biochemical, and immunologic grounds (Raviola 1971; Swan *et al.* 1978; Streeton *et al.* 1980), we anticipate improved understanding of the dynamics of these important connective

191

tissue elements based on research concerning *in vivo* modulation of the zonule by lid suture and cycloplegia.

Furthermore, demonstration of developmental changes caused by atropine administration is consistent with our proposal that accommodation is the physiologic visual phenomenon at which paradoxical developmental processes (refractive changes vs. axial elongation) intersect (McKanna and Casagrande 1978; 1980). As described above, blockage of accommodation seems to inhibit axial elongation and to increase zonule development. Such results complement the lid-suture myopia data in suggesting that accommodation influences ocular development, and thereby support the intersecting feedback loop hypothesis.

REFERENCES

McKanna, J.A. and Casagrande V.A. Reduced lens development in lid-suture myopia. Exp. Eye Res., 26: 715–723 (1978).

McKanna, J.A. and Casagrande V.A. 1980 Zonular dysplasia in myopia. In: 2nd Int. Conf. on Myopia, Proc. Ed. R. Yamaji, Kannehara Shuppan, Ltd. Tokyo, (1980 in press).

McKanna, J.A., and Lempka T. Phase separation in alcohol/liquid carbon dioxide solvent systems facilitates critical point drying. J. Micros. 118: 1–4. (1980).

Raviola, G. The fine structure of the ciliary zonule and ciliary epithelium with special regard to the organization and insertion of the zonular fibrils. Invest. Ophthalmol. 10: 851–869. (1971).

Sato, T. The Causes and Prevention of Acquired Myopia. Kanehara Suppan Co., Ltd., Tokyo, (1957).

Sorsby, A., B. Benjamin, and Sheridan M. Refraction and its components during the growth of the eye from the age of three. (Medical Council Special Report Series No. 301). Her Majesty's Stationery Office London (1961).

Streeton, B.W., and Licari, P.A. Immunohistochemical comparison of zonular fibrils and elastic tissue microfibrils. ARVO, 255. (1980).

Swann, D.A., and B.W. Streeton Amino acid and peptide composition of zonular fibers. ARVO: 209. (1978).

van Alphen, G.W.H.M. On emmetropia and ametropia. Ophthalmologica, 142 (suupl): 1–92. (1961).

Senior author's address:
J.A. McKanna, Ph.D.
Department of Anatomy, Vanderbilt University School of Medicine,
Nashville, Tennessee, 37232,
U.S.A.

EXPERIMENTAL VISUAL DEPRIVATION AND MYOPIA

A. SHAPIRO, M.D.

(Jerusalem/Israel)

ABSTRACT

Eye lid closure in chicks during the first three months of life created myopia, flatness of the cornea and enlargement of the axial length. Suturing of only one eye provoked myopic changes in the closed eye, while the untreated eye remained unaffected. It is concluded that a component in the eye plays a role in the patho-physiology of myopia, and refractive errors may occur independently in either eye.

INTRODUCTION

Lid closure in animals, whether mono- or binocularly, may cause refractive changes in the sutured eye(s). In cats and shrews, only mild myopia developed (Wilson and Sherman 1977; Sherman *et al.* 1977) while in monkeys a greater degree of myopia, mainly due to enlargement of the axial length, has been described (Wiesel and Raviola 1977; Raviola and Wiesel 1978).

METHODOLOGY AND RESULTS

The experiments in this study were started on one-day old chicks. Refractions, curvatures of the cornea and axial length of mono- and binocularly sutured eyes were compared to the eyes of normal chicks. The lids were released after three months and retinoscopy, keratometry and A-mode ultrasound were carried out. There were no statistically significant differences in the measurements between the monocularly and binocularly closed eyes, nor were such differences found between the monocularly unsutured eyes and the control group.

In the image-deprived eyes, myopia of more than 6 D was found, while mild hypermetropia (up to + 1.00 D) was noted in the unsutured eyes. Keratometry revealed a flattened cornea (an average difference of 5.82 D) in the sutured eye, which makes the high myopia even more significant.

The myopic eye also displayed increased axial length (average difference of 2.03 mm by A-scan ultrasound). The axial difference by itself does not explain, however, the difference in refractive power. Most probably, the lens position, too, has an affect on the degree of myopia (Yinon et al. 1980).

DISCUSSION

Visual space restriction in monkeys (Young 1961; Young 1963) and cats (Belkin et al. 1977) caused myopia in these animals. Does experimental restriction simulate the environment of domestic animals? The latter are known to be more short-sighted than their wild counterparts (Vakkor and Bishop 1963; Vakkor et al. 1963; Duke-Elder 1970; Glickstein and Millodot 1970; Young and Leary 1973; Rose et al. 1974). In humans, near work during childhood and adolescence may lead to myopia (Young et al. 1969; Morgan and Munro 1973; Richler and Bear 1980). These findings even induced a trial to prevent myopia by means of accommodation paralysis with daily drops of atropine sulfate 1% (Gruber 1979).

The fused lids in the present study produced a thin, translucent membrane covering the eye, which prevented accurate image imprint on the retina. These findings correlate well with the myopia described in chicks that were constantly kept in surroundings with low intensity of light, a myopia which was due mainly to eye enlargement (Lauber and Kinner 1979).

Lid closure in a monkey during the neonatal period had no effect on the refractive status or axial length of the eye when the animal was kept in a dark environment. However, when the animal was transferred to illuminated quarters (while the lids remained fused), myopia and elongation of the eye developed (Raviola and Wiesel 1978). These results emphasize that myopia in lid closure is partly due to the lack of accurate image formation on the retina.

Lid fusion of neonate monkeys, whether mono- or binocularly, caused myopia due to elongation of the axial length (Wiesel and Raviola 1977). As the elongation occurred mainly in the post-equatorial hemisphere, no significant changes were present in the corneal curvature. In our studies, the sutured lids created myopia and flatness of the cornea in the chicks' eyes. The corneal flatness was not due to pressure of the lids, as the fused lids did not press on the cornea. This corneal flatness was caused by enlargement of the entire globe.

Near work and lid closure both create myopia. In near work, the pathology may be attributed to the process of accommodation. In lid closure, however, when no accurate image is formed on the retina, no accommodation is provoked. It is therefore postulated that different mechanisms are involved in the creation of myopia in lid closure and in near work.

The current study showed that monocular lid closure in chicks led to the same refraction, corneal curvature and axial length as in binocular closure. The monocular unfused eye presented with the same refraction, corneal curvature and axial length as found in the untreated eyes of the control

194

chicks. These experimental results suggest that the pathophysiology of myopia is locally determined, in the eye itself. Thus myopia may develop independently in either eye.

REFERENCES

Belkin, M., Yinon, U., Rose, L. & Reisert, I. Effect of visual environment on refractive error of cats. Docum. Ophthalmol. 42: 433–437 (1977).

Duke-Elder, S. System of Ophthalmology, Vol. V. Ophthalmic Optics and Refraction, Henry Kimpton, London, pp. 238–239 (1970).

Glickstein, M. & Millodot, M. Retinoscopy and eye size. Science 168: 605–606 (1970).

Gruber, E. The treatment of Myopia with Atropine: A Clinical Study. XXIII Concilium Ophthalmologicum, Pars II, Excerpta Medica, Amsterdam-Oxford, pp. 1212–1216 (1979).

Lauber, J.K. & Kinnear, A. Eye enlargement in birds induced by dim light. Can. J. Ophthalmol. 14: 265–269 (1979).

Morgan, R.W. & Munro, M. Refractive problems in northern natives. Can. J. Ophthalmol. 8: 226–228 (1973).

Raviola, E. & Wiesel, T.N. Effect of dark rearing on experimental myopia in monkeys. Invest. Ophthalmol. 17: 485–488 (1978).

Richler, A. & Bear, J.C. Refraction, near work and education. A population study in Newfoundland. Acta Ophthalmol. 58: 468–478 (1980).

Rose, L., Yinon, U. & Belkin, M. Myopia induced in cats deprived of distance vision during development. Vision Res. 14: 1029–1032 (1974).

Sherman, S.M., Norton, T.T. & Casagrande, V.A. Myopia in the lid sutured tree shrew (Tupaia glis). Brain Res. 124: 154–157 (1977).

Vakkur, G.J. & Bishop, P.O. The schematic eye in the cat. Vision Res. 3: 357–381 (1963).

Vakkur, G.J., Bishop, P.O. & Kozak, W. Visual optics in the cat including posterior nodal distance and retinal landmark. Vision Res. 3: 289–314 (1963).

Wiesel, T.N. & Raviola, E. Myopia and eye enlargement after neonatal lid fusion in moneys. Nature 266: 66–68 (1977).

Wilson, J.R. & Sherman, S.M. Differential effects of early monocular deprivation on the binocular and monocular segments of cat striate cortex. J. Neurophysiol. 40: 891–903 (1977).

Yinon, U., Rose, L. & Shapiro, A. Myopia in the eye of developing chicks following monocular and binocular lid closure. Vision Res. 20: 137–141 (1980).

Young, F.A. The effect of restricted visual space on the primate eye. Am. J. Ophthalmol. 52: 799–806 (1961).

Young, F.A. The effect of restricted visual space on the refractive error of the young monkey. Invest. Ophthalmol. 2: 571–577 (1963).

Young, F.A. The distribution of refractive errors in monkeys. Exp. Eye Res. 3: 230–238 (1964).

Young, F.A., Baldwin, W.R., Leary, G.A., West, D.C., Box, R.A., Harris, E. & Johnson, C. The transmission of refractive errors within Eskimo families. Am. J. Optom. & Arch. Am. Acad. Optom. 46: 676–685 (1969).

Young, F.A. & Leary, G.A. Visual optical characteristics of caged and semi-free ranging monkey. Am. J. Physiol. Anthropol. 38: 377–382 (1973).

Author's address:
A. Shapiro, M.D.
Department of Ophthalmology
Hadassah University Hospital
Kiryat Hadassah
P.O.B. 12 000
il-91120
Jerusalem, Israel

ROLE OF ACCOMMODATION AND DEVELOPMENTAL ASPECTS OF EXPERIMENTAL MYOPIA IN CHICKS

J. WALLMAN, D. ROSENTHAL, J.I. ADAMS,
J.N. TRACHTMAN and L. ROMAGNANO
(New York, New York, U.S.A.)

ABSTRACT

We have previously shown that extreme axial myopia (often more than 40 D) could be produced by raising chicks with their field of view restricted to the frontal visual field.

Since animals raised with their vision restricted to the lateral visual field do not become myopic, it is the specific visual experience that is important. Since chicks use the frontal visual field for near vision and the lateral for distance vision, it is possible that the amount of near vision is the relevant variable.

We have now completed a series of developmental studies on this experimental myopia. The results can be summarized as follows: (1) The myopia can be reversed, in most subjects, by removing the visual field restriction. (2) This recovery process is extremely rapid for young animals, but much slower for older animals. (3) The experimental myopia develops very rapidly, being substantial at one week of age and maximal at two weeks. (4) The myopia shows some spontaneous reversal even with the visual field restrictors still in place. This result seems consistent with a hypothesis implicating accommodation in the etiology of myopia, since severely myopic animals would presumably have little need to accommodate, and thus the myopia would decrease. (6) Normal chicks have rather variable refractions at hatching. These change in the direction of emmetropia over approximately the same time period that the myopia develops in the experimental chicks.

Taken together, these studies argue that although this experimental myopia, and the recovery from it, can both occur over a substantial period of the animals development, the extent of susceptibility to both processes changes greatly as the animal develops. The similarity in the developmental time course of the refractive changes in normal and myopic chicks argues that the experimental myopia may be the result of the same developmental regulatory mechanisms that normally cause the eye to grow toward correct refraction.

Longitudinal studies of the anatomical changes associated with the experimental myopia and recovery from it are in progress.

INTRODUCTION

The substantial controversy that has surrounded myopia for centuries may reflect the complexity of its etiology. The usefulness of experimental models of myopia lies not only in providing the opportunity for animal tests of potential therapeutic approaches but also in the possibility of understanding the relation of myopia to normal ocular development, and particularly the interactions of the environmental and experimental factors involved. The recent interest in animal models of myopia has risen from the findings that neonatal lid closure produces myopia in monkeys (Wiesel and Raviola 1977), tree shrews (Sherman, *et al.* 1977; MacKanna and Casagrande 1978), and cats (Wilson and Sherman 1977) and that a long period of close vision produces less severe myopia in monkeys (Young 1961) and cats (Belkin, *et al.* 1977).

We have been exploring an experimentally induced myopia in chicks that has the following features: (1) It is clearly related to the specific type of visual experience the animal has, rather than simply to the presence or absence of vision. (2) There is a defined developmental period of susceptibility to the myopia. (3) The myopia can be reversed within the susceptible period. (4) The anatomical changes that result in the myopia involve increased axial length of the eye and changes in corneal curvature. (5) These refractive changes occur extremely rapidly. (6) Finally, there is substantial evidence that ocular accommodation is a causative factor in the myopia.

FRONTAL VISION MYOPIA

The principal experimental manipulation we use to produce myopia in chicks is to restrict their vision to the frontal visual fields by means of translucent plastic occluders for the first one to four weeks of life. This produces approximately 20 D of myopia.[1] Although myopia can also be produced in chicks by total restriction of form vision by means of lid closure or translucent occluders (Wallman, *et al.* 1978; Yinon, *et al.* 1980), the frontal vision myopia is not simply a consequence of visual field restriction per se, since restricting vision to the lateral field does not produce myopia (Wallman, *et al.* 1978).

Frontal vision myopia is associated with increased axial length of the eye. In our earlier study we showed by measurement of enucleated formalin-perfused eyes that the eyes of frontal-vision animals are statistically significantly longer than those of normal animals. We have now investigated this more rigorously by raising animals with one eye restricted to frontal vision and the other eye normal. We measured the differences in the axial length and the spacing of the refractive surfaces by A-scan ultrasonography, recording the reflections with a Nicolet digital storage oscilloscope. This

---

[1] Refractions were done by streak retinoscopy on anesthetized animals under cycloplegia; cycloplegia was obtained by corneal application of a curare-benzalkonium chloride-atropine solution.

TWO WEEKS

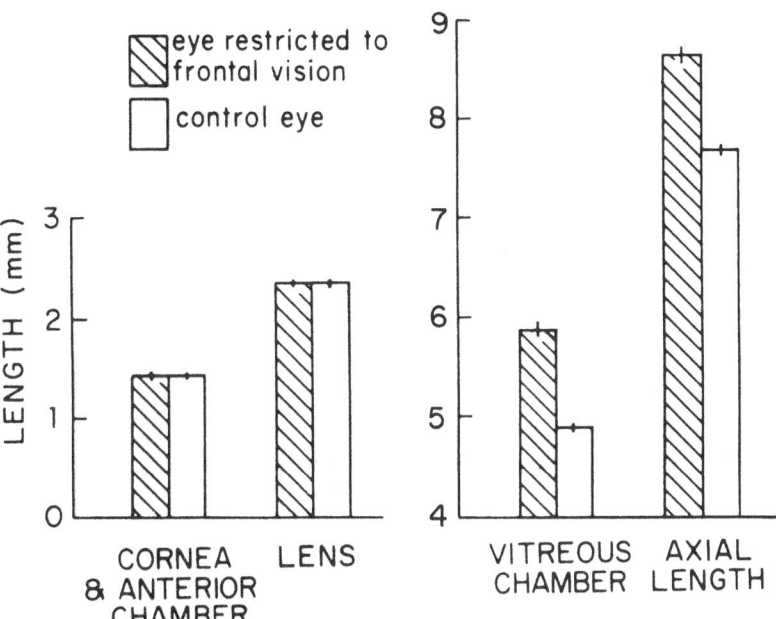

Fig. 1. Ultrasound measurements of axial distances in eyes of animals raised with vision of one eye restricted to the frontal field. Mean ± standard error is plotted.

permitted measuring all spacings from the echoes of the same pulse of ultrasound. To compute the actual distances, we determined the velocity of sound in the lenses and vitreous of several 6-week-old chicken eyes; we assumed the velocity of sound to be equal in the aqueous and vitreous humours.

The results of these measurements are that in 2-week-old animals, in each one of our ten cases, the axial length of the eyes with frontal vision is increased, because of the increased length of the vitreous chamber (Figure 1). A similar result is found in lid-closure myopia in primates (Wiesel and Raviola 1977) and chicks (Yinon, *et al.* 1980). It is interesting that these differences in 2-week-old animals are so small, since our earlier work on 4-to 6-week-old animals showed larger differences, and that of Yinon, *et al.* (1980) on lid closure myopia in chickens several months old showed even larger effects. As we will show below, the axial length increase is not the only cause of the myopia observed.

DEVELOPMENTAL COURSE OF SUSCEPTIBILITY TO MYOPIA

Two of the remarkable characteristics of frontal vision myopia are how rapidly it develops during the period of maximum susceptibility and how

199

clearly defined this period is within the life of the animal. We have shown that restriction to frontal vision starting at hatching produced a median change after only one week of -25 D; the maximum myopia was reached after two weeks. In contrast, three weeks of restriction to the frontal visual field beginning at nine weeks of age produced a change of only -1.1 D (Wallman, Trachtman and Ledoux, submitted manuscript).

If the restriction to frontal vision is removed, recovery from the myopia proceeds rapidly. The rate of recovery is age-dependent in a fashion similar to the susceptibility to myopia. For example, the median decrease in myopia when the visual restriction is removed at two weeks of age is 22 D in the first week, whereas it is 3 D at six weeks (Wallman, *et al.* MS.).

The speed of this recovery seems too rapid to be accounted for by changes in overall growth of the globe. We will show below that some of this recovery may be produced by changes in corneal curvature. The other factors involved are unknown.

RELATION OF FRONTAL VISION MYOPIA TO NORMAL CHANGES IN REFRACTION

Like other authors in this volume we are interested in what clues myopia can give to the developmental processes at work in the normal development of the eye. Since we found a clear period of susceptibility to changes in refraction that seemed similar both for induction of and recovery from myopia, we investigated what changes in refraction normal eyes undergo during this period. In particular, we were interested in the hypothesis that frontal vision myopia results from interference with a vision-dependent developmental regulatory mechanism that works postnatally to correct errors in refractive state. If such a mechanism did exist one would expect that older animals would all be nearly emmetropic whereas newly hatched animals would have more variable refractions.

We did cycloplegic refractions on 242 different eyes at ages from hatching to 8 weeks of age and found dramatic confirmation of these hypothesized results (Wallman, *et al.* 1981). In newly hatched animals the refractions were very variable (6 D between first and third quartile) and quite hyperopic (median = 9 D); over the next 8 weeks the variability and hyperopia declined continuously (at 8 weeks, .25 D between first and third quantile, median = 1.8 D).[2] These results do not necessarily implicate a postnatal regulatory mechanism, since the same pattern of changes could result from the continuation of embryological processes independent of vision. It is interesting, however, that the variability declines sharply near hatching and then much more slowly by eight weeks, the same time course shown by the susceptibility to myopia. A similar postnatal decline in variability of refractions has been shown in human infants by Mohindra and Held (this volume).

---

[2] The decline in hyperopia is due at least in part to an artifact of retinoscopy that results in an error in the direction of hyperopia that is inversely proportional to eye size. This artifact would be largest in the newly hatched animals.

Since these results argue for the existence of a postnatal growth regulatory mechanism that makes the eye grow toward emmetropia, they raise the question of what error signal would guide this mechanism. The most compelling answer seems to be a signal related to the average level of accommodation, since this would directly provide a measure of how well suited the eye's refractive state is to its visual demands. If accommodation in excess of some set point caused growth in the myopic direction, or if a deficit in accommodation caused growth in the hyperopic direction, the eye would tend toward the refractive state best suited to its environmental circumstances.

IS ACCOMMODATION INVOLVED IN THE ETIOLOGY OF FRONTAL VISION MYOPIA?

The argument just presented shows the plausibility of an excess of accommodation resulting in myopia. In this connection we are intrigued by the possibility that the explanation for the dramatic and rapid development of myopia with brief periods of frontal vision may be related to the fact that chicks appear to use their frontal visual fields for the very close (2–5 cm) visual inspection that precedes pecks. Perhaps being deprived of the use of their lateral visual fields usually employed in distance vision encourages more close vision, a possibility supported by evidence that the frontal and lateral visual fields cannot be used interchangably (Nye 1973).[3]

To evaluate more directly the possibility of accommodation playing a role in frontal vision myopia we tested whether cutting the ciliary nerve to one eye would protect that eye from the myopia. The surgery was performed on newly hatched animals; the ciliary nerve on one side was cut just distal to the ciliary ganglion; a sham operation consisting of the same incision and manipulation without nerve section was performed on the other side. To avoid interference with healing of the incision, the animals were left for a week before their vision was restricted to the frontal field. They were tested at two weeks of age. The results are clear: in 21 out of 24 cases, the eye with ciliary nerve section is less myopic than the companion, sham-operated, eye. The distribution of refractions is shown in Figure 2. The median refraction of the nerve-cut eyes was -4 D, compared to a median of -22 D for the fellow eyes, a significant difference (Mann-Whitney U test, $p < 0.01$). These results constitute strong evidence for the role of accommodation in frontal vision myopia.

Interestingly, although the nerve section reduced the myopia resulting from restriction to the frontal visual field, it did not abolish it. This might indicate another mechanism unrelated to accommodation being involved in the etiology of this myopia. An alternative possibility is that the regenerating ciliary nerve, which starts to reinnervate the muscle after a week

[3] Alternatively, there are other possible causal links between accommodation and frontal vision myopia. For example, if deprivation of form vision in the lateral field induced excess accommodation, this would account for both frontal vision myopia and lid-closure myopia.

201

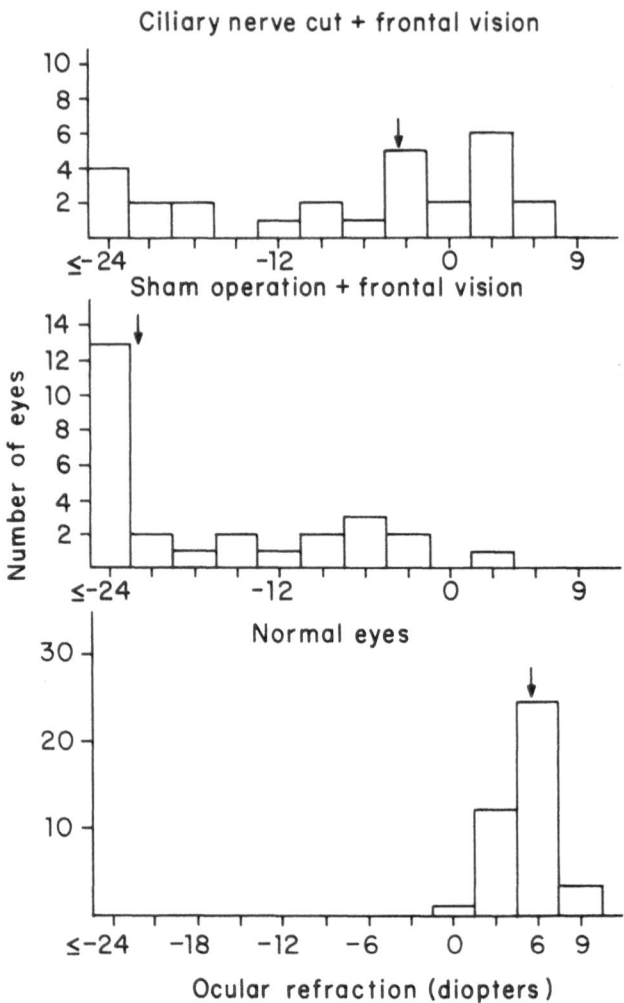

Fig. 2. Cycloplegic refractions of eyes with monocular section of ciliary nerve. Arrows indicate medians. Each of the three distributions shown is significantly different from the other two (Mann-Whitney U test; p < 0.01).

(Pilar, *et al.* 1980), might produce some accommodation, although we do not observe evidence of any accommodative or pupillary function within the post-operative two weeks. Another possibility is that the nerve section has some secondary effects that confound the effect of absence of accommodation. For example, the extremely dilated pupil in the nerve-sectioned eyes may interfere with aqueous drainage and thereby cause changes in intraocular pressure leading to increased eye size and myopia.

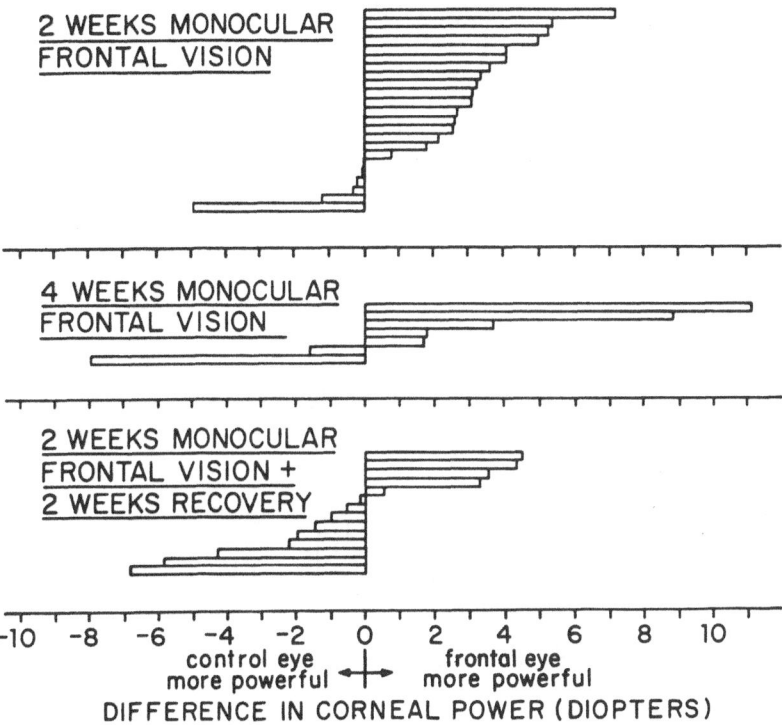

2 WEEKS MONOCULAR
FRONTAL VISION

4 WEEKS MONOCULAR
FRONTAL VISION

2 WEEKS MONOCULAR
FRONTAL VISION +
2 WEEKS RECOVERY

-10 -8 -6 -4 -2 0 2 4 6 8 10

control eye
more powerful ◄──┼──► frontal eye
more powerful

DIFFERENCE IN CORNEAL POWER (DIOPTERS)

Fig. 3. Corneal power differences associated with the presence of and recovery from frontal vision myopia. Each horizontal bar represents the corneal power of the eye with frontal vision minus the control eye. Only comparison of the top and third distribution yielded statistically significant results (Mann-Whitney U test; p < 0.01).

CHANGES IN CORNEAL CURVATURE

There are two obvious roles that changes in the curvature of the cornea could play in the results presented here: Increases in corneal curvature could account for part of the myopia observed; decreases in corneal curvature during recovery from myopia might explain the dramatic and rapid recoveries described above. The latter suggestion is similar to emmetropization in human eyes, in which eyes of greater than normal axial length tend to have corneas and lenses less curved than normal (Sorsby 1976). Yinon, *et al.* (1980) report a similar association for chickens made myopic by lid suture. It is generally difficult to know in such cases as these whether the less curved corneas and lenses in fact represent an active growth process or whether they are simply the consequence of larger eyes having larger corneas and lenses, these having proportionately larger radii of curvature.

We examined corneal curvature during three experimental situations: Induction of monocular myopia by restricting one eye to frontal vision; recovery from two weeks of monocular myopia induced by removal of the

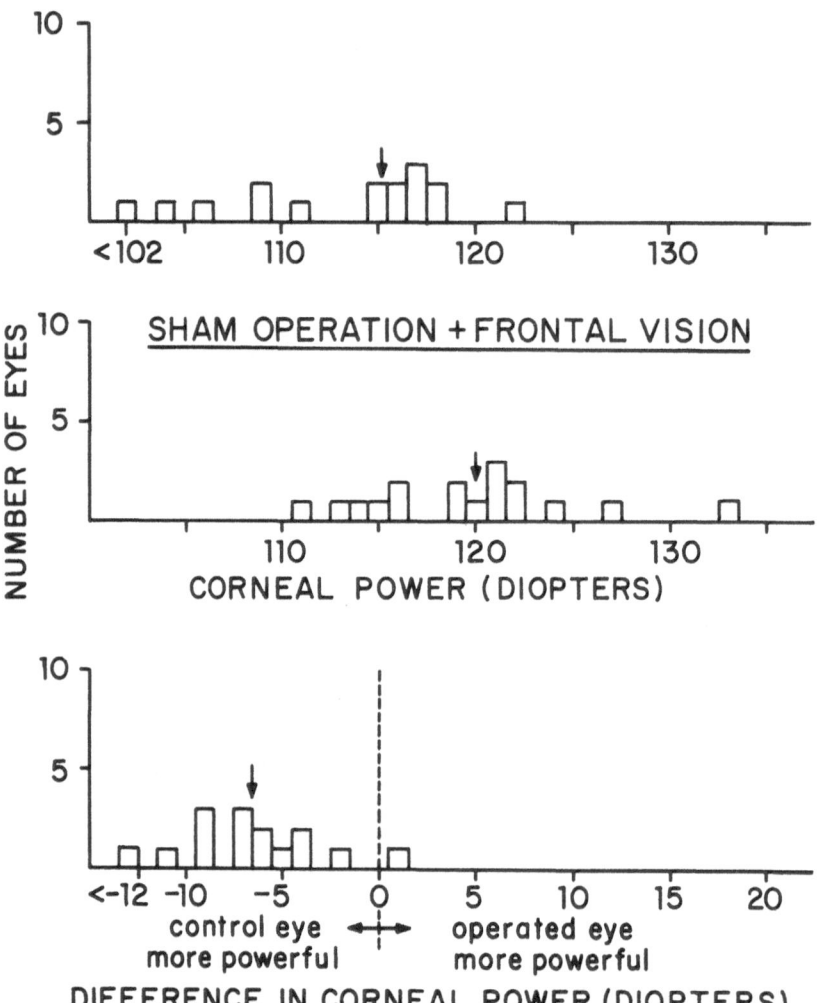

Fig. 4. Effect of monocular ciliary nerve cut on corneal power in animals binocularly restricted to frontal visual fields. Arrows indicate medians. The upper two distributions are significantly different (Mann-Whitney U test, P < 0.01). Lower distribution is of the difference between each nerve-cut eye and its sham-operated companion; its median is significantly less than 0 (Binomial test, p < 0.01).

visual restriction; and ciliary nerve cut plus restriction to frontal vision. Corneal curvature was assessed by photographing the eyes with a circular flash tube centered on the pupil. Measurements of the resulting corneal reflection were compared to similar photographs of calibrated steel spheres to yield the radius of corneal curvature. The refractive power of the anterior corneal surface was estimated from this by using the refractive index of chicken cornea (Sivak, *et al.* 1978).

The results (Figure 3) showed that when frontal vision myopia was induced in one eye the corneal curvature of that eye became significantly greater, thereby contributing to the myopia observed. This change is opposite from what would be expected as a passive result of the increased eye size in this condition reported above. Conversely, during recovery from myopia the difference in corneal curvature decreased, thereby reducing the myopia. In the animals with ciliary nerve section of one eye, that eye had lower corneal power than the companion eye (Figure 4), suggesting that accommodation may be required for the increases in corneal power found in myopic animals.

It is easy to imagine a mechanism to account for this effect of lack of accommodation on corneal growth, at least in birds. The ciliary muscles of birds are attached in such a manner that, during contraction, forces are exerted on the corneal margin tending to move it centripetally, thereby decreasing its radius of curvature (Gundlach, *et al.* 1945). We have measured this change in corneal power during pharmacologically induced accommodation to be approximately 11 D (Rosenthal and Wallman, manuscript in preparation). One can envision frequent stress of the cornea in this manner provoking corneal growth that permanently alters the corneal radius of curvature.

Thus changes in corneal curvature can occur either in a direction that compensates for or in a direction that augments the refractive changes produced by axial length increase. It therefore appears that corneal curvature is dynamically controlled at least during the first weeks of life to help adjust the refractive power of the eye.

CONCLUDING REMARKS

More generally, we have shown that there is a period of plasticity of the refractive condition of the chick eye during which restriction to the frontal visual field produces severe myopia, and the removal of the restriction produces amelioration of the myopia. The myopia is associated with axial length increase and corneal curvature increase; however, comparison of the magnitude of these changes with the severity of the myopia suggests that part of the refractive error may be due to lenticular changes. The fact that ciliary nerve section significantly reduces the effect of restriction to the frontal visual field argues that accommodation is a mediating variable.

It is interesting that the susceptible period for refractive changes resulting from these experimental manipulations is the same developmental period during which the eye grows in such a way as to reduce the high variability of neonatal refractions. We propose that the mechanism for this growth toward emmetropia is probably the same as that responsible for frontal vision myopia and that this mechanism uses accommodation or accommodative demand as an error signal to regulate the harmonious growth of globe, cornea and lens, leading to a refractive condition suited to the organism's visual requirements.

REFERENCES

Belkin, M., Yinon, U., Rose L. & Reisert, I.: Effect of visual environment on refractive error of cats. Documenta Ophthalmol. 42: 433 (1977).

Gundlach, R.H., Chard, R. & Skahen, J.R.: The mechanism of accommodation in pigeons. J. Comp. Psychol. 38: 27 (1945).

McKanna, J.A. & Casagrande, V.A.: Reduced lens development in lid-suture myopia. Exp. Eye Res. 26: 715 (1978).

Nye, P.W.: On the functional differences between frontal and lateral visual fields of the pigeon. Vision Res. 13: 559 (1973).

Pilar, G., Landmesser, L. & Burstein, L.: Competition for survival among developing ciliary ganglion cells. J. Neurophysiol. 43: 233 (1980).

Sherman, S.M., Norton, T.T. & Casagrande, V.A.: Myopia in the lid-sutured tree shrew (Tupaia glis). Brain Res. 124: 154 (1977).

Sivak, J.G., Bobier, W.R., & Levy, B.: The refractive significance of the nictitating membrane of the bird eye. J. Comp. Physiol. 125: 335 (1978).

Sorsby, A.: Biology of the eye as an optical system. In: Clinical Opthalmology, Vol. 1, Ed. T.D. Duane New York, Harper and Row (1976).

Wallman, J., Adams, J.I. & Trachtman, J.N.: The eyes of young chickens grow toward emmetropia. Invest. Ophthalmol. Vis. Sci. 20: 557 (1981).

Wallman, J., Turkel, J. & Trachtman, J.: Extreme myopia produced by modest change in early visual experience. Science. 201: 1249 (1978).

Wiesel, T.N. & Raviola, E.: Myopia and eye enlargement following neonatal lid fusion in monkeys. Nature. 266: 66 (1977).

Wilson, J.R. & Sherman, S.M.: Differential effects of early monocular deprivation on binocular and monocular segments of cat striate cortex. J. Neurophysiol. 40: 891 (1977).

Yinon, U., Rose, L. & Shapiro, A.: Myopia in the eye of developing chicks following monocular and binocular lid closure. Vision Res. 20: 137 (1979).

Young, F.A.: The effect of restricted visual space on the primate eye. Am. J. Ophthalmol. 52: 799 (1961).

Authors' address
Biology Department, City College,
City University of New York,
New York, New York 10031
U.S.A.

THE NATURAL HISTORY OF POSTERIOR STAPHYLOMA DEVELOPMENT

B.J. CURTIN, M.D.

(New York, N.Y., U.S.A.)

ABSTRACT

Posterior staphyloma is the most important lesion of pathologic myopia (which ranks as the seventh cause of adult blindness in U.S.A.). A knowledge of the evolution of the most common form of staphyloma, that involving the posterior pole (type 1), is indispensable for the understanding and eventual treatment of this disease.

A total of 400 eyes with type 1 staphyloma were involved in this cross-sectional and longitudinal study using binocular ophthalmoscopy. The present survey is based on 350 consecutive patients aged 1–82 years. Five ophthalmoscopic stages of the disease can be distinguished.

Two principal factors are involved in the progression of the ectatic process: scleral resistance and intraocular pressure. Prophylactic and therapeutic possibilities are discussed on this background.

INTRODUCTION

The posterior staphyloma is found with increasing frequency as the degree of myopia becomes greater (Curtin and Karlin 1971). Its presence is also associated with substantial reductions in visual acuity (Curtin 1976, Curtin 1977). In spite of the obvious importance of this lesion, little is known of its natural history. This study was undertaken to determine the manner in which the most common type of primary posterior staphyloma, (Type 1), evolves (Figure 1) (Curtin 1977).

SUBJECTS AND METHODS

A total of 350 consecutive patients who demonstrated a posterior pole staphyloma (Type 1) or its compound, multilevel variants (Types 6 through 10) were included in this cross-sectional and longitudinal study. Each patient was given a complete ophthalmologic examination including binocular indirect ophthalmoscopy. There were 208 female and 142 male patients who ranged in age from one to 82 years.

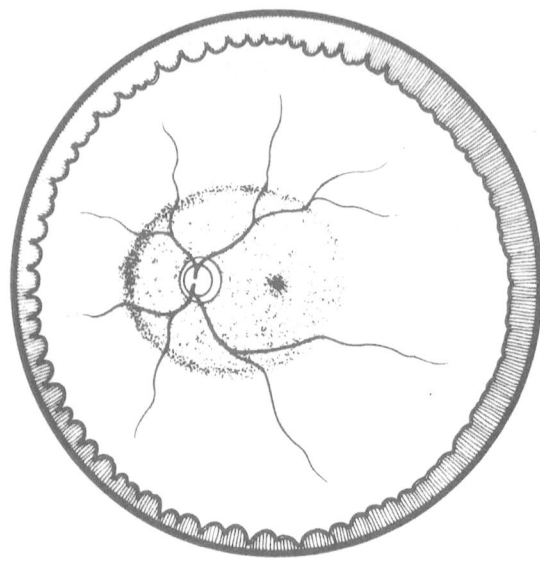

TYPE I

Fig. 1. The primary Type 1 (posterior pole) staphyloma.

RESULTS

Five grades or stages of posterior staphyloma development could be discerned. Longitudinal studies verified the progression of the posterior staphyloma from each grade to the next. In some eyes the progression was extremely rapid and the most advanced grade five could be found in eyes of patients as young as eight years.

Grade 1. These eyes evidence mild tesselation and pallor involving the fundus in an oval or circular area. This area extends from two to four disc diameters nasal to the optic nerve temporally to the macular region. Crescent formation is seen on the temporal margin of the disc and peripapillary extention may also be present. Ectasia of this area is not apparent (Figure 2). 236 eyes of 142 patients presented with these fundus changes. 82 were female and 60 were male. The age range extended from one to 71 years with a median age of 8.5 years.

Grade 2. The area and degree of tesselation and pallor is usually somewhat greater than in grade 1 in these eyes. A shallow sloping ectasia of the nasal margin can now be detected (Figure 3). 54 eyes of 34 patients were seen with these findings. The age range was from three to 67 years and the median age was 10 years.

Grade 3. These eyes show a distinct, sharp ectasia of the nasal staphyloma margin in addition to a soft sloping of the balance of the staphyloma

208

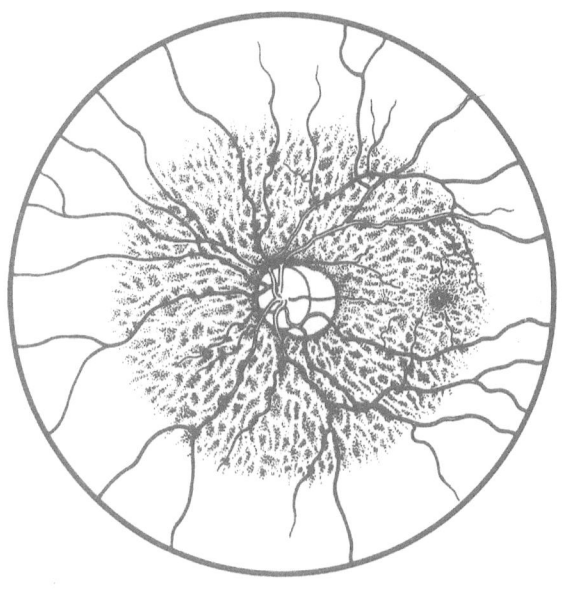

Fig. 2. Posterior pole staphyloma; Grade 1.

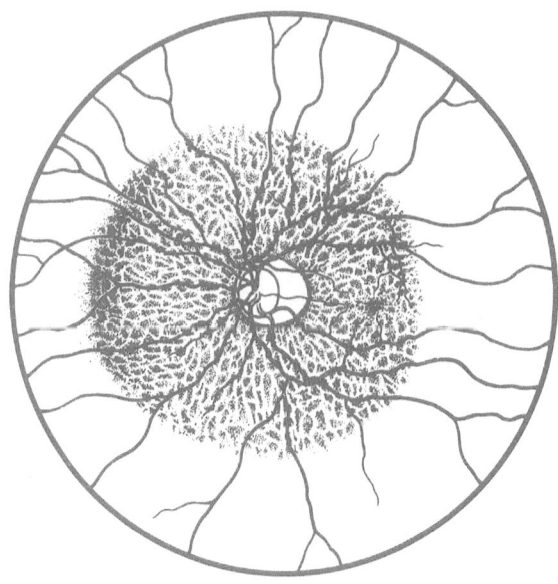

Fig. 3. Posterior pole staphyloma; Grade 2.

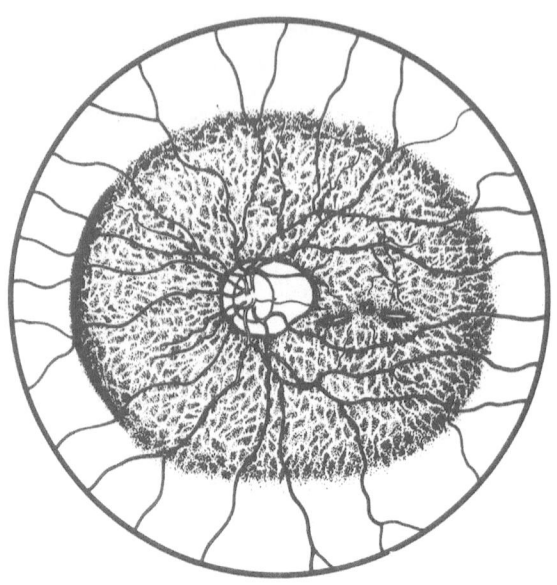

Fig. 4. Posterior pole staphyloma; Grade 3.

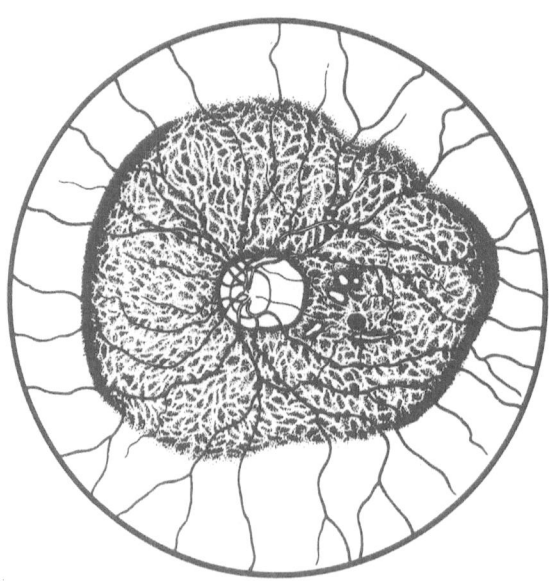

Fig. 5. Posterior pole staphyloma; Grade 4.

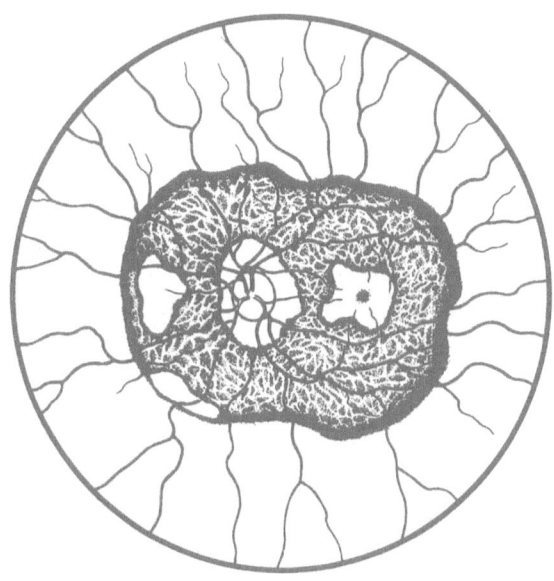

Fig. 6. Posterior pole staphyloma; Grade 5.

perimeter. The staphyloma area may also be increased in size (Figure 4) and the pallor and tesselation further accentuated. In the eyes of individuals 40 years and above, the presence of degenerative fundus changes within the staphyloma can be detected. These preferentially affect the peripapillary area and the macular region. 167 eyes of 111 patients showed these changes. Their age ranged from four to 75 years. The median age was 26 years.

Grade 4. The presence of an abrupt edge extending over 180° but not the complete circumference of the staphyloma marks the distinctive fundus picture in this group. The sharp staphyloma edge rarely extends about the margin from the nasal side, however. Rather a new abrupt margin appears on the temporal aspect of the staphyloma. This is usually well temporal to the macula due to the expansion of the staphyloma. Tesselation, pallor and degenerative changes are somewhat greater at this level (Figure 5). 49 eyes of 32 patients showed such fundi. Their age range was from eight to 75 years and the median age was 46 years.

Grade 5. In these eyes sharp or abrupt borders can be seen over the entire circumference of the staphyloma or the multileveled, compound types of staphyloma emerge. These latter types may feature staphylomas within staphylomas (Types 6 and 7), terraced or steplike ectasia of the nasal staphyloma wall (Type 8) or unusual septa or plicae which compartmentalize the staphyloma (Types 9 and 10) (Figure 6) (Curtin 1971). 112 eyes of 69 patients were found with these changes. Their age ranged from eight to 82 years and the median age was 52 years.

211

DISCUSSION

This study indicates that the posterior staphyloma is a progressive developmental lesion. It can be detected in its earliest form before ectasia is demonstrable and has its most significant development from the median age of 8.5 to 26 years. This study also indicates that, while any grade of staphyloma development can be an end stage in itself, there is a strong tendency for these lesions to undergo continued ectasia. Increasing axial length, as well as age, have been demonstrated to be important factors in the production of myopic chorioretinal degeneration (Curtin and Karlin 1971). In view of these facts it is apparent that an effective treatment, instituted at grade 1, could have a beneficial effect upon the course of pathologic myopia with posterior staphyloma.

Two cardinal factors are involved in scleral ectasia, the intraocular pressure and scleral resistence. Ocular hypertension should be carefully controlled in these patients. The recent additions of timolol maleate and dipivephrine to our pharmacologic armamentarium makes available effective means of controlling the intraocular pressure without the risk that the use of miotics pose to the myopic eye.

Animal experiments have found scleral reinforcement to be an effective means of increasing scleral resistence (Curtin 1960, Johnson, et al. 1962). Numerous clinical studies have reported excellent results in the stabilization of progressive high myopia with this procedure (Borley and Snyder 1958, Curtin 1961, Miller and Borley 1964, Nesterov and Libenson 1967, Nesterov and Libenson 1970, Nesterov, et al. 1976). The results of this study indicate that most of these efforts would seem to be misdirected. The macular area, the object of these supporting procedures, appears to be involved secondarily in the expanding ectatic process which originates nasal to the optic nerve. Attempts have been made to support both the macula and nasal areas using either a horizontal graft (Barraquer and Barraquer 1956) or a segment of donor scleral shell (Zardova and Negoda 1970, Whitwell, 1971). In general, scleral reinforcement surgery has failed to gain widespread acceptance as an effective treatment of progression in high myopia. It would seem that fresher approaches to reinforcement of the posterior sclera, especially the area about the optic nerve, should be made. These procedures must not damage the ciliary nerves, blood vessels or the optic nerve. The scleral application of biocompatible synthetics is one possibility, another would be the transplantation of normal fibroblasts into the defective sclera. These materials are presently available and their effective use would not appear to be beyond the capabilities of modern ophthalmic science.

REFERENCES

Barraquer, T. and Barraquer, J.: Nueva orientation terapeutica en la miopia progressiva. Arch. Soc. Oftal. Hisp-Amer. 16: 1137–1144 (1956).
Borley, W.E. and Snyder, A.A.: Surgical treatment of high myopia. Trans. Am. Acad. Ophthalmol. & Otolaryng. 62: 791–802 (1958).

Curtin, B.J.: Surgical support of the posterior sclera. Part I. Experimental results. Am. J. Ophthalmol. 49: 1341–1350 (1960).

Curtin, B.J.: Surgical support of the posterior sclera. Part II. Clinical results. Am. J. Ophthalmol. 52: 853–862 (1961).

Curtin, B.J.: Visual acuity in myopia. In: Clinical low vision, Ed. Faye, E.E. Little, Brown and Co., Boston, pp. 295–300 (1976).

Curtin, B.J.: The posterior staphyloma of pathologic myopia. Trans. Am. Ophthalmol. Soc. 75: 67–86 (1977).

Curtin, B.J. and Karlin, D.B.: Axial length measurements and fundus changes of the myopic eye. Am. J. Ophthalmol. 71: 42–53 (1971).

Johnson, W.A., Henderson, J.W., Parkhill, E.M. and Grindlay, J.H.: Transplantation of homographs of sclera. Am. J. Ophthalmol. 54: 1019–1030 (1962).

Miller, W. W. and Borley, W.E.: Surgical treatment of degenerative myopia; Scleral Reinforcement. Am. J. Ophthalmol. 57: 796–804 (1964).

Nesterov, A.P. and Libenson, N.B.: Strengthening of sclera with a strip of broad fascia in progressing myopia. Vest. Oftal. 46 (1): 15–19 (1967).

Nesterov, A.P. and Libenson, N.B.: Strengthening the sclera with a strip of fascia lata in progressive myopia. Br. J. Ophthalmol. 54: 46–50 (1970).

Nesterov, A.P., Libenson, N.B. and Svirin, A.V.: Early and late results of fascia lata transplantation in high myopia. Br. J. Ophthalmol. 60: 271–273 (1976).

Whitwell, J.: Scleral reinforcement in degenerative myopia. Trans. Ophthalmol. Soc. U.K. 91: 679–686 (1971).

Zarkova, M.V. and Negoda, V.I.: Grafting of homologous sclera in progressive myopia Vest. Oftal. 49 (4): 16–20 (1970).

Author's address:
B.J. Curtin, M.D.
Myopia Clinic of the Manhattan Eye, Ear and Throat Hospital
New York, New York
U.S.A.

213

NATURAL HISTORY OF FUCHS' SPOT: A LONG-TERM FOLLOW-UP STUDY

M. FRIED, A. SIEBERT, G. MEYER-SCHWICKERATH and
A. WESSING

(*Essen, West-Germany*)

ABSTRACT

Basic data on 206 eyes of 145 patients with Fuchs' spot and follow-up results on 55 eyes of 36 patients were reported to elucidate the nature and natural course of this condition.

Fuchs' spot is not a rare occurence, affecting 5–10% of myopes over − 5. D. Sex bears an influence on incidence, women being twice as often affected as men. Fuchs' spot tends to develope in both maculas in a considerable percentage (20–50%) during a short interval. There is a marked effect of age, refraction and axial length on incidence with peaks of manifestion between 40–50 years, around − 12,0 D and between 26,5 to 31,4 mm of axial length.

In unilateral cases affected eyes are usually more myopic than non-affected eyes. Anisomyopia is no protection for the less myopic eye against Fuchs' spot. In unilateral cases usually the higher myopic eye will be affected. There is a tendency to earlier manifestation with rising degree of myopia. Patients with Fuchs' spot are almost exclusively juvenile myopes with a high percentage of myopia in their families.

The follow-up study revealed in general a relatively benign visual prognosis, especially for near vision. Fuchs' spot seems to be largely a non-progressive, relatively stationary condition for about 2/3 of patients. The high percentage of spontaneous scarring of subretinal neovascularisation (SRN) is of favourable prognostic significance. SRN in high myopes seem to posses a less active potential than SRN in emmetropes, probably due to the atrophic changes that take over. The course of this condition is mostly self-limited. Spontaneous cicatrization of SRN and stabilization or slight improvement of vision in 2/3 of cases characterize the natural course of Fuchs' spot.

INTRODUCTION

The ophthalmoscopic appearance of a pigmented lesion of the macula in highly myopic eyes is well known since its first description by Förster (1862) and its detailed analysis by Fuchs (1901). In their honour it has been termed

Table 1. Study population of patients with Fuchs' spot from the Essen University Eye Hospital during the years 1957 to 1980.

	No. of patients	No. of eyes
Group A*	145	206
Group B**	36	55

*Includes all patients documented to have Fuchs' spot.
**Patients answering to a follow-up call in 1980.
Group B is part of Group A.

Förster-Fuchs' spot. Its histologic features have first been studied by Lehmus (1875) and valuable clinical reports have been produced by various authors (Aiello and Master 1953; Lloyd 1954; Campos 1957, D'Hoine *et al.* 1974). Gass (1967) first interpretated this lesion as a disciform, neovascular process associated with breaks in Bruchs' membrane. This notion gained universal acceptance and has found confirmation in further fluorescein angiographic studies by Levy, *et al.* (1974, 1977). Ultrasonic data of eyes with Fuchs' spot were first produced by Curtin and Karlin (1971).

However, the question regarding the visual prognosis and natural course has received little systematic attention. We report herein the findings in this regard based on a retrospective follow-up study with a final reexamination at the end of the observation period.

The purpose of this study was to evaluate the natural course of visual acuity, changes in fundus appearances, frequency of recurrencies and involvement of the second eye.

SUBJECTS AND METHODS

For this purpose the fundus slides and records of all patients with the diagnosis Fuchs' spot at the Essen University Eye Hospital were reviewed in 1980. 206 eyes of 145 patients were documented to have Fuchs' spot (Group A) and up to date 36 patients living within a reasonable travel distance answered to our follow-up call (Group B). (Table 1). A complete ocular examination, including fundus photography, fluorescein angiography and ultrasonic biometry was performed. Follow-up ranged from three to 15 years, with a median of five years. A follow-up of at least three years was considered sufficient to meet the natural history criteria.

RESULTS AND DISCUSSION

Women were twice as often affected as men, the female – male ratio being 2:1. One explanation for the predominance of females is that women are more prone to higher degrees of myopia (Duke-Elder 1976).

Patients with Fuchs' spot are almost exclusively juvenile myopes (94,4%), myopia developing before the age of 15 years (mean 9,6 ± 5,2 years).

216

Table 2. Frequency of unilateral and bilateral cases of Fuchs' spot.

	Unilateral	Bilateral
Group A	86/145 (59,3%)	59/145 (40,7%)
Group B	17/36 (47,2%)	19/36 (52,8%)

At the same time, the frequency of myopia in their first degree relatives is quite high, reaching 29,68%. 58,3% of their parents were myopic.

Age of manifestation of Fuchs' spot varies largely in individual cases. In our series the youngest was a 14-year old boy and the oldest men and women 66 years of age. There is a strong predilection for the 30 to 60 years age group, the median being 41 years. Males and females show no significant differences regarding age at manifestation.

Bilaterality

The frequency of Fuchs' spot in both eyes was 40–52% in our series, which is higher than in other reports. (Fuchs (1901) = 24%; Campos (1957) = 28–42%; Curtin and Karlin (1971) = 18,2%). This figure depends very much on length of follow-up and reflects the fact that referral centers see the more desperate cases. (Table 2).

The follow-up group revealed rising bilaterality with length of follow-up. The time interval between involvement of the first eye and the second eye may vary largely from days to many years. The average time interval in this study was 2.4 years, with a range from 0–8 years and the median being one year. Fuchs (1901) in his original article mentioned a time interval of up to five years. We confirm, that in the majority of susceptible individuals both maculas may be affected during a short course.

Refraction

This study corroborates that Fuchs' spot affects mainly moderately high myopes around $-12,0$ D.

However, a comparison with the refraction curve of Betsch (1929) shows that the incidence of myopia decreases as the degree of myopia increases. In other words, excessive high myopes are infrequent and so are Fuchs' spot in such eyes as well.

The importance of degree of myopia in the pathogenesis of Fuchs' spot becomes apparrent in that affected eyes are significantly more myopic than non-affected eyes in the same individuals ($-12,47 \pm 5,08$ D vs $-10,52 \pm 5,5$ D; $p < 0.01$).

Anisomyopia as such is no protection against Fuchs' spot, since 44,6% of anisomyopes were bilaterally affected. On the other hand, in anisomyopia the more myopic eye is significantly more frequently affected than the less myopic eye ($p < 0.05$).

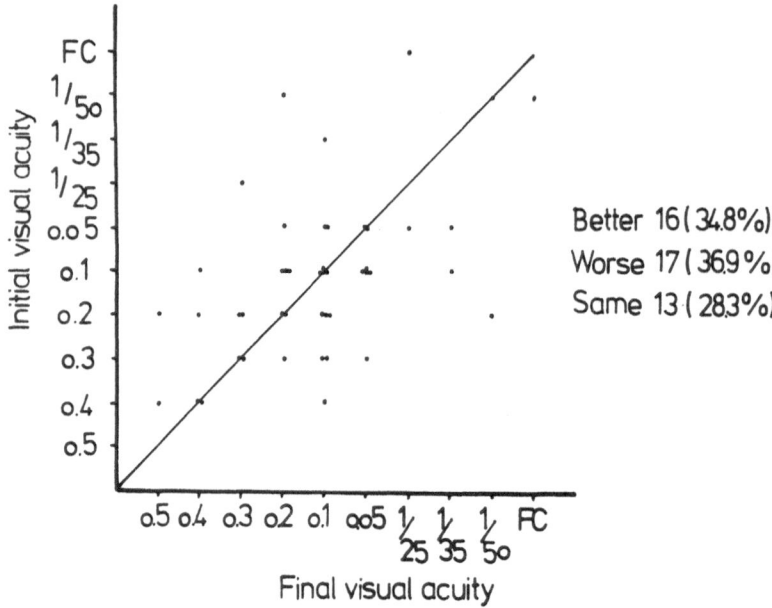

Fig. 1. Scattergram comparing initial visual acuity and final visual acuity in the follow-up group.

Age of onset of Fuchs' spot and degree of myopia are significantly related in such a way, that manifestation tends to occur earlier with rising degree of myopia, the correlation coefficient being $r = -0,44; p < 0,001$.

The same relation exists between age of onset of Fuchs' spot and axial length ($r = -0,33; p < 0,05$).

All this proofs the fundamental role of the degree of myopia in the pathogenesis of Fuchs' spot.

Visual prognosis

When initial visual acuity is plotted against final visual acuity apparently 34,8% of eyes improve, 36.9% deteriorate and 28,3% retain unchanged visual acuity (Figure 1). This is to say, that in about 2/3 or 63% of eyes visual acuity was stabilized or improved untreated during follow-up. Almost as many eyes improved spontaneously as deteriorated. The overall distribution of visual acuity changes very little during follow-up. Median visual acuity at begin and at end of study was unchanged 0,1.

Visual prognosis is slightly better in the younger age group ($r = -0,36; p < 0,01$). Visual prognosis is not related to the degree of myopia. Unilateral and bilateral cases do not differ in their visual outcome.

218

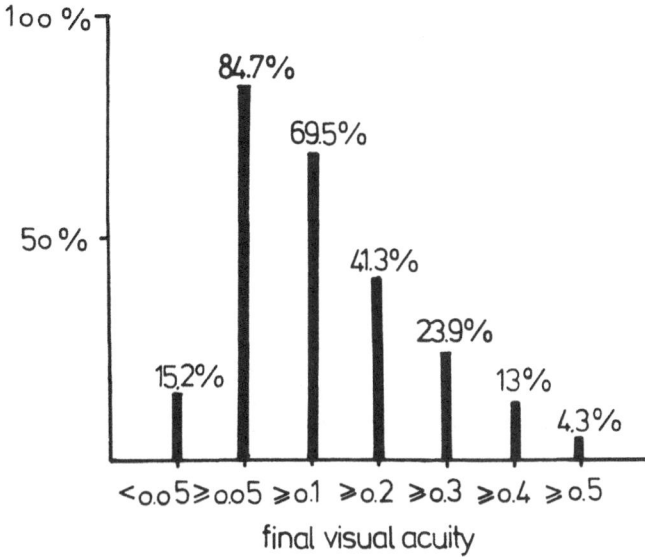

Group B   n = 46 eyes

Fig. 2. Histogram showing the cumulative final visual acuity in the follow-up group.

Interestingly, near visual acuity recorded at the most favourable reading distance is usually better than distance visual acuity (67,3% of eyes; $p < 0,001$). Most eyes with Fuchs' spot retain some reading vision ability. This reflects the fact, that in most cases not the whole fovea is involved and that myopes benefit from their own magnification as they approach the reading text.

On the whole, Fuchs' spot seems to carry a relatively benign visual prognosis. Visual acuity of 0,2 or more was retained by 41,3% of eyes, of 0,1 or more by 69,5% and of 0,05 or more by 84,7% of eyes. Legal blindness resulted in three out of 46 eyes (6,5%) (Figure 2).

Regarding visual prognosis Fuchs' spot seems to be a non-progressive, relatively stationary condition. After the initial visual impairment chances for moderate improvement or stabilization are good.

Morphology

Fuchs (1901) in his original article gave a distinctive clinical description of the typical pigmented lesion of the macula, which he thought was due to the accumulation of pigment and not related to hemorrhage. Fuchs had observed hemorrhage in only nine of his 50 cases and considered it to be a merely accidental association. He stressed to have seen many macular hemorrhages in myopes not resulting in a pigmented lesion.

219

In this report we were able to detect fresh macular hemorrhage in 78% and subretinal neovascularization (SRN) on fluorescein angiography in 77% of macular lesions. We also noted lacquer cracks in 54,5% at the posterior pole. Lacquer crack lesions are due to rupture of Bruchs' membrane and may provide the entry for subretinal neovascularization. (Klein and Curtin 1975). The high percentage of chorioretinal atrophy found (90,9%) is another clue to the pathogenesis.

The course of these fresh hemorrhagic macular lesions due to SRN is, however, quite variable. During the subsequent course the clinical appearance is to a high degree changeable. Many turn into this heavily pigmented, sharply demarcated black lesion. Others tend to develop pigment dispersion as the acute hemorrhage resolves. Increase in chorioretinal atrophy (75%) during the course is a prominent feature, sometimes dissolving the typical Fuchs' spot.

When visual prognosis is related to morphology the single most important variable is foveal involvement. Involvement of the fovea was defined as an area roughly equivalent to the normal retinal avascular zone using a transparent overlay grid. Involvement of the fovea was noted initially in 26 of 46 eyes reducing visual acuity to 0,1 or less. As the acute lesion resolved seven eyes regained visual acuity above 0,1 (range 0,2–0,4; mean 0,25). There is a decent chance of improvement as the acute lesion resolves. On the other hand ten of 46 eyes with an extrafoveal lesion initially developed foveal involvement during follow-up reducing visual acuity to 0,1 and less.

A second factor of significance is recurrent hemorrhage which we observed in 15 of 55 eyes (27,3%). Such recurrency led to further deterioration in eight of 15 eyes (53,3%), while in five of 15 eyes acuity improved and in two of 15 eyes remained unchanged despite recurrency of bleeding.

A third factor of significance regarding visual acuity is persistence of SRN (as documented by fluorescein angiography) with or without recurrent hemorrhage. Persistent SRN were detected in 11 of 29 eyes (37,9%). In such cases vision deteriorated further in 72,7% (8 of 11 eyes).

Spontaneous scarring of SRN was seen in 72,4% (21 of 29 eyes) and increase in chorioretinal atrophy in 75% (22 of 29 eyes) of eyes. In such eyes vision improved in 50% and stabilized in 60–80% in due course. Spontaneous scarring of SRN coincident with increase in chorioretinal atrophy is frequent and turned out to be of favourable prognostic significance. SRN in high myopic eyes seem to possess a less active potential than in emmetropic eyes, probably due to atrophic changes that take over. In no case did we note such enormous disciform responses as may be seen in the presumed ocular histoplasmosis syndrome or in senile disciform macular degeneration (Junius Kuhnt).

This might explain the relatively benign course Fuchs' spot has. Progressive visual loss, recurrent hemorrhage and persistent growth of SRN are absent in about 2/3 of all patients. Spontaneous cicatrization of the SRN and stabilization or slight improvement of visual acuity in about 60% characterize the natural course of Fuchs' spot.

REFERENCES

Aiello, J.S., Master, S.: Fuchs' spot in the macula. A rare lesion in myopic patients. Am. J. Ophthalmol., 36: 1126–1128 (1953).

Campos, R.: La tache de Fuchs. Mod. Probl. Ophthalmol., 1: 364–373 (1957).

Curtin, B.J., Karlin, D.B.: Axial length measurements and fundus changes of the myopic eye. Am. J. Ophthalmol., 71: 42–53 (1971).

D'Hoine, G., Turut, P., Francois, P., Hache, J.Ch.: L'atteinte maculaire des myopes. Bull. Soc. Ophthal. Fr., 74: 821–826 (1974).

Duke-Elder, S.: System of Ophthalmology. Vol. V: Ophthalmic optics and refraction. Henry Kimpton, London pp. 300–362 (1970).

Förster, R.: Ophthalmologische Beiträge. p. 55, T.C.F. Enslin, Berlin (1862).

Fuchs, E.: Der zentrale schwarze Fleck bei Myopie. Z. f. Augenheilk., 5: 171–178 (1901).

Gass, J.D.M.: Pathogenesis of disciform detachment of the neuro-epithelium. VI.: Disciform detachment secondary to heredogenerative neoplastic and traumatic lesions of the choroid. Am. J. Ophthalmol., 63: 689–711 (1967).

Klein, R.M., Curtin, B.J.: Laquer crack lesions in pathological myopia. Am. J. Ophthalmol., 79: 380–392 (1975).

Lehmus, Die Erkrankungen der Macula lutea bei progressiver Myopie. Inaug. Diss., Zürich (1875).

Lloyd, R.I.: Clinical studies of the myopic macula. Trans. Am. Acad. Ophthalmol. Otolaryngol., 51: 273–284 (1954).

Levy, J.M., Pollock, H.M., Curtin, B.J.: The Fuchs' spot: an angiographic study. In: Ed. Shimizu, K. Fluorescein angriography. Proc. Int. Symposium 'Fluorescein Angiography', Tokyo pp. 182–186 (1972), Igaku Shoin, Publ. Tokyo (1974).

Levy, J.H., Pollock, H.M., Curtin, B.J.: The Fuchs' spot: an ophthalmoscopic and fluorescein angiographic study. Ann. Ophthalmol., 9: 1433–1443 (1977).

Authors' address:

Prof. A. Wessing, M.D.
Essen University Eye Hospital
Hufelandstrasse 55
D-4300 Essen 1
West-Germany

DIFFUSE CHOROIDAL ATROPHIES AND HIGH MYOPIA

A. GIOVANNINI and S. COLOMBATI

(*Bologna, Italia*)

ABSTRACT

After having classified the atrophies of the choroid and of the pigment epithelium, which can be found in cases of high myopia, three cases of widespread atrophy of the choroid and of the pigment epithelium are presented: these atrophies cover more than half of the retina, 5/8 and 7/8 of the total area of the retina.

INTRODUCTION

Atrophic changes of the choroid and of the pigment epithelium represent a common trait of high myopia.

They can be classified in a manner analogous to non-myopic choroidal atrophies as regional choroidal atrophy (RCA) and diffuse choroidal atrophy (DCA).

The RCA's can be defined, according to their location, as central or peripheral, and, according to their extension, as total or segmentary.

The DCA's can be complete or incomplete depending on their extension.

Moreover, both RCA's and DCA's can involve only the pigment epithelium and the choriocapillaris, or they may affect almost the entire choroid.

REGIONAL CHOROIDAL ATROPHY (RCA)

(a) *Central RCA's* are most frequently *partial.*

The finding of *almost total* atrophies in the peri-para-papillary and macular regions is typical in high myopia.

Sometimes, these atrophies can have a long and wave-like shape, and spare the macular region, while in other instances they can be of limited extension but affect the macular region.

Within these atrophies it is easy to recognize those secondary to seroushaemorrhagic detachments of the pigment epithelium and of the macular neurosensorial retina, which we will therefore separate from the others to be considered primary.

Doc. Ophthal. Proc. Series, Vol. 28,
ed. by H.C. Fledelius, P.H. Alsbirk and E. Goldschmidt
© *1981 Dr W. Junk Publishers, The Hague*

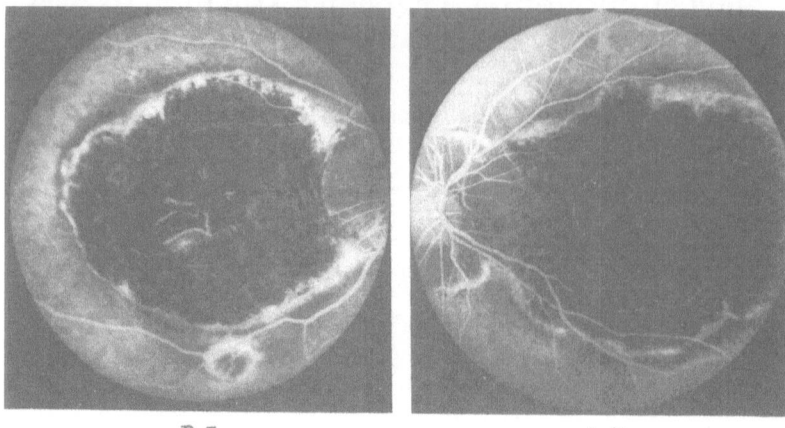

R.E.   L.E.

Fig. 1. Total regional choroidal atrophy (RCA) in high myopia, shown by fluorescein angiography.

The *total RCA's,* also frequent in high myopia, can be extremely characteristic, as in the case shown in Figure 1.

Their frequent bilateral nature and the clinical characteristics (which allow their differentiation from the related Amalric major ovalar syndromes) suggest a nosologic entity and a pathogenesis at variance with those found in non myopic eyes (true Amalric syndromes), which are clearly acquired and secondary to vascular accidents to the ciliary vessels.

(b) As for *peripheral RCA's,* the *total* forms are also typical of myopia, even though the *incomplete* forms are very frequent as well.

As already mentioned, they can involve total atrophy of the choroid (the so-called gyrate atrophies of the myopic eye, Figure 2), or only of the pigment epithelium.

A large part of the equatorial and peripheral retinic degenerations give rise to segmentary forms, which are therefore not specific of high myopia.

As with the central forms, one can of course find 'secondary' atrophies among peripheral RCA's, as shown in the following case in which one can see a wide band of mixed atrophy, in part only of the pigment epithelium and of the choriocapillaris, in part of the whole choroid.

Such mixed atrophy, which is secondary to a giant retinoschisis, the profile of which it interrupts, describes a wide arch in the inferior hemiretina, from the nasal to the temporal periphery and affects part of the macular area (Figure 3).

DIFFUSE CHOROIDAL ATROPHY (DCA)

While some of the *complete* forms of DCA (choroideremies) are unrelated to myopia, the gyrate atrophies of the choroid and retina are found in association with myopia in 80–90% of the cases. In our experience however, the

224

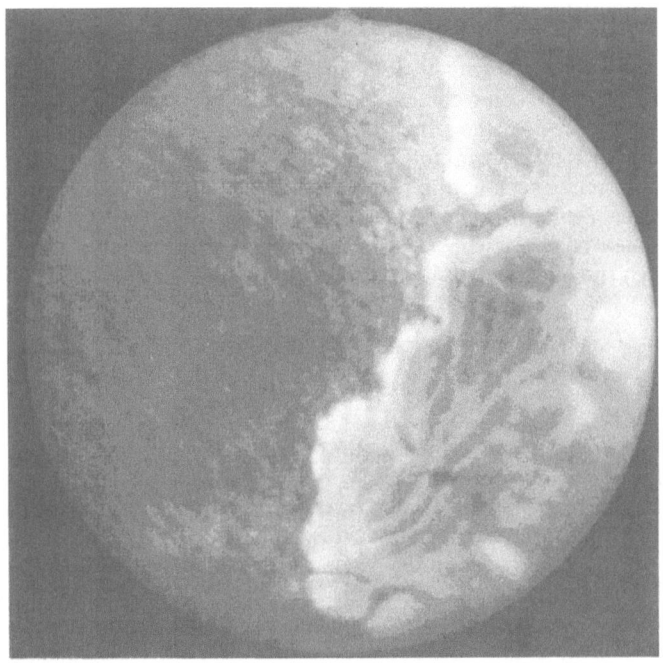

Fig. 2. Peripheral regional choroidal atrophy (RCA) in a myopic eye, total form.

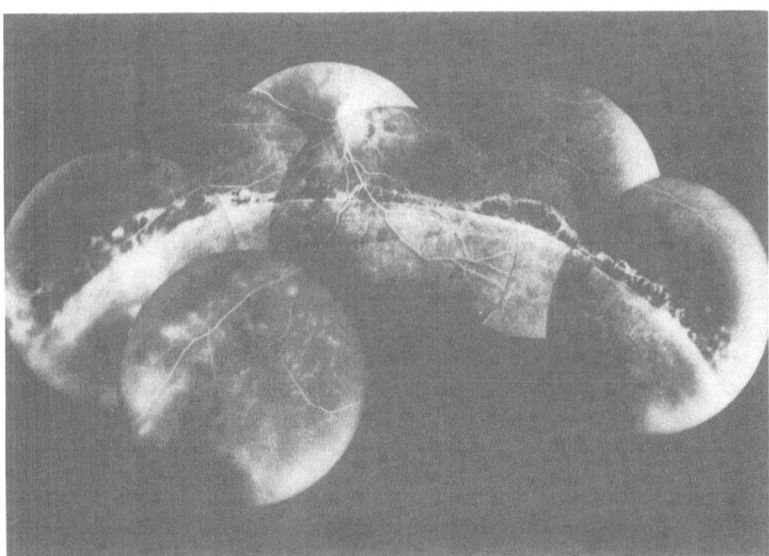

Fig. 3. Mixed atrophy (in part only of pigment epithelium + choriocapillaris, in part of the whole choroid) secondary to giant retinoschisis.

atrophies appearing in strict association with myopia are mostly *incomplete* forms of DCA.

There are extensive forms which can affect from half to 6/8 of the entire retinal surface and which we have observed only in cases of high myopia.

They always involve the whole of the inferior hemiretina, sometimes part of the superior retinal quadrants, including almost always the optic disc and always the macular region: the fovea can be spared so that no serious impairment of visual acuity is present.

Sometimes however, the superior margin of this atrophy, always sharp even though the limit is wave-like, reaches the fovea.

CLINICAL EXAMPLES

Case No. 1:

A 43-year-old female had eight diopters of myopia and a visual acuity RE of 0.1 and LE of 0.7. Her mother was myopic.

Retinal fluorescein angiography showed the presence of an extensive atrophy affecting 5/8 of the retinal surface (Figure 4, RE). More precisely, atrophy of pigment epithelium and choroid involved 4/8, while 1/8 showed deeper choroidal atrophy.

The upper margin of the lesion included the whole optic disc, as also the macular region, including the fovea. Note the clear-cut upper margin, wave-like in the temporal region, linear in the nasal area. The superior retina did not show alterations worth noting, and neither did the other eye.

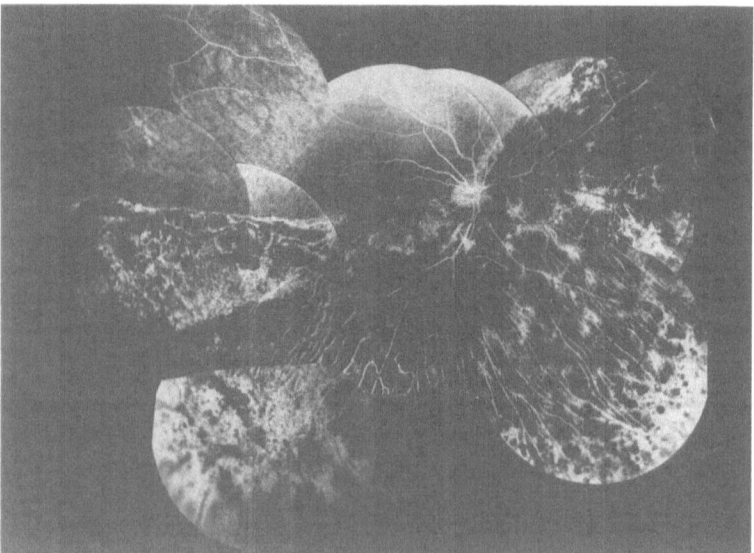

Fig. 4. Fluorescein angiography in case No. 1, right eye, cf. text.

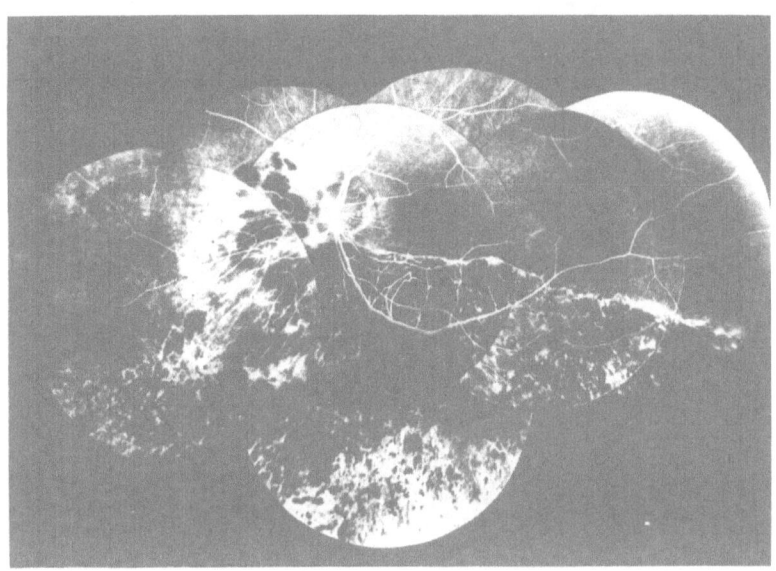

Fig. 5. Fluorescein angiography in case No. 2, left eye, cf. text.

Case No. 2:

A 43-year-old female with high myopia, again with a myopic mother.

Retinal fluorescein angiography (Figure 5) indicated the presence of an extensive atrophy affecting almost half of the retino-choroidal surface; here too, the optic disc was included in the atrophy; the upper retina did not show any relevant changes.

Case No. 3:

A 46-year-old male with visual acuity of 1/50 and with 18 diopters of myopia in both eyes. His mother was myopic.

Retinal fluorescein angiography (Figure 6) indicated an atrophy involving 7/8 of the retinal surface, and not sparing the macula. There is only a small island of partly trophic retinal tissue.

In this case too, the edges of the atrophic areas are sharp and clear-cut. The atrophy involves only the pigment epithelium and the choriocapillaris in the central areas, whereas it affects the choroid more deeply at the periphery.

CONCLUDING REMARKS

To conclude, chorio-retinal degenerative changes are extremely frequent in cases of high myopia.

To be separated from the more frequent manifestations appropriately

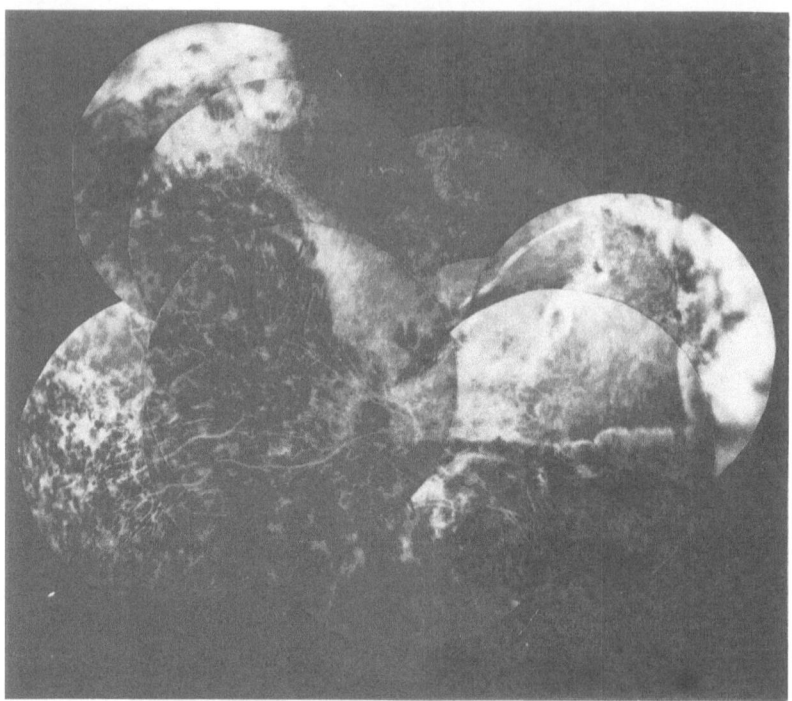

Fig. 6. Fluorescein angiography in case No. 3, cf. text.

considered secondary to the progressive elongation of the bulb, we have described other types of atrophies which we encountered only in association with high myopia (but without relation to the above-mentioned pathogenetic mechanism): namely a central RCA, and an incomplete DCA, to which the three presented cases belong.

The RCA was bilateral, the DCA was monolateral, and always affecting the most myopic eye. A myopic family history through three generations was present in all cases.

These associations suggest that the origin is probably due to the pleiotropic effects of the same gene as proposed by Krill (1977).

REFERENCE

Krill, S.. Hereditary retinal and choroidal diseases. Harper & Row Publ., Hagerstown, Maryland pp. 1, 17 (1977).

Author's address:
S. Colombati, M.D.
Clinica Oculistica I
University of Bologna
Via Massarenti, 9
40100 – Bologna
Italia

228

NASAL MYOPIA

D. RIISE
(Hamar, Norway)

ABSTRACT

An eye anomaly is described, consisting of several characteristics. As name for the disorder 'nasal myopia' or 'nasal fundus ectasia' has been selected.

Infero-nasal crescent, dysversion of the optic disc, inverse vessel emerge, myopia, astigmatism and nasal fundus ectasia belong to the symptom complex. Special attention has been paid to the bitemporal visual field defects, which can easily lead to suspicion of tumour in the region of the optic chiasm.

INTRODUCTION

The posterior segment of the eye usually forms an approximately spherical surface. However, several forms of ectasia can be found. The most common is the staphyloma of the macular area in high myopia.

In 115 eyes in 66 patients I found an ectasia of the fundus lying *nasally* and a bit downward from the optic disc. The literature referring to the subject is comparatively sparse, and the terminology somewhat confusing. Names as Fuchs coloboma, posterior staphyloma, situs inversus of the optic disc, dysversion, inverse myopia, refraction scotoma and nasal fundus ectasia have been used since Fuchs described it in 1882.

I have felt it worthwhile here to report on the findings in this disorder, which in my opinion makes up a clinical entity.

ETIOLOGY

The etiology of the disorder is not known. Histologically there is thinning of the sclera, choroid and retina nasally and downwards from the optic disc. The location, which corresponds to the eye's embryonic cleft, has led many to interpret the anomaly as a form of coloboma. The disorder cannot, however, be a pure coloboma because there are neither duplications, nor defects.

Well-founded suggestions regarding the disorder as a malformation in the 'papilla epithelialis primitiva', or a developmental disturbance in the secondary eye vesicle, can not be dismissed. What does seem clear is that the (mal)development must be seen in connection with the formation of the posterior part of the sclera in the fifth fetal month. At this stage the retina's pigment epithelium has been shown to exert a decisive influence upon the growth of the sclera.

Genetically a family concentration is found. Probably there is a polymeric mode of inheritance similar to that of refraction anomalies.

CLINICAL PICTURE

Clinically the nasal fundus ectasia has a series of characteristics but does not in itself give rise to typical symptoms. The patient is most often led to the ophthalmologist due to problems with glasses in connection with myopia or astigmatism.

The anomaly occurs in presumably about 1% of the population, with equal incidence in men and women. The condition must be regarded as congenital, but progresses during adolescence. In 75% of the patients, the disorder is bilateral.

Myopia is found in 90% of the cases, mostly in the range of 0 to -8 D. *Astigmatism* of more than 1 D occurs in 70% of the cases. The majority have the negative cylinder axis in the vicinity of 0°.

Visual acuity with optimum correction is moderately reduced since only 25% have visual acuity 1.0, the majority lying within the range 0.33 to 1.0. This may be due to the Stiles-Crawford effect as the retina stands obliquely in relation to the visual axis.

The ophthalmoscopic picture contains a series of characteristic findings, not all of which are necessarily present in all patients. In more than 50% of the eyes in the present series, there was a distinct *inferior-nasal crescent,* and the majority of the remainder had a scleral ring most marked in the corresponding place. Tilting of the optic disc in a downward nasal direction

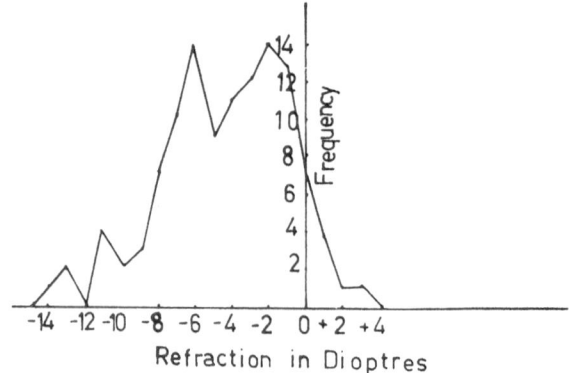

Fig. 1. Curve of refraction in 115 eyes with nasal myopia.

230

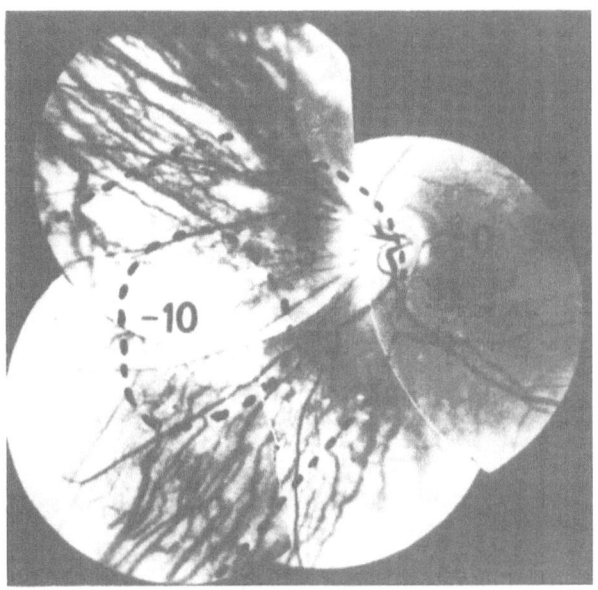

Fig. 2. Ectasia of the fundus with tilted disc, left eye.

occurred in 65% of the eyes, and in 80% there was a somewhat *nasally directed vessel emerge.*

Nasal ectasia of the fundus was − by definition − the most characteristic feature. The optic disc was usually situated within, but not at the bottom of the ectasia. The *depth of the fundus ectasia* was judged by ophthalmoscopy, and in some cases also by retinoscopy, refractometry and ultrasonic examination. By far the easiest and most practical method was point ophthalmoscopy, but all methods gave fairly consistent results. The ectasia was usually 4 to 8 D deep, but could reach 15 D. In the ectasia, the fundus was of *light colour*, had *poor choroidal circulation* and *hypopigmentation*. In some cases *degenerations* were seen, most often in elderly patients. The most important changes were thus confined to the posterior part of the eye, but the fact that the astigmatism was to a large extent *corneal* suggests that the whole eye is involved in the anomaly. The material gave no grounds to suppose that nasal fundus ectasia is part of any general disease. Moderate exophthalmos was found in 5% of the cases. Presumably, this corresponds to the slightly protruberant eyes found in high myopia. *Retinal detachment* was found in four eyes with nasal fundus ectasia. The retinal holes did not lie within the ectasia, but in the upper temporal quadrant. It is probable that the disorder, similarly to other myopia, predisposes to detachment. Monolateral fundus ectasia appears to predispose to *squint* and *amblyopia*.

Visual fields: Familiarity with the entity is of great practical interest because it involves bitemporal hemianopia, which by mistake can suggest the presence of tumours in the region of the optic chiasm. Three patients of the present material had thus been subjected to exploratory craniotomy for

231

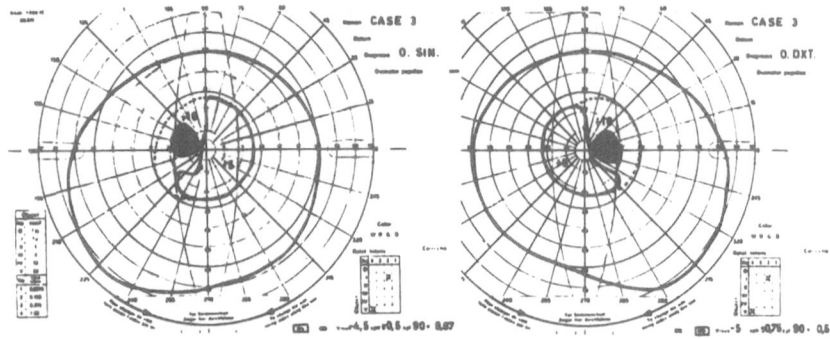

Fig. 3. Relative bitemporal visual field defects disappear with corrective glasses corresponding to the fundus ectasia.

suspected pituitary tumour, and another six had undergone extensive investigation in neurosurgical departments (9/66 = 14%). Familiarity with the nasal fundus ectasia can spare such patients from great inconvenience, but it must not be forgotten that the combination of pituitary tumour and nasal fundus ectasia can occur, and has been described; nor can this be surprising keeping in mind that about 1% of the population has fundus ectasia.

The most important investigation consists of perimetry of the patients with corrective glasses corresponding to the bottom of the fundus ectasia. If the visual field defects then disappear they must be attributed to the fundus ectasia.

REFERENCE

Riise, D. The nasal fundus ectasia. Acta ophthalmol. (Kbh.) suppl. 126 (1975).

Author's address:
D. Riise, M.D.
Eye dept., Hamar Sykehus
N-2300 Hamar
Norway

CLINICAL FEATURES IN HIGH MYOPIA

A ten-year follow-up of a representative sample of young adults

E. GOLDSCHMIDT, H.C. FLEDELIUS AND F. ERLIN LARSEN

(Odense and Copenhagen, Denmark)

ABSTRACT

On the basis of a follow-up study of 29 young persons with unilateral or bilateral high myopia (> 6 D) clinical and oculometric results are presented. 50 eyes had high myopia, average almost 10 D, while eight fellow eyes had either low myopia or emmetropia and were used as a reference group.

The well-known association between refractive value and axial length is demonstrated. The anterior eye segment is nearly identical in low and high myopia, except the latter group has a higher degree of corneal astigmatism. The enlargement of the globe seems to follow the main dimensional rules of the eye, even in the marginal group of high myopia.

The time at onset and the progression in these myopic cases vary considerably, some being stationary from early childhood. Only very few eyes show a heavy progression between the ages of 14 to 24; the highest progression is demonstrated in an amblyopic eye.

The study includes fundus photos taken at the age of 14 and again at the age of 24, and though the changes in this age group are minor some characteristic posterior pole changes have developed. The visual acuity has not decreased much during the follow-up period.

The study indicates that even high myopia is a heterogeneous condition.

INTRODUCTION

The present study deals with ocular findings in high myopia in young adults ($n = 29$) aged 24. The exceptional age homogeneity is explained by the fact that the material derives from an earlier epidemiological study on myopia in Danish school children (Goldschmidt 1968). Although the sample is small the investigation is of interest due to the age homogeneity and the representativity.

MATERIAL AND METHODS

In the previous epidemiological study of 9.243 Copenhagen school children, aged 13–14 years, 877 were recorded as myopic (9.5%). Thirtynine – or

0.4% of the total sample – had high myopia (above 6 D) in one eye or both.

The basic examination included subjective and objective assessment of refraction, determination of visual acuity, keratometry, exophthalmometry, ophthalmoscopy and fundus photography. In addition, relevant data were collected from practising ophthalmologists with a view to determining the progress of the myopia. At initial assessment, ultrasound facilities were not available.

The 39 high-myopia cases now make up the target group of a 10 year ophthalmic follow-up; 29 were able to attend.

The present sample thus consists of 29 young adolescents, now 24 years old, with high myopia in both eyes (21 persons) or only in one eye (eight persons). The eight fellow eyes had either low myopia or emmetropia; in the following they will be used as a within-material reference group called 'low myopia'.

Of the 50 eyes with high myopia 33 were female and 17 male eyes.

The following eye examinations were carried out:

Determination of visual acuity

Refraction
(a) subjectively for each eye with glasses, and
(b) by retinoscopy.
By diverging results the subjective was chosen in eyes with a good visual acuity. The refractive value is given as the spherical equivalent.

Keratometry (Javal-Schiøtz), measuring
(a) the corneal curvature radius in the main meridians (in mm) using the mean in the following, and
(b) the corneal astigmatism, in dioptres.

Optical pachymetry with the Haag-Streit 900 devices in the slit lamp measuring
(a) central corneal thickness (CTT), and
(b) anterior chamber depth (ACD).

Ultrasound oculometry (TAU), with a methocel-filled contact glass, Kretztechnik 7000 and Ultrasonolux 10 Mc transducer, as described in detail elsewhere (Fledelius 1976). ACD, lens thickness, vitreous length and axial length (AL) are given in mm.

Exophthalmometry (Hertel), values in mm.

Applanation tonometry, IOP, values in mm Hg.

Ophthalmoscopy and fundus photography.

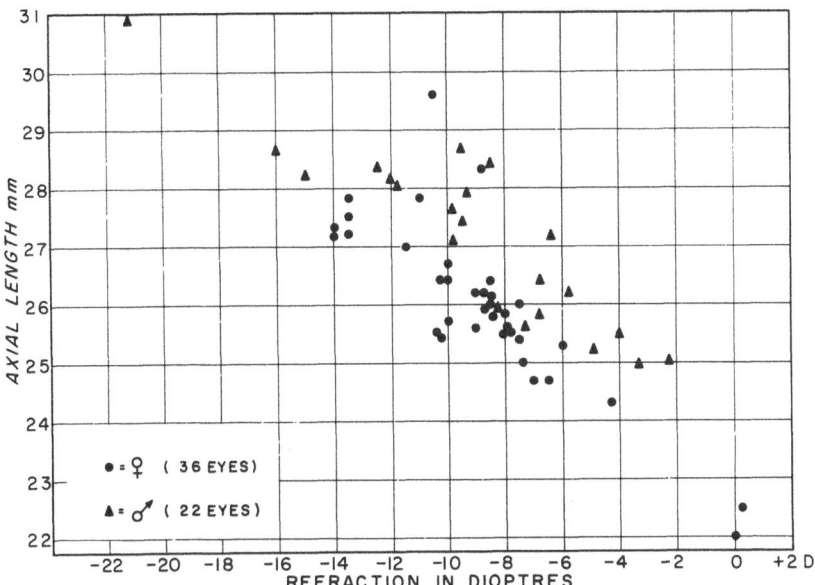

Fig. 1. Axial length and refractive values in 58 eyes of 29 persons with uni- or bilateral high myopia.

Statistical evaluation. Because of the marked right-left differences in the sample (refraction, degree of change in refraction, axial length) all 58 eyes are included (and not merely one eye per individual). Further, the current computer program for Spearman's rank correlation analysis has given one-tailed P-values. Obviously, both factors contribute to a higher number of significant findings than if two-tailed analyses and number of persons are used. However, the size of the material is small due to selection. If possible correlations shall appear, or 'tendencies' be suggested, it has therefore to be on the statistically least critical grounds. The results to be presented should be assessed on this background. Finally, non parametric evaluation is to be preferred, because the sample is 'marginal' on the refractive curve, but parametric mean values will be given on some occasions. This is done primarily for the sake of comparison with the results of other studies on the subject.

RESULTS

The 58 eyes (18 females, 11 males) are presented in Figure 1, showing the association between axial length and refractive value, and in Table 1, with mean values, SD, and ranges of the various ocular parameters.

1. High and low myopia, progression during adolescence.

There are 50 eyes with high myopia (above 6 D) and eight 'fellow eyes' with so-called 'low myopia', cf. Material and Methods. In addition, Table 1 shows the group of high myopia divided by sex (33 female and 17 male eyes).

235

Table 1. Refractive and oculometric parameters in 58 eyes from 29 young adults with high myopia (uni- or bilaterally) divided by degree of myopia (left) and sex (right, high myopia only). Mean values and ranges, standard deviation in brackets.

	Low myopia n = 8 fellow eyes	High myopia n = 50 eyes	High myopia n = 33 female eyes	High myopia n = 17 male eyes
Refractive value (sph. equivalent, D)	− 3.0 (2.22) 0.25 to − 5.75	− 9.9 (2.89) − 6.0 to − 21.3	− 9.5 (2.20)	− 10.2 (3.88)
Progression of myopia over 10 years, in D	1.2 (1.30) 0–4.0	2.2 (1.70) 0–9.3	2.0 (1.10)	2.8 (2.44)
Keratometry (a) curv. radius (mean, in mm)	7.69 (0.28) 7.15–8.08	7.69 (0.28) 7.12–8.30	7.60 (0.27)	7.87 (0.20)
(b) corneal astigmatism (D)	0.7 (0.41) 0–1.25	1.4 (0.98) 0–4.0	1.3 (0.87)	1.7 (1.13)
Astigmatism (D) (glass correction)	0.5 (0.66) 0–2.0	0.9 (1.11) 0–4.5	0.6 (0.81)	1.4 (1.43)
Optical pachymetry (a) Central corneal thickness (mm)	0.543 (0.027) 0.51–0.59	0.550 (0.037) 0.49–0.62	0.554 (0.033)	0.542 (0.044)
(b) Anterior chamber depth (mm)	3.75 (0.19) 3.5–4.0	3.72 (0.24) 3.2–4.1	3.71 (0.26)	3.75 (0.18)
Ultrasound oculometry (a) anterior chamber depth (mm)	3.88 (0.22) 3.5–4.1	3.88 (0.26) 3.3–4.3	3.86 (0.27)	3.90 (0.23)
(b) lens thickness (mm)	3.74 (0.18) 3.5–4.0	3.82 (0.23) 3.4–4.5	3.85 (0.20)	3.74 (0.20)
(c) vitreous length (mm)	16.9 (1.44) 14.1–18.4	19.0 (1.24) 16.4–22.0	18.6 (1.0)	20.0 (1.14)

Table 1. (continued)

	Low myopia n = 8 fellow eyes	High myopia n = 50 eyes	High myopia n = 33 female eyes	High myopia n = 17 male eyes
(d) axial length (mm)	24.5 (1.48) 22.0–26.2	26.8 (1.32) 24.7–30.8	26.3 (1.09)	27.7 (1.29)
Exophthalmometry (Hertel value, mm)	14.8 (2.32) 12–18	15.4 (2.52) 12–20	15.5 (2.44)	15.2 (2.73)
IOP, applanation value (mm Hg)	15.5 (1.73) 14–18	14.2 (2.98) 7–20	14.1 (2.10)	14.5 (4.47)

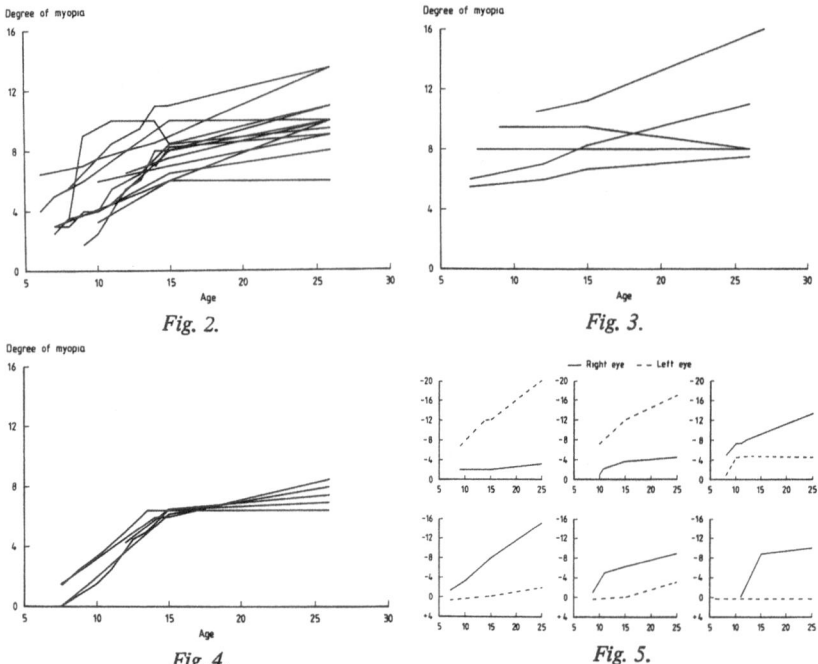

Fig. 2. Progress of myopia in 13 bilateral cases with mean annual progress above 1/3 D (average of both eyes) up to the age of 14.

Fig. 3. Progress of myopia in five bilateral cases with mean annual progress below 1/3 D up to the age of 14.

Fig. 4. Progress of myopia in the most myopic eye of five cases with > 6 D in one eye and 4.5 to 6 D in the other at the age of 14.

Fig. 5. Progress of myopia in six unilateral cases.

The *progression of myopia* over ten years averages 1.2 D in low myopia (median value 0.8 D), and 2.2 D (median 2.0 D) in high myopia.

The range was 0–9.3 D. The progression pattern of 23 cases from their documented onset are depicted in Figures 2, 3, and 4. In some cases the myopia is stationary during the decade under study, or may even decrease. In others, the increase continues also after the end of bodily growth, however decelerating.

The (intra-individual) side difference in progression was below 1 D in 16 and above 1 D in the remaining 13. All considered, they ranged from zero to 8 D. The latter extreme occured in a male who progressed from − 2.0 to − 3.25 D in his less myopic eye, and from − 12.0 to − 21.25 D in that with high myopia. This case is among the six, which are shown graphically in Figure 5.

Astigmatism was most pronounced in high myopia. Correspondingly there is a negative correlation between refractive value and corneal astigmatism (Table 2).

238

Table 2. Non-parametric correlations (Spearman rank) between some oculometric parameters in the material. Asterisks designate significance (p < 0.05, however one-tailed only, cf. Methods).

x		y	r_s	p value
Refraction (in D)	and	Corn. curv. radius	− 0.14	0.15
(n = 58)		Corneal astigm.	− 0.29*	0.013
		Central corn. th.	− 0.24*	0.033
		ACD (optically)	− 0.03	0.42
		ACD (ultrasound)	− 0.01	0.48
		Lens thickness	− 0.20	0.07
		Vitr. length	− 0.77*	zero
		Axial length	− 0.76*	zero
Axial length	and	Corn. curv. radius	0.44*	0.0003
(n = 58)		Corneal astigm.	0.30*	0.01
		CCT	0.11	0.21
		ACD (opt.)	0.16	0.11
		ACD (ultrasound)	0.20	0.07
		Lens th.	0.13	0.16
		Vitr. length	0.97*	zero
Intraocular pressure	and	Refraction	0.30*	0.022
(n = 46)		Axial length	− 0.02	0.44
		CCT	0.30*	0.021
Exophthalmometry	and	Refraction	− 0.07	0.30
(Hertel value, n = 58)		Axial length	0.19	0.08
		Ratio ACD:Ax. L.	0.08	0.29

Summing up the differences between low and high myopia (Table 1), the main finding is the longer axial (and vitreous) length of the latter. The mean values of lens thickness and Hertel values are only slightly elevated in high myopia, IOP a little lower, while CCT, central corneal curvature, and ACD are almost identical in the two myopic subgroups.

2. Sex differences

Sex differences are included in Table I, comprising female and male eyes with high myopia. The male group has a significantly longer mean axial length and a less curved cornea (P < 0.01), while mean lens thickness and CCT seem to be a little lower than in female eyes. Otherwise, sex differences are not conspicuous.

3. Anisometropia

A side difference in refraction of at least one diopter is seen in 17 of the 29 myopic eye-pairs. Anisometropia is of a low order (1–3 D) in ten, while it exceeds 5 D in the remaining seven (with refractive side differences ranging from 5.8 to 18 D, median value 10.5 D).

Within each anisometropic eye-pair, the only marked oculometric difference (except the definitory refractive) is that between axial (and vitreous) lengths. In the subgroup of high anisometropia (n = 7) a summed-up 74.3 D difference corresponds with a 23.7 mm axial length difference, or 3.1 D:1 mm The corresponding mean ratio in low anisometropia (10 eye-pairs) is 3 D:1 mm.

The more myopic eye in anisometropia thus invariably has the longer axial length. Concerning the other intra-pair differences (corneal curvature radius, CCT, ACD, lens thickness, Hertel value), they all group closely around zero.

4. Correlations

Table 2 gives some oculometric correlations in the sample. Significant rank correlation coefficients ($r_s \neq$ zero at $p < 0.05$; NB one-tailed, cf. Methods) are marked with asterisks. In brief, the following correlations are found:

(a) *The more myopic the eye,* the longer the axial and vitreous length, the thicker the cornea centrally, the larger the corneal astigmatism, and the lower the IOP.

(b) *The longer the eye axially,* the longer the vitreous length, the less curved the cornea, and the larger the corneal astigmatism.

(c) *The thicker the cornea centrally,* the higher the IOP.

Close to significance ('tendencies', $0.05 < p < 0.10$) came the following associations:

(d) *The more myopic the eye,* the thicker the lens.

(e) *The longer the axial length,* the deeper the ACD (at least as measured by ultrasound).

(f) *The longer the axial length,* the higher the Hertel value.

5. Visual acuity and fundus changes.

Visual acuity with correction was good ($\geq 6/12$) in 42 out of 50 eyes with high myopia. The acuity decreased somewhat by increasing degree of spherical myopia, but seemed to decrease particularly in cases of high astigmatism with oblique axes, or in cases with an axial length above 28 mm. The visual acuity was poor in three eyes due to amblyopia, a rather low frequency considering the many cases of anisometropia. However, the finding is not embarrassing, because myopic anisometropia usually develops in later childhood where 'lazy eye' is exceptional.

Fundus changes were of the diffuse myopic type, with pallor of the fundus etc. Severe fundus changes such as demarcated posterior pole degenerations, posterior staphylomas, Fuchs' spot, and retinal tears were not observed at follow-up, probably because the subjects are still so young.

We further looked for clinical correlations by way of arbitrarily sub-dividing the sample into thirds, according to degree of myopia, axial length, IOP readings, etc. Fundus changes were then evaluated in such high versus low-risk groups, but we could not point out particular clinical types on these grounds.

Figures 6–8 show some fundus pictures, documenting changes during adolescence in three eyes with marked progression of myopia.

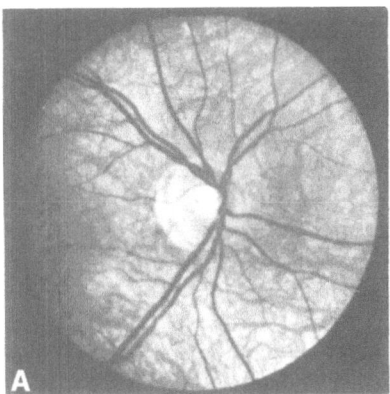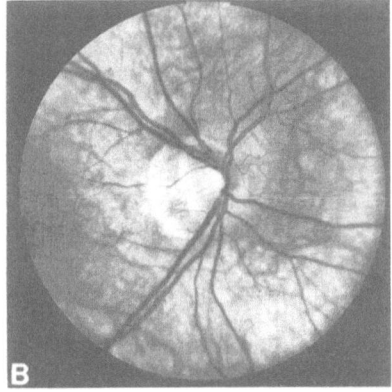

Fig. 6AB. Right fundus of a female eye with v.a. 6/9 − 10 (AL: 25.5 mm, progress: 4 D) and enlargement of the temporal crescent (A = 1964; B = 1974).

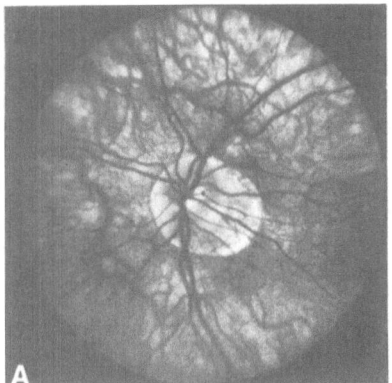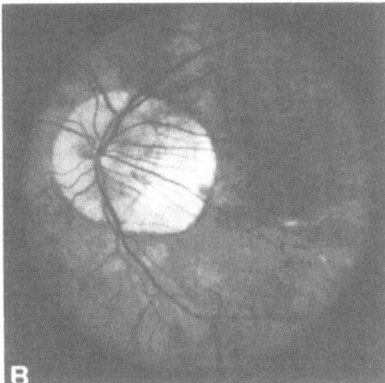

Fig. 7AB. Left fundus of a male eye with v.a. 6/36 − 20−2.5 × 170° (AL: 30.8 mm, progress: 9 D) with enlargement of conus, stretching of retinal and thinning of choroidal vessels and some neovascularisation and macular degeneration (A = 1964; B = 1974).

DISCUSSION

The present results are in accordance with those of previous studies of high myopia (e.g. Franceschetti and Gernet 1965, François and Goes 1973) and anisometropia (Franceschetti *et al.* 1968). The increased axial (and vitreous) length is the outstanding exception to the rule, that oculometric parameters in high myopia by and large show distributions like those found around emmetropia. We also confirm the usual correlations between refraction and axial length and between the latter and corneal curvature. Another normal feature, the sex difference, is retained as well. Male eyes are longer axially, and keratometrically less curved, than female eyes. Though

241

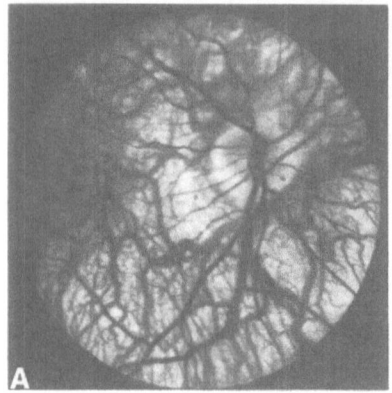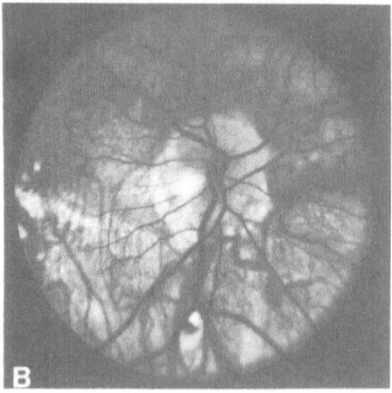

Fig. 8AB. Right fundus of a male eye with v.a. 6/18 − 15 (AL: 28.2 mm, progress: 7 D) with enlargement of conus and choroidal breaks (A = 1964; B = 1974).

'stretched' beyond norms, the eyes belonging to the marginal (and potentially pathological) refractive group with high myopia seem to follow the 'dimensional rules' of the eye.

Further comments concern aspects of ocular stretching in high myopia. Von Bahr (1956) found thinner corneae in high myopia than in markedly hypermetropic eyes, suggesting a myopic stretching and thinning also of the anterior eye segment. This gets no support from the present sample, in which thicker corneae seem to be a feature of more myopic eyes (Table 2). The significance levels are, however, low regarding correlation between CCT and refraction and other ocular parameters. This is suggested also from the fact that the present CCT values (of high myopia) are not far from those of other Danish materials, dominated by refractions around emmetropia (Kruse Hansen 1971, Ehlers and Kruse Hansen 1976, Alsbirk 1978).

Some features of Table 2 may be discussed in relation to the hypothesis of near-work and accommodation as factors in myopia pathogenesis. Among the 'tendencies' is lens thickening with increasing degree of myopia, a possible indication of an (otherwise balanced) hyperaccommodative state which might − earlier − have led to increased intraocular pressure of the posterior eye segment and mechanical enlargement of the still plastic juvenile globe.

Although they have been advanced primarily in relation to low myopia, such theories may be tested also by data from the present high myopia sample. To this aim, correlations of Table 2 have been analysed, e.g. refraction-IOP, refraction-CCT, and IOP-CCT. Some of the actual cross-correlations seem mutually inconsistent, but (again) this probably indicates only that the associations under study are indeed weak (cf. Ehlers *et al.* 1975, Alsbirk 1978). Further, the sample is small.

The balance between anterior and posterior eye segment stretching in high myopia (cf. von Bahr 1956, above) was viewed from an exophthalmometry angle by Bertelsen, also in 1956. He found that the degree of ocular protrusion might reflect this balance (with a more 'healthy' posterior segment in case of anterior stretching, giving more protrusion). In the present material, the ACD:AL ratio (another expression of the same 'balance') showed no correlation to Hertel values, a conclusion which was also arrived at in an earlier study by Fledelius 1971.

The exceptional age-homogeneity of the present sample was emphasized in the introduction. Such samples are hard to collect and therefore rare in ophthalmic literature. This is unfortunate, because possible oculometric features may be obscured in samples with a wide age range. In particular, this has bearing to the structures of the anterior eye segment, with its continued thickening of the (healthy) lens with age, and the corresponding shallowing of the ACD (Delmarcelle *et al.* 1976, Fledelius and Bruun Laursen 1979).

CONCLUDING REMARKS

In the above presentation emphasis is laid on progression patterns and oculometric features of high myopia. Social aspects are deliberately omitted from discussion, primarily because till now there have been no severe problems caused by the refractive disorder. All have retained their 'social vision' (visual acuity of best eye $\geq 6/12$, with glasses or contact lenses) and have not (yet) suffered from disabling complications.

Considering oculometry results, we must regret that measuring by ultrasound was not possible at initial assessment, at the age of 14. Nevertheless we find it justified to state that increase in axial and vitreous length are by far the strongest determining factors in myopia progression.

How and why this comes along is not equally obvious. The discussion is centered upon the possible role of accommodation and intraocular pressure in myopic eye-stretching. The near work evaluations being retrospective, and the oculometric tendencies vague, the present investigation of high myopia does not lend support to the current near work theories, advanced in relation to juvenile myopia of lower order.

Finally we shall stress the need of further research into the various aspects of high myopia. One reason is that information in literature derives mainly from hospital materials, which are skew, attendance usually being prompted by some kind of eye disease. We therefore intend to contribute with future longitudinal data from the present representative (and age-homogeneous) sample of individuals with high myopia.

REFERENCES

Alsbirk, P.H. Corneal thickness. I, Age variation, sex difference and oculometric correlations. Acta Ophthalmol. (Kbh.) 56: 95–104 (1978).

Bahr, G. von. Corneal thickness. Its measurement and changes. Amer. J. Ophthalmol. 42: 251–266 (1956).

Bertelsen, T.I. The difference in exophthalmometric values on the two eyes in persons with high degree of myopia in one eye. Acta Ophthalmol. (Kbh.) 34: 69–72 (1956).

Delmarcelle, Y., François, J., Goes, F., Collignon-Brach, J., Luyckx-Bacus, J. & Verbraeken, H. Biométrie oculaire clinique, Masson, Paris pp. 198–205 (1976).

Ehlers, N., Kruse Hansen, F. & Aasved, H. Correlations of corneal thickness. Acta Ophthalmol. (Kbh.) 53: 652–659 (1975).

Ehlers, N. & Kruse Hansen, F. Further data on biometric correlations of central corneal thickness. Acta Ophthalmol. (Kbh.) 54: 774–778 (1976).

Fledelius, H. Ultrasound oculometry and exophthalmometry in high myopia, with reference to the occurrence of retinal detachment. Acta Ophthalmol. (Kbh.) 49: 707–714 (1971).

Fledelius, H. Prematurity and the eye. Ophthalmic 10-year follow-up of children of low and normal birth weight. Acta Ophthalmol. (Kbh.) Suppl. 128 (1976).

Fledelius, H. & Bruun Laursen, A. Cataract and lens thinning. An oculometric-biomicroscopical study of unilateral cataract cases and of normal controls. In Ed. H. Gernet Diagnostica Ultrasonica in Ophthalmologia Münster, pp. 184–189 (1979).

Franceschetti, A. & Gernet, H. Über die optischen Grössen bei leichter und höher Myopie auf Grund echographischer Befunde. Graefes Arch. Ophthalmol. 168: 1–16 (1965).

Franceschetti, A.T., Linder, A. & Franceschetti, A. New results concerning the problem of axial lengths of the eye in anisometropia. In Ed. Vanysek Diagnostica Ultrasonica in Ophthalmologia Brno pp. 235–238 (1968).

François, J. & Goes, F. Biométrie de la myopie. Ophthalmologica 167: 49–65 (1973).

Goldschmidt, E. On the etiology of myopia. Acta Ophthalmol. (Kbh.), suppl. 98 (1968).

Kruse Hansen, F. A clinical study of the normal human central corneal thickness. Acta Ophthalmol. (Kbh.) 49: 82–89 (1971).

Senior author's address:
E. Goldschmidt, M.D.
Odense Sygehus, Eye Dept. E
DK-5000 Odense C
Denmark

TREATMENT OF MYOPIA

Results and clinical findings

T. HARA

(Ishikawa-ken, Japan)

ABSTRACT

A treatment of myopia is described based on the viewpoint that a sclero-choroiditis of the posterior pole, due to paranasal sinusitis, is an important pathogenetic factor. Effective treatment results, based on improvement of visual acuity, was obtained in 80% of about 900 patients of all ages. They were treated by antibiotic-steroid-adrenalin nasal drops plus orally given antibiotics, antiphlogistic enzymes and vitamine B_1 as well as chondron injected into Tenon's capsule. Attempts were made to reduce risk factors in diet and nearwork habits. Chinese excercises were used pressing the fingers of the patient against seven points around each eye, corresponding to the paranasal sinuses.

INTRODUCTION

The cause of myopia is still obscure. A. von Graefe in 1854 drew attention to sclerochoroiditis as one of the causes. Hallett (1931) stressed that chronic paranasal sinuitis was the primary lesion weakening the posterior pole of the eye through sclerochoroiditis. In the following results of myopia treatment are given based on such ideas.

MATERIAL

During 1978 915 myopia patients were treated among a total of 2639 patients seen at our clinic. Of the myopia patients 893 visited more than twice. They had a total of 1759 treated eyes (as 15 patients had a blind eye and 12 a hyperopic eye). The majority of the patients were women (62%). The age distribution ranged from five to 88 years.

METHODS OF TREATMENT

The following principles of treatment were used:
(1) *Nasal drops aiming at the paranasal sinus apertures.* A mixture

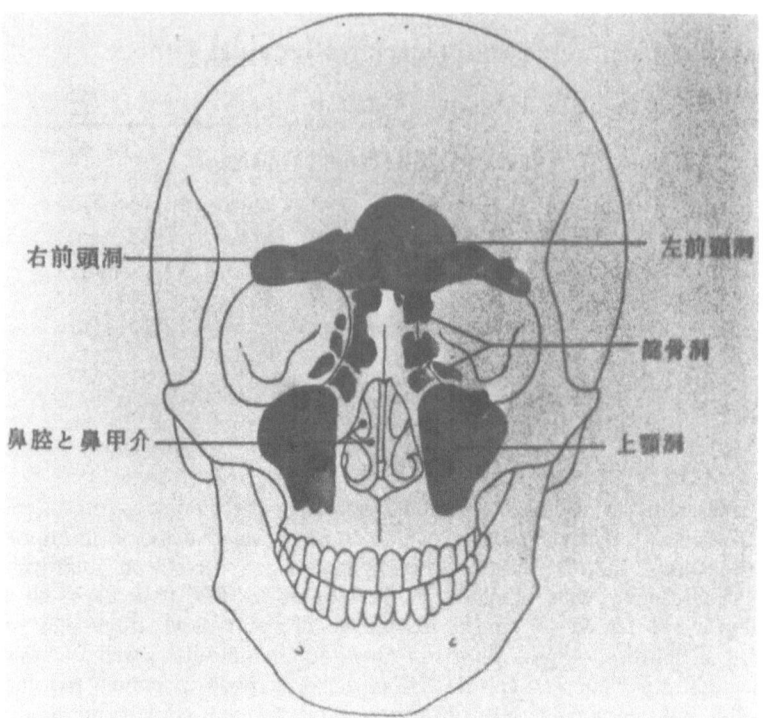

右前頭洞

左前頭洞

篩骨洞

鼻腔と鼻甲介

上顎洞

Fig. 1. Pressure points in the Chinese ophthalmo-sanitary exercise method, indicated by black spots.

of a broad spectrum antibiotic (Lilacillin, SB-PC) 1.0 g, cortisone acetate 25 mg/ml 2.0 ml, adrenalin 0.1% 5.0 ml and physiological saline 50 ml was used. During the first week a dose of 0.25 ml twice a day was dripped on to the lateral upper part of the nasal wall, into the meatus nasi medius. Through the next three weeks the drops were given without cortisone. Such four-week treatment series were repeated until sufficient effect was obtained.

(2) *Oral administration* of a broad spectrum *antibiotic* (Pacetocin, AM-PC) 125–250 mg, 3 T; an *antiphlogistic enzyme* (Pronase 7.5 mg, Pancreatin 60 mg/caps) 3 caps; active *vitamine B_1* (Alinamin F 5-25 mg) 3 T. This combination was administered for 3–4 consecutive days a week.

(3) *Injection of chondron* 1%, 0.5–1.0 ml into Tenon's capsule, once or twice a week until sufficient effect was obtained.

(4) *Elimination of risk factors* such as

    (a) Unsuitable diet, e.g. diet of refined cereals or high carbohydrate intake, especially sugar.

    (b) Heavy exercise, hard work, insufficient sleep, hot baths, swimming, drinking, pregnancy, diseases or operations.

    (c) Near work under insufficient luminosity (refractive myopia especially).

Table 1. The treatment results of myopia. Total no. of *cases* = 1269, because one patient was counted as two cases, if the eyes differed. Total no. of *patients* 893 and *eyes* 1759.

Grade of myopia	Result	Effective	Ineffective
Myopia initialis (− 0.25 to − 3.0 D)	Cases	794 (83.1%)	162 (16.9%)
	Eyes	1.112 (82.8%)	232 (17.2%)
	Mean duration of treatment	15.0 weeks	16.3 weeks
Myopia generalis (− 3.0 to − 5.0 D)	Cases	112 (70.9%)	46 (29.1%)
	Eyes	154 (73.7%)	55 (26.3%)
	Mean duration of treatment	15.0 weeks	13.4 weeks
Myopia excessiva (− 5.0 to − 10.0 D)	Cases	74 (67.3%)	36 (32.7%)
	Eyes	104 (72.2%)	40 (27.8%)
	Mean duration of treatment	28.3 weeks	24.2 weeks
Myopia gravissima (above − 10.0 D)	Cases	29 (64.4%)	16 (35.6%)
	Eyes	44 (71.0%)	18 (29.0%)
	Mean duration of treatment	51.3 weeks	27.7 weeks
Total	Cases	1.009 (79.5%)	260 (20.5%)
	Eyes	1.414 (80.4%)	345 (19.6%)
	Mean duration of treatment	16.7 weeks	17.6 weeks

(5) *Chinese ophthalmo-sanitary excercises,* so-called *'Tsubo'* in *Japanese.* The finger-pressure points are shown in Figure 1. Their locations correspond to sinus frontales, ethmoidales and maxillares (on each side 3, 2 and 2 points respectively).

SUMMARY OF RESULTS

Table 1 shows that the treatment given was found to be more or less effective in about 80% of the patients. The highest efficiency was observed in myopia below 3 D but even in myopia greater than 10 D 71% of the eyes showed improvement.

The effectiveness of treatment was judged by the number of lines' improvement of (uncorrected) visual acuity at Ishihara's visual chart. Of the 1759 eyes treated a *conspicuously effective* treatment result (improvement ⩾ 7 Ishihara lines) was found in 22%. *Effective results* (4–6 lines) were found in 19% and *slightly effective* results (1–3 lines improvement) appeared in 39%. Only 9% were unchanged and 11% of the eyes degraded.

The average number of weekly attendances for treatment is shown in the Table 1. Most treatment series were concluded in about 15 weeks, but excessive myopes were treated for longer periods.

Association between anisometropia and side difference of the nasal cavities.

An anterior rhinoscopy was performed in 76 myopes showing anisometropia. The eye with higher acuity (= lower myopia) was found on the side with the *narrower* nasal cavity in 53 patients, on the side with the *wider* nasal cavity in (only) 13 patients, while ten anisometropes had right and left nasal cavities of equal size. The nasal assymmetry was due to deviating nasal septa and/or to more or less hypertrophic chonchae.

Author's address:
T. Hara, M.D.
Hara Clinic,
Otemachi
Nanao, Ishikawa
Japan

THE ARREST AND PROPHYLAXIS OF EXPANSION GLAUCOMA (MYOPIA)

T. STUART-BLACK KELLY
(Bath, England)

ABSTRACT

The various forms of treatment to bring about arrest of Expansion Glaucoma, including the adult onset, and established adult malignant myopia types are described. The details of offset lenses, manufacture, fitting, use and after care are described. Prophylaxis is discussed involving scleral rigidity, single and bifocal systems, collimation, Japanese exercises and Living Guidance, racial and environmental effects, and damage by television.

PROPHYLAXIS AND ARREST OF EXPANSION GLAUCOMA (MYOPIA)

In expansion glaucoma, bifocals arrest most of the temporary self-inflicted myopias caused by pressure increase in the vitreous due to zonular block. Contact lenses arrest most of the long acting increase in the anterior chamber due to the schisis block. The effects can overlap, so success depends mainly on bifocals first, then contacts with bifocals, with or without eye drops.

BIFOCAL GLASSES

Consistent use of bifocals is the basis of success in children. So instructions regarding use of bifocal glasses are of great importance in early myopia, even with contact lenses. The failure to wear bifocals all the time when inside school or home is the most difficult to overcome.

(a) *The prescription.* For the distance correction, use the best result found by testing to the red side of duochrome test, reduced by $+ 0.5$ D. This roughly reduces the accommodation required from 20 ft to the area of the bifocal segment range. The bifocal segment has a flat top as recommended by Oakley and Young (1975), with the addition of $+ 1.5$ D. The top of the segment is placed passing through the center of the pupil, which allows for the drop sliding down on the nose often seen in children. This flat top prevents the accommodation being used in looking down sideways to some extent. If prisms are needed the weight must be reduced as much as possible. Plastic lenses are recommended. A special pair for cricket without reduction can be allowed but must only be used for that purpose.

(b) *Bifocal Instructions.* A detailed written instruction is essential, describing what happens in myopia in very simple terms: the reason for the two lenses; why the top of one is reduced; the similarity of the eye to a balloon and camera; the relief of focussing by the lower segment thus preventing increase of IOP, and instructions when to wear them, such as always indoors etc.. They must stress that 'Your eyes will become worse if you do not wear your bifocals, so you may have to wear glasses for life later on!'.

You may also give a sheet of general instructions copied from the Japanese called 'Living Guidance' on the optical care of the eyes: Positions for reading; TV-instructions, such as one hour a day at 10 feet; developing distance viewing habits etc. There are also some Japanese exercises provided by Nakajima (1976) ind Ichichi (1976) that are still on trial. Re-check after one month to see if the instructions are being carried out, and to support the parents! Adjust the glasses etc., and then check at three or six months.

(c) *If the Bifocals fail by 0.25 D in three months.* Check carefully and correct; use of the bifocals and distance vision habits (living guidance), add Japanese exercises or eye-drops as advocated below.

THE USE OF DROPS

(a) *Atropine.* If possible, as Otsuka and Sato advise (1968), use atropine 1% three times a day for seven days, after the first visit. Give an instruction sheet. Atropine has several uses: It will expose any spasm. It cures the Caucasian but many Orientals go on to myopia (Yamaji 1967). Check IOP with a Mydriacyl trial (for angle closure attacks) before using atropine in Orientals.

If atropine reduces the myopia by + 1.0 D., continue once per day (at bed-time) for one month or more, until no further scleral shrinkage occurs. Then use that refraction as the distance correction without any reduction. A reduction in myopia can happen even at 18 years; the effect can vary depending on whether the drops are given nightly, twice or three times per day (some clinical examples are given (slides)).

Congenital myopia is extremely rare, and illustrated only by accidental findings; by using atropine 1% nightly, the myopia can be reduced by several dioptres over some months.

Most commonly the myopia is reduced by + 0.5 D.. When it does so, give that refraction as the distance refraction. This is just the same as reducing the distance correction when no atropine is used, but spasm may be missed if atropine cannot be used. If the atropine refraction is level with the first refraction, bifocals alone will probably have no effect, and contact lenses will be needed because the block is probably a schisis block.

If you are ever in doubt, use atropine nightly for even a month or two until you have made up your mind.

Continuous atropine is best used for these special circumstances but is only needed for a few months. No child enjoys atropine, and it has to be limited anyway only to part of the 'progressive' years, whereas the correct type of bifocal can be used into adult years.

When used in early years, atropine in both eyes (or even in alternate eyes monthly) is always followed by some progression, which may be enough to make glasses necessary for driving. However, Dr Simmons has told me, at the present conference, that he finds atropine in alternate eyes for only two to three days each week can stop this progression.

(b) *Eye drops other than atropine.* Phenylephrine 5% (nocte up to a year or more) was the most successful drug in reducing myopia, out of nine types of drops tried by Dr Toki, under Professor Otsuka 20 years ago. It probably acts by constricting the ciliary body vessels, thus opening the lens gap. They can be used to prevent slow increase with bifocals as long as the child does not find that they smart too much.

Timoptol ® 0.5% twice daily may be used alone or with atropine. Before this is used on a large scale its safety in children should be ascertained for a six month period. The great advantage is that accommodation can be used. Ganda ® has not yet been tried, but it is safe according to the manufacturers.

Simplene ® acts quickly but does not last long enough after each drop.

CONTACT LENSES, VARIOUS TYPES

If bifocals fail $-0.5\,D.$ *or more in six months,* fit offset or aspherical or continuous curve contact lenses combined with the use of plano bifocals. Do not use multicurve or soft lenses. A keratometer is unnecessary. I usually fit 7.5 R and 7.4 L and change each lens until the apical pool is as wide and shallow as possible. Reduce the final Power by 0.5 as in the bifocal distance correction and explain to the children why you are reducing their acuity. Use plano bifocals + 1.5 as for contact lens wearers bifocals.

The lenses usually hang from the upper lid. On blinking the lens slides upwards under the lid to the upper part of the corneal surface, depressing it sufficiently on its' return to boost the 'milking out' of the aqueous, for, as Goldman (1946) stated, 'slight pressure on the cornea increases the output of the aqueous veins'.

The offset contact lens is so free that the margin of the lens can lift off the cornea to 1 mm in some in extreme version. The reason for the mobility is that the second (and only other) curve is centered on a much longer radius (24 mm) which is offset from the center line. The two curves are fitted together on exactly the same plane, so the entire edge lift is an almost 'flat curve'. This allows the lens to ski over the cornea governed by the position of the upper lid.

The essential contact lens

Eye surgeons, medical ophthalmologists, and many opticians are eventually involved with contact lenses in fitting, or in rescuing an eye that has not had the essential after-care. The offset hard lens is particularly important because it is, as are the other aspheric lenses, the best for myopia and, since it will be needed in 5% of myopias, it may be the most commonly used in a practice. As mentioned, multicurves only act slowly and soft lenses do not act at all in arresting myopia. They can be fitted in a short time without a keratometer. A 9.0 or 10.0 mm lens can be used in offset form instead of the old small thin lenses which had to be in multicurve form.

Many of our myopic *children* used their original PMMA lenses for ten to 15 years of daily wear without any trouble. In my view, offset lenses and other aspheric lenses should replace other types of contact lenses.

Most new *adult* myopes are under 30 years and are *zonular* types. They are always arrested by bifocals but with a + 1.0 D addition instead of + 1.5. The lenticular ones, extremely rare, are usually diabetic, and need investigation. Adults can use the same bifocal (adding + 1.0 for age 20–30) and contact lens scheme, but before using atropine, a trial with Mydriacyl (angle closure glaucoma!) is necessary. Lowering the pressure towards 10 mm by drops such as Timoptol, to maintain normal tissue exchange would seem wise in all axial myopes over − 10.0 D, or any which are still increasing. The importance is that the tangential scleral stress is reduced from its very high level.

GENERAL CONSIDERATIONS

Do not be surprised if a child who is stabilised on bifocals begins to 'progress'. It may be due for example, to lack of wearing bifocals, due to adolescent consciousness, plus increased physical activity, close work for exams, but particularly to someone else giving them a full distance correction with no bifocal. The best line may be to change to contact lenses with plano/bifocals, for both schisis and vitreous increased pressures must be treated together in some cases.

When atropine 7-day refraction comes up to level with the normal refraction, a contact lens is indicated.

If the child's myopia has risen at the rate of one dioptre a year before the first appointment with you, a schisis block is probably the cause and contact lens should be started as soon as possible.

Hallucinations are the only side reaction we have had. They have been rare, one in 500, and last for one night (the child enjoys visions of cars etc.). Only the parents are worried. The instruction sheet is used each time. The drops or ointment should be stopped if the parents have any anxiety.

Lastly, treatment is continued or changed depending on success.

Prophylaxis

This part of the presentation has been shortened in the written version, as has previous details concerning contact lens types.

Prophylaxis is based on Japanese exercise, living guidance, and on selection of children especially at risk (racial factors, heredity, high IOP, high level of nearwork − also other than reading!).

In summary, it is recommended that we watch for the so-called schisis block anatomy, and prevent the zonular type.

A more detailed account, as in the original papers read at the conference, can be achieved by personally addressing the author.

CONCLUDING REMARK

In Europe about 50,000 children become myopic each week, resulting in a generation with 60 million of which 6 million are severely damaged. So while the problem of arrest is enormous the benefits would be too. We must not fail our children.

REFERENCES

Dallos J., The myth of oxygen permeability. J. Br. Contact Lens Soc. (April 1980).

Goldman H., Quote in System of Ophth. Duke-Elder 4: 127 (1968).

Ichichi, Mrs. Jurake School, Kyoto. personal communication (1976).

Kelly T. S-B., Chatfield C., and Tustin G., Clinical assessment of arrest of myopia. Br. J. Ophthalmol. 59 (1975).

Kelly T. S-B., and Butler D. Changing view on senile uniocular aphakic contact lenses. Trans. Ophthalmol. Soc. U.K. p. 75 (1971).

Nakajima, Prof. A., Juntendo University. Tokyo. personal communication (1976).

Oakley K.H., and Young F.A., Bifocal control of myopia. Am. J. Optom. and Physiol. Optics 52 (11) (1975).

Otsuka, Prof. J. Personal help with Sato's helpful experience (1968).

Ruben M., Br. J. Ophthalmol. 50 (1966).

Simmons Richard E., Ohio State University, Columbus. Personal communication (1980).

Toki J., from Otsuka J., Acta Soc. Ophthalmol. Japan. (1967).

Yamaji R. et al., Group therapy against Pseudo-Myopia. Bull. Osaka Medical School 13 (1967).

Author's address:
Dr. T. S-B. Kelly, M.D.
Linden
Weston Road
Bath
England